Ulla Kriebernegg
Putting Age in Its Place

Cultural Perspectives on Age(ing) | 14

Ulla Kriebernegg is the director of the Center for Interdisciplinary Research on Aging and Care (CIRAC) and full professor of Cultural Aging and Care Research at Universität Graz in Austria. In her research and teaching she focuses on North American literary and cultural studies, aging and care studies, and health humanities. She has taught internationally and has won several teaching and research awards.

Ulla Kriebernegg

Putting Age in Its Place

Long-Term Residential Care in Contemporary Film and Fiction

[transcript]

Open Access publication co-funded by the University of Graz and the State of Styria.

Bibliographic information published by the Deutsche Nationalbibliothek
The Deutsche Nationalbibliothek lists this publication in the Deutsche Nationalbibliografie; detailed bibliographic data are available online at https://dnb.dnb.de

transcript Verlag | Hermannstraße 26 | D-33602 Bielefeld | live@transcript-verlag.de

Cover design: Maria Arndt
Cover illustration: Hartmut Wilkening, "Vrij Geestig" (2010), ("Michel Foucault in the Nursing Home")
Printing: Elanders Waiblingen GmbH, Waiblingen
Korrektorat: Urša Marinšek
https://doi.org/10.14361/9783839464120
Print-ISBN: 978-3-8376-6412-6 | PDF-ISBN: 978-3-8394-6412-0
ISSN of series: 2702-8011 | eISSN of series: 2702-8038

Printed on permanent acid-free text paper.

Contents

Acknowledgments

This book grows out of my long-standing work on care home stories and is a revised and expanded version of my habilitation monograph, submitted to the University of Graz in 2015. I remain grateful to my generous reviewers, Walter Grünzweig and Rüdiger Kunow, whose thoughtful feedback helped shape this expanded version.

My initial inspiration for this book came from Sally Chivers's chapter, "'Here, Every Minute Is Ninety Seconds': Fictional Perspectives on Nursing Home Care," in her monograph *From Old Woman to Older Women* (2003). Sally's scholarship in Age Studies, which I have long admired, encouraged me to explore this topic in greater depth. I am grateful to her not only for her intellectual generosity and encouragement but also for her friendship over the years.

My understanding of Age Studies has also been shaped by Stephen Katz, whose mentorship and conversations continue to challenge and inspire me. With his and Sally Chivers' support, I was able to spend several months of research time at Trent University and the University of Toronto's Institute for Life Course and Aging—enriching experiences that shaped this book.

Warm thanks go to Maureen and Peter Goggin at Arizona State University for providing a true home away from home, sustaining me both intellectually and personally during several months of research and writing through their hospitality, conversations, and Peter's exceptional cooking. Their friendship, open-mindedness, and generous care were invaluable during the more challenging phases of this project and will always remain close to my heart.

In addition to his foundational contributions to the field, I am deeply grateful to Thomas R. Cole for the insightful conversations we shared during my visit to the McGovern Center for Humanities and Ethics at UTHealth Houston. He listened with extraordinary care and understanding, offering support that meant more than he knows. The cowboy hat he gave me now hangs in my office as a lasting reminder of his generosity and spirit.

My work has also greatly benefited from the expertise, collaboration, and support of my colleague-friends Annette Leibing, Heike Hartung, Amelia DeFalco, Kate de Medeiros, and Anita Wohlmann, who encouraged me to move forward with this publication. I am also grateful to the community of like-minded researchers of ENAS and NANAS. The collegial spirit in both networks has strengthened my commitment to the field.

Within the Age Studies community at the University of Graz, I am especially grateful to my colleagues Dagmar Gramshammer-Hohl and Juliane Jarke for the enriching perspectives they contribute from their respective disciplines. I also wish to acknowledge Roberta Maierhofer's support in the earlier stages of my career, when she introduced me to Age Studies and its academic community.

My gratitude goes to all my colleagues at the Center for Interdisciplinary Research on Aging and Care (CIRAC), past and present, for their support, enthusiasm, and the team spirit that shapes our shared vision for Aging and Care Research at the University of Graz. I especially thank Sarah Bindar, whose warmth, positivity, and creativity have enriched our collaborations and brought sunshine to the office; Regina Brunnhofer, for her experience, insight, honesty, and humor; and Urša Marinšek, for her meticulous editing and reliability, which greatly improved this manuscript. I also thank Klaus Wegleitner, Eva-Maria Trinkaus, and Anna-Christina Kainradl for their valuable collegial friendship and ongoing support.

My thanks go to my friends Ursula Mindler-Steiner and Gerald Lamprecht. Sharing similar stages of our projects, we had open conversations and a friendship that sustained me along the way. I also thank my dear friend Annette Sprung for her unwavering support—her honesty, encouragement, and timely nudges kept me grounded and brought this book to completion.

Most of all, I am deeply grateful to my parents, Inge and Franz Gartler, my husband, Sepp, and our daughter, Lena, who has grown up with this project. Their patience, love, and steady support have carried me through every stage.

Acknowledgment of Prior Publications

A condensed article version of the main ideas presented in this book appeared in "Putting Age in Its Place. Representations of Institutional Eldercare in Contemporary Film and Fiction." *Virus: Beiträge zur Sozialgeschichte der Medizin*, vol. 16, 2017, pp. 251–71.

Chapter 2.3 is an adapted version of my previously published chapter "'It'll Remain a Shock for a While': Resisting Socialization into Long-Term Care in Joan Barfoot's *Exit Lines*." *Methoden der Alter(n)sforschung: Disziplinäre Positionen und transdisziplinäre Perspektiven*, edited by Andrea von Hülsen-Esch, Miriam Seidler, and Christian Tagsold, transcript, 2013, pp. 189–208.

Chapter 2.4 previously appeared, in a slightly different form, in "Defeating the Nursing Home Specter? Celebrations of Life in the Canadian Short Film *Rhonda's Party*." *Crossroads in American Studies: Transnational and Biocultural Encounters*, edited by Frederike Offizier, Marc Priewe, and Ariane Schröder, Winter, 2016, pp. 489–506.

Chapter 3.3 contains revised parts of my journal article "Putting Age into Place: John Mighton's *Half Life* and Joan Barfoot's *Exit Lines*." *Age, Culture, Humanities: An Interdisciplinary Journal*, vol. 2, Jan. 2015, pp. 159–83, https://doi.org/10.7146/ageculturehumanities.v2i.130742 and is republished here with permission from Coastal Carolina University.

Chapter 3.4 is an extended version of my article "'Time to Go. Fast Not Slow': Geronticide and the Burden Narrative of Old Age in Margaret Atwood's 'Torching the Dusties.'" *European Journal of English Studies*, vol. 22, no. 1, 2018, pp. 46–58, https://doi.org/10.1080/13825577.2018.1427200, © Informa UK Limited, trading as Taylor & Francis Group, reprinted by permission of Informa UK Limited, trading as Taylor & Francis Ltd, http://www.tandfonline.com.

Chapter 4.2 previously appeared in parts as my book chapter "A Man Should Be Able to Take a Trip If He Wants: Oscar Casares' *Amigoland*." *Senior Tourism: Multi- and Interdisciplinary Perspectives*, edited by Simone Francescato, Roberta Maierhofer, Valeria Minghetti, and Eva-Maria Trinkaus, transcript, 2017, pp. 50–75.

Chapter 4.3 contains revised texts from my journal article "Transgressing Borders: Intersectionality and Genre in Thom Fitzgerald's *Cloudburst* (2010)." *Oltreoceano: Transatlantic Transition*, vol. 11, 2016, pp. 41–48. The subchapter on *Flee, Fly, Flown* has previously been published in parts in the book chapter "Forget, Forgot, Forgotten? Cultural Constructions of Dementia in Janet Hepburn's Care Home Novel *Flee, Fly, Flown* (2013)." *Kulturen der Sorge: Wie unsere Gesellschaft ein Leben mit Demenz ermöglichen kann*, edited by Harm-Peer Zimmermann, Campus, 2018, pp. 361–83.

Introduction

The sun goes down. The trees bend,
they straighten up. They bend.
At eight the youngest daughter comes.
She holds his hand.
She says, Did they feed you?
He says no.
He says, Get me out of here.
He wants so much to say please,
but won't.

After a pause, she says—
he hears her say—
I love you like salt.

— Margaret Atwood, "King Lear in Respite Care"

Most had pleasant-sounding names referring to a valley or a view, a rest or a happy mood, like Sunset Manor or Pine View Hills or Merry Rest.

— Timothy Diamond, *Making Gray Gold*

Issues of aging, demographic change, and care dependency have become increasingly urgent across the United States, Canada, and Europe. As the North American baby boomer generation reaches retirement, the so-called "silver tsunami"—an ageist metaphor describing the anticipated demographic change (Charise)—has sparked widespread concern about economic stability and the sustainability of health care infrastructures. Consequently, considerations about how to grow old and where to live in old age have grown more pressing, emerging not just as matters of public policy but also as deeply personal anxieties. These societal debates resonate within contemporary literary and cinematic representations, where narratives of aging, caregiving, and institutionalization critically engage with, and often challenge, prevailing cultural perceptions of later life. In literature, these concerns have given rise to a distinct new genre, the *care home novel,* which focuses specifically on the emotional, social, and psychological experiences tied to relocating oneself or loved ones into a nursing home or similar care facilities. While moving to a care home can be rewarding experience that opens up new opportunities for social engagement and improved health, most fictional representations of institutional life are still rooted in a narrative of failing to age well (Chivers, "Blind" 134). Through such representations, film and fiction participate in the discursive construction of aging and old age and invite readers to re-imagine what eldercare could or should look like. The spatial setting of the care home often functions symbolically—as a metaphorical space embodying the experiences, fears, and uncertainties associated with old age. By literally and figuratively "putting age in its place," the care home highlights the marginalized social position of older adults, yet it can also facilitate agency and a reimagination of the protagonists' life-course narratives. A metaphorical reading of the care home thus shifts our focus from concrete realities to more abstract considerations, encouraging us to reflect on existential questions and whether, and how, an "ideal place" to live and grow old truly exists.

This book contributes to the interdisciplinary field of Age Studies, particularly its exploration of reimagining long-term residential care. Through a close reading and critical analysis of novels, short stories, plays, and films, it investigates how spaces and places designed to house the oldest old are simultaneously shaped by—and actively shape—the experience of old age. What underlying fears, hopes, and assumptions can be traced in such cultural representations? How do aspects of space and place influence the narrative construction of the life course and old age? Furthermore, what do such representations (and blanks that are not narrated) reveal about prevailing imaginations of aging and especially old age, in Canada and the United States, and the cultural assumptions surrounding care homes? Drawing on Susan Braedley's conceptualization of "ruling metaphors" (57) in care home design—namely the hospital, hotel, and home, as well as the prison metaphor proposed here within fictional contexts—this study seeks to contribute to a typology of the "care home novel."

It explores the spatial dimensions of late life and potentially uncovers new, forward-looking metaphors that may redefine conversations about aging, old age, and care practices. Anita Wohlmann's work on metaphor dovetails with this idea when she argues that "even when a metaphor appears problematic and limiting, it can in fact be reused and reimagined in unexpected and creative ways [...] we can repair it, or we can repurpose it (if need be) and thereby—in the spirit of upcycling—discover new value" (1).

While aging has traditionally been conceptualized as a temporal phenomenon, I argue—building on the work of cultural geographers of aging such as Glenda Laws, Gavin Andrews, and others[1]—that it must also be understood through the lens of spatiality. The experience of aging is not only a passage through time but also a movement through space—an idea explicitly embedded in common metaphors of aging. The metaphorical and literal marginalization of older adults as a separate population group, the notion of "the big move"[2] to a care home that severely disrupts everyday routines both temporally and spatially, as well as the prevailing ideal of "aging in place" all underscore the spatial dimensions inherent in discourses on later life. The room of the care home and even the old body itself can be read as converging time and space, intertwining personal histories, memories, and identities with immediate physical surroundings to continuously reshape experiences of selfhood. Recognizing how spatial and temporal dimensions intersect helps us understand how cultural narratives around aging, identity, and care are influenced by the physical spaces older adults live in, move through, and embody in their later years.

By linking Age Studies with approaches used by cultural geographers, this book analyzes how care home narratives rewrite the institution as a textual space in which stereotypical notions of old age can be challenged and deconstructed. Arguing for the centrality of the intersection of age, space, and place to increase our understanding of what it means to grow old, this study uses contemporary anglophone North American texts to illustrate how cultural constructions of especially old age are embedded in spatial practices. Entering the

---

1 For an excellent overview of approaches in geography, see Enßle-Reinhardt and Helbrecht.

2 Anne M. Wyatt-Brown, Helen Q. Kivnick, Ruth Ray Karpen, and Margaret Morganroth Gullette reflect on the transition into a Continuing Care Retirement Community in *The Big Move: Life Between the Turning Points*, Indiana UP, 2016.

fictional space of narrated long-term care facilities opens a terrain largely unexplored by Age Studies scholars. As the analyzed examples will show, cultural representations of the nursing home may open up theoretical and experiential dialogues about the role of space and place in relation to experiences of aging and the life-course.

This book situates itself in the field of literary Age Studies, or literary gerontology,[3] which has flourished during the past decades. In addition to the successful relaunch of the journal *Age, Culture, Humanities*, edited by Aagje Swinnen and Anita Wohlmann, two significant publications highlight the development and latest advancements in the area: *The Bloomsbury Handbook to Ageing in Contemporary Literature and Film* (2023), edited by Sarah Falcus, Heike Hartung, and Raquel Medina, and *The Palgrave Handbook of Literature and Aging* (2024), edited by Valerie Lipscomb and Aagje Swinnen. Both volumes showcase the diverse range of critical approaches employed in literary Age Studies, encompassing perspectives from environmental studies and cultural geography to critical race theory, postcolonialism, and queer studies. The intersection of space, place, and age is an underrepresented category in this field. The newly emerging genre of care home narratives has also not yet been addressed from an Age Studies perspective that includes spatial theory. Reflecting the *Spatial Turn*, I therefore suggest adding the dimension of space as a lens to a literary Age Studies approach in order challenge prevailing assumptions of the care home as merely a place of decline, disease, and death. Focusing on the importance of spatiality as a framework through which contemporary cultural constructions of home, embodied subjectivity, and old age can be understood, this book addresses cultural representations of institutional eldercare to showcase the complex spatial dynamics that are at play with regard to the construction and redefinition of life-course narratives.

Cultural depictions of care homes in literature and film consistently stress that they function as complex sites where architectural design, institutional organization, and social relationships intersect, shaping both lived experiences and broader perceptions of aging (Katz, *Cultural* 204; Buse et al. 1436). Far from neutral spaces, care homes reflect and reinforce ideologies of care, health, and wellbeing through the practices they make possible. Scholars across disciplines—from sociology and health geography to social policy and gerontology—have examined these institutions as sites where questions of

3 For a detailed discussion of the terms "Age Studies," "Aging Studies," and "Literary Gerontology," see Lipscomb and Swinnen, pp. 2–4.

identity, autonomy, and belonging are negotiated (Andrews 61). Yet the diversity of cultural, political, and economic contexts makes theorizing the care home difficult, underscoring the need for interdisciplinary approaches that can account for both material realities and cultural representations (Chivers, *From*; Chivers and Kriebernegg).

When confronted with the increasingly common imagery of aging and old age in popular culture, film, and literature, we are, as Mike Featherstone and Mike Hepworth argue, in our age-conscious society encouraged to scrutinize physical appearance and focus on the age characteristics of the bodies presented (29). Many such images display older people who have preserved their active lifestyle, beauty, fitness, health, and energy, focusing on "successful aging" (Rowe and Kahn), a term which is still used, but has been critically challenged by Age Studies scholars (Cruikshank, "Successful"; Stowe and Cooney; Katz and Calasanti). However, there are also disturbing images of people who are less successful, people who have "failed"—those "whose bodies have betrayed them and, whether through neglect, illness, accident, or fate, face a future in which they have been accorded the negative status of a dependent [...] old age" (Featherstone and Hepworth 29). Cultural representations of nursing homes usually highlight this "failure," not only in terms of the individual's failing body, but also in terms of the families' failure to take care of their loved ones, and society's failure to offer adequate care-giving structures for older adults, as Sally Chivers points out (*From Old Woman* 57).

Margaret Atwood's poem "King Lear in Respite Care," cited in the epigraph, exemplifies the perception of the care home as a site of failure, highlighting both familial guilt and societal neglect. The poem begins with the line, "The daughters have their parties" (85), immediately evoking a sense of abandonment. Like Lear's daughters in Shakespeare's play, they have left their aging father behind. The old man, disoriented and helpless, questions his surroundings: "How did this happen, this cave, this hovel?" (85), emphasizing his alienation. His youngest daughter, likened to Cordelia, visits him and holds his hand, yet her presence only reinforces his unfulfilled longing to return home. The poem suggests that she, too, carries a sense of guilt, embodying the societal expectation that his daughters should provide care. Here, the poem not only points to unresolved intergenerational conflicts and the wish for (re-)connection, but has also been read to reveal the pressure often felt, especially by women, to adhere to traditional gender roles and meet cultural expectations to act as the forgiving, caring, nurturing female (S. Jamieson 3). "King Lear in Respite Care" not only exposes unresolved intergenerational tensions, but also critiques the cultural and structural inadequacies that frame institutional care as both a personal and collective failure. As the poem's title indicates, the old man is in "respite care," a model of short-term institutional care developed to provide temporary relief for family members or other caretakers. How long "King Lear" will be in the nursing home is left open in the poem, but he obviously does not feel "at home" there. At the very least, the reference to Shakespeare's play insinuates a tragic ending.

As film and fiction not only reflect, but also create reality, an analysis of care home narratives might contribute to a new understanding of old age and, consequently, to cultural and social change with regard to care-giving institutions. John Bender, Stanford professor of English and Comparative Literature, shows in his seminal work *Imagining the Penitentiary* that attitudes toward prison that were formulated in eighteenth-century English literature in fact enabled the conception and construction of actual penitentiary prisons and prison reform: "The earlier eighteenth century novel bore the form within which the seeming randomness inside the old prison boundaries would later be restructured into a new penal order. Fabrications in narrative of the power of confinement to reshape personality contributed to a process of cultural representation whereby prisons were themselves conceived and thereby ultimately reinvented" (1). Following Bender, who considers "literature and the visual arts as an advanced form of knowledge, as cognitive instruments that anticipate and contribute to institutional formation" (1), I argue, perhaps boldly, that the recent emergence and rapidly increasing visibility of the care home narrative, together with its Age Studies analysis, could potentially be seen as anticipating and contributing to reform in the area of long-term institutional care. Several of the texts that are analyzed in the following chapters actually counteract the predominant narrative of decline (Gullette, *Declining*) and offer narratives of possibility, agency, and a good life until the very end.

When discussing my research with others, I often noticed that as soon as the term "care home" was mentioned, people felt compelled to share personal stories of visiting or placing a loved one in long-term care—stories often marked by difficult decisions, guilt, and a sense of loss or sadness. Sally Chivers offers an explanation for this reaction when she writes that nursing homes invite fear "partly because they house a conglomeration of what people often dread about old age. If old age were not necessarily to conjure up negative opinion, nursing homes may, in turn, not seem or be as threatening" (From 57–58). I hope that empowering fictional narratives can help reshape these negative perceptions of old age, ultimately fostering a vision of long-term care as a space of community, perhaps even joy, where a meaningful life is possible.

This project follows in the footsteps of my earlier collaboration with Sally Chivers, whose work on fictional representations of long-term care (Chivers, "Reimagining"; Chivers, *From Old Woman*; Adams and Chivers, "Architecture") has had a huge impact on my thinking, inspiring me to dig deeper into this genre. In 2017, Sally and I collaboratively edited *Care Home Stories: Aging, Disability, and Long-Term Residential Care*, a volume that aimed at highlighting the individual experiences of what it means to grow old in such facilities. Together with our authors, we aimed to challenge stereotypes of institutional care for older adults, illustrate the changes that have occurred over time, and illuminate the continuities in the stories we tell about nursing homes. By bringing together diverse perspectives, our volume sought to deepen the understanding of care homes as complex social and cultural spaces, emphasizing the need for more diverse and empathetic narratives about aging and long-term residential care. We explored various ways in which long-term residential care in later life might become desirable rather than merely necessary. What if institutional long-term care became a place not to fear but to look forward to—a milestone celebrated rather than dreaded, worthy of marking positively, even with a greeting card?

Finally, a quick note on terminology: in the context of this book, the term "long-term care facility" comprises all forms of institutionalized eldercare such as nursing homes, assisted living facilities, or retirement homes. A plethora of different definitions exist that not only depend upon country and region, but also upon individual institutional policies and funding schemes, and although I am aware of the differences, I use the terms "care home," "long-term-care facility," or "retirement home" interchangeably, and am only more specific if the exact type of institution is relevant for the argument upon which I base my interpretation. Sally Chivers and I agreed on a similar solution in our introduction to *Care Home Stories*, where we argue that the term "care homes" is complex enough to warrant discussion. While "nursing home" is commonly used in North America, its meaning varies by jurisdiction. Not all spaces explored in this book involve nursing, though all relate to paid or unpaid care work. Sally and I acknowledge the institutional legacy of these residences but avoid overemphasizing it, as "long-term residential care" can carry difficult connotations, especially for Indigenous people in Canada. With this in mind, I chose to use "care home" for its broader implications while incorporating other terms where relevant. After all, as Baldwin, Harris, and Kelly have noted, "'institutionalization' may occur regardless of the care setting" (qtd. in Andrews and Phillips, "Changing" 65).

Chapter Outline

In Chapter One, "Over the Hill to the Margins: The Spatial Politics of Age and Care," I briefly trace the development of institutional eldercare in North America. This is not to be understood as a detailed historiography of care-giving institutions, but serves to establish the context within which cultural narratives appearing in care-home literature and film are embedded. The chapter begins by tracing the historical stigma associated with the institution's history from poorhouses to modern care facilities. The enduring fear of nursing homes, described by Betty Friedan as "death sentences" (510) is linked to their historical roots in poor relief systems and their continued portrayal as spaces of decline and dependency. Building on this historical context, the chapter delves into the spatiality of age relations, emphasizing how care homes are more than just physical structures; they are shaped by intersecting social, economic, and ideological forces. Drawing on theorists such as Stephen Katz, Gavin Andrews, and Glenda Laws, the discussion highlights how spatial organization within these institutions influences the lived experiences of residents, caregivers, and family members. Institutional spaces, rather than being neutral, actively contribute to the construction of aged identities through their design, regulations, and the discourses surrounding them.

The second part of this chapter puts contemporary spatial theory, especially the work of Michel Foucault, Henri Lefebvre, Doreen Massey, John Urry, and Mikhail Bakhtin in dialogue with Age Studies in order to elucidate how these approaches and methods can enrich one another and to set the stage for my analysis. The third part of the chapter introduces the genre of the "care home narrative" and discusses the themes that have thus far guided its interpretations. The emergence of the "care home novel" as a distinct genre signals a growing engagement with the complexities of later life in fiction. While many narratives reinforce fears of institutionalization through depictions of neglect and confinement, others present more refined portrayals that emphasize autonomy, resilience, and community within care homes. By integrating historical analysis, spatial theory, and a typology of the care home novel, this chapter underscores the importance of viewing long-term care through a spatial lens.

The first part of Chapter Two, "Home, Hotel, Hospital: The Care Home at the Nexus of Public and Private," establishes the care home as a liminal space that exists between institutional and domestic realms, drawing comparisons to hospitals, hotels, and even airplanes to highlight its structured yet ambiguous nature. While efforts to design care homes with homelike aesthetics seek to soften their institutional character, the chapter interrogates the limitations of these approaches, questioning whether spatial design alone can counteract the loss of autonomy, identity, and agency experienced by residents—laying the foundation for the literary analysis that follows. I then explore the symbolic and concrete dimensions of spatial identity by focusing on fictional characters who, as residents or workers of an institution discursively lodged within decline, search for new progress narratives that emphasize their individuality. Patients/residents and caregivers alike must redefine their identities in the homogenizing place situated at the crossroads of hotel and hospital, a place that is commonly seen as the opposite of "home." With Edna Alford's short story cycle *A Sleep Full of Dreams* and the Caribbean-Canadian writer Shani Mootoo's novel *Cereus Blooms at Night* as touchstones, the first part of this chapter discusses narratives in which care-givers function as focalizers, introducing readers to the world of the care home from the perspective of two nurses. *A Sleep Full of Dreams* focuses on Nurse Arla, a young woman who finds it terribly difficult, even threatening, to deal with old age, frailty, and dying. In vignettes that are simultaneously brutal, grotesque, comically absurd, and sad, readers are presented with a nightmarish hospital-like institution that is diametrically opposed to any notion of what it means to be "at home." The cycle reveals the powerlessness, vulnerability, and loneliness of the old in the world of the care home, and crystallizes the conflicts central to the struggle to maintain one's sense of self in an institutional space that interpellates, in the words of Louis Althusser (28), everyone (i.e., both caregivers and recipients of care) into their respective roles.

The second text, *Cereus Blooms at Night*, explores intersectional identity, memory, and resilience by examining the entanglement of personal histories, spatial belonging, and the legacies of colonial violence. Through the narrative of Tyler, a homosexual Afro-Caribbean nurse at Paradise Alms House on the Caribbean island of Lantanacamara, readers learn the life story of his patient, an old woman named Mala Ramchandin. The almshouse, literally a "home over the hill," and its adjacent garden constitute the setting of the story's frame narrative and function as a productive literary "third space" (Bhabha 37) in which both Mala's and Nurse Tyler's life course narratives can be re-written, enabling the marginalized characters to come to terms with their traumatic pasts.

In the second part of chapter two, I juxtapose Joan Barfoot's novel *Exit Lines* and Ashley McKenzie's short film *Rhonda's Party*. These two narratives depict institutional care from the point of view of residents who challenge the "nursing home specter." In contrast to phenomenological studies of care home narratives that explore transformation processes of individuals into "institutional bodies" (Wiersma and Dupuis), I show how fictional characters (both patients and care-givers) can be transformed and themselves transform the institution in what I see as counter-narratives of long-term institutional care. They demonstrate how subversive protagonists manage to maintain a sense of self in seemingly unconquerable institutional settings.

In Chapter Three, "Captives of Care—Prisoners to the Palsy: Resisting Confinement from Within," I reconsider the representation of spatial exclusion of frail, old people in the context of institutional care by offering a close reading of four texts that interpret the care home as an institution of confinement. These serve as examples that illustrate how care home residents, or inmates, each in their own way, rebel more or less successfully against their confinement from within the care home. The first part establishes confinement as a central metaphor in representations of aging, positioning the nursing home as a synecdoche for broader anxieties about bodily decline and loss of autonomy. Drawing on Bakhtin's concept of the chronotope, as well as literary and cultural narratives that frame old age as imprisonment, the discussion highlights how spatial metaphors—whether the aging body as a restrictive space or the care home as a site of entrapment—shape perceptions of aging, thereby setting the stage for the literary analysis that follows. I then juxtapose May Sarton's *As We Are Now* (1973) with Leslie Larson's *Breaking Out of Bedlam* (2010), two *Reifungsromane* (Waxman, "From") in which the old and strong female protagonists document their struggle against homogenization and marginalization in institutional long-term care by means of keeping a journal. Both women find a way to maintain their agency and individuality and figuratively shake off the shackles of institutional confinement. While Sarton's main character Caro Spencer chooses to commit suicide by burning down the care home, Larson's protagonist Cora Sledge opts for life and moves back into her old house.

In the third text discussed in this chapter, John Mighton's play *Half Life* (2005), the space of a prison-like long-term care facility is represented as a "total institution" (Goffman, *Asylums* xiii) in which the "geriatric gaze" (Hepworth, "Images" 12) prevents a romantic relationship between two residents, Clara and Patrick, from developing. Patrick, who is locked away on a closed ward, keeps cracking the door code in order to see his beloved Clara, who has dementia, but seems to remember very clearly that she and Patrick were lovers during the war. However, both her son and Patrick's daughter have difficulties accepting the old couple's romance. Life inside the limits of institutional space is, as the title of the play indicates, only a "half life;" the nursing home is a world separated from the outside, where different rules and regulations apply that contribute to interpellating individuals into their roles as patients, stripping them of their personal freedom and choice.

This choice is entirely obliterated in Margaret Atwood's dystopian short story "Torching the Dusties," which portrays a violent movement systematically incinerating elder care facilities across North America. Returning to Michel Foucault's concept of "heterotopia," I explore the marginalization of old age and the ageism manifested in spatial segregation. The short story can be read as a satirical burden narrative of old age that reveals how the rhetoric of crisis disaffiliates the oldest old (in discursive and spatial terms) from the young, establishing a binary opposition that affects the nursing home inmates' identity construction.

Chapter Four, "Fugitives and Escapees: A Gendered Reading of the Spatiality of Resistance," explores the care home escape narrative, a genre that has gained increasing popularity in recent years. Using the road narrative as a template, these stories contrast the freedom of the open road with the limited world of the care home, presenting escape as an act of resistance against the institutionalization of old age, and old age itself. The journeys undertaken by care home "escapees" are both physical and psychological, allowing protagonists to challenge spatial confinement, reclaim agency, and reevaluate their identities in ways that would not have been possible within the restrictive context of institutional care. Framing these narratives within spatial theory, particularly Doreen Massey's argument that space is inherently shaped by gendered power relations, the chapter examines how care homes function as sites of coerced immobility (Urry), where older individuals—especially women—are positioned as passive subjects rather than autonomous agents. The decline narrative of old age is counteracted by the escape narrative, which reconfigures the spatiality of aging in complex and ambivalent ways. Gendered power structures remain deeply embedded in these narratives: female escapees, as seen in *Cloudburst* (Fitzgerald, 2010) and *Flee, Fly, Flown* (Hepburn, 2013), often encounter obstacles and are perceived as being "out of place" when transgressing spatial and social boundaries. Hepburn's protagonists, for example, find their newfound mobility overwhelming and "disconcerting" (172), whereas male escapees, such as those in *Amigoland* (Casares, 2009), tend to navigate their newfound autonomy with greater self-determination. By integrating theories of mobility (Urry), agency, and the gendered spatiality of the road (Ganser; Sletedahl Macpherson), this chapter interrogates the ways in which care home escape narratives challenge dominant discourses on aging and institutionalization. It also considers the increasing popularity of these narratives and their potential to subvert traditional representations of old age—not by denying its limitations, but by reimagining aging as a site of resistance and self-assertion.

1 Over the Hill to the Margins

The Spatial Politics of Age and Care

Over the hill to the poor-house—my child'rn dear, good-bye!
Many a night I've watched you when only God was nigh;
And God'll judge between us; but I will al'ays pray
That you shall never suffer the half that I do to-day!

— Will Carleton, "Over the Hill to the Poorhouse"

As of now, we all know what to expect, but their generation
is the first to fade like this, not at home, but assigned
to a numbered frequent ward, stowed out of conscience
as unpopular luggage.

— W. H. Auden, "Old People's Home"

While institutional eldercare has advanced considerably over the past century, the transition into a care facility often remains fraught with fear and uncertainty. As Chivers observes ("Blind" 134), this move is still frequently regarded as "a fate worse than death." Similarly, Betty Friedan's discussion of the "nursing home specter" in *The Fountain of Age* underscores how deeply such anxieties persist in cultural memory, continuing to shape societal perceptions of long-term institutional care. Friedan characterizes nursing homes as "death sentences, the final interment from which there is no exit but death" (510), capturing the hopelessness, fear, and threat emanating from such institutions. The dread associated with nursing homes arises, in part, from their inextricable link to decline, decrepitude, and death, and the often bleak, neglectful conditions documented in some facilities. It is no coincidence that the term "nursing home" holds a significant place in the 2016 edition of the *Encyclopedia of Ageism*. Additionally, the institution remains burdened by its historical roots in the poorhouse system, reinforcing its enduring stigma.[1]

Already in 1872, when Will Carleton published his poem "Over the Hill to the Poorhouse," institutional care was a dreaded fate for older adults. The poem, later adapted into a popular song (1874), features an old woman lamenting her destiny: "Many a step I've taken a-toilin' to and fro / But this is a sort of journey I never thought to go," she complains (30). She is unable to comprehend why none of her six children will care for her. In her youth, she never faced marginalization: "Once I was young an' han'some—I was, upon my soul— / Once my cheeks was roses, my eyes as black as coal: / An' I can't remember, in them days of hearin' people say / For any kind of reason, that I was in their way" (30). Now, in old age, she has nowhere to go but the poorhouse, a fate she describes as 'horrid and queer'" (30).

The Spatiality of Age Relations

When care homes are represented in novels or films, such depictions always place an emphasis on the fact that such a home is more than just a simple building. Rather, it is "a micro-complex of architectural, administrative, financial, clinical, familial, symbolic, and emotional interactions and power relations" (Katz, *Cultural* 204).[2] These institutions are neither neutral nor static spaces; rather, they are socially constructed—both as physical environments and as fictional representations—shaped by intersecting and sometimes conflicting social imaginaries and discursive frameworks. As Buse et al. explain, "More than simply acting as repositories of symbolic power or ideological meaning (Jones 2011), buildings help to enact ideologies – of care, health and wellbeing – through the social practices they enable and encourage" (1436). These different frameworks shape not only the design of such institutions and the care they provide but also reflect and reinforce societal perceptions of aging, an idea Susan Braedley theorizes in her work on "ruling metaphors" ("Reinventing").

Although it is quite difficult to theorize the care home due to the vast differences not only in terms of geographical, cultural, socio-political and

---

1 For a comprehensive history of the nursing home as an institution, see Michael B. Katz; Stephen Katz (*Disciplining*); Foundation Aiding the Elderly (FATE) as well as Holstein and Cole.

2 Similar observations that interpret the home and other total institutions as mini-cosmoses of society have been made by Caudell.

economic contexts, (Chivers, *From;* Chivers and Kriebernegg) the last decades have witnessed the production of institutional ethnographies and socio-gerontological studies that deal with the conditions of living and working in institutional, residential, and community-care spaces (Arber and Ginn; Arber and Evandrou; Diamond, *Making;* Diamond, "Nursing;" Gubrium, *Speaking;* Gubrium, *Living*). A vast body of work has been produced on the nursing home and its relation to aging and identity by sociologists and critical gerontologists (Dyck et al.; Kontos, "Resisting;" Kontos, "Rethinking"), as well as by cultural gerontologists and cultural geographers (McHugh, "Generational;" Andrews). Health geographer Gavin Andrews maintains that "[r]esearch interest in residential homes has occurred across a number of academic subdisciplines including medical/health geography, medical sociology, environmental psychology, social policy and health economics, as well as across health professional research disciplines including nursing, occupational therapy and social work research" (61). Andrews is particularly interested in the spatial aspects of aging and how space shapes the experience of later life, considering, for example, how the built environment, institutional organization, and social relationships within care homes influence older adults' sense of identity, autonomy, and belonging. Andrews's review notably omits the humanities, despite the growing body of work examining how literature and film engage with aging, space, and institutional care. This gap underscores the need for an interdisciplinary approach that integrates literary analysis into discussions of the spatial dimensions of aging. Building on this need, my book examines how contemporary anglophone literature and film narrate the care home as a complex and often contested space, demonstrating how fiction both reflects and reshapes cultural understandings of old age and institutional care.

The spatiality of identity, particularly in its intersections with time and experience, serves as a productive starting point for analyzing care home narratives. Cultural geographer Glenda Laws, referencing Edward Soja's concept of the "socio-spatial dialectic," maintains that space and place not only reflect but also actively shape social practices and identities, including aging and care. She emphasizes that "places, like retirement communities or nursing homes, are obviously created by social practices. For example, once nursing homes were created, attitudes about the appropriate locus of care for certain categories of older people changed" ("Spatiality" 92). Her work illustrates how institutionalized spaces influence both individual and collective perceptions of aging. Age is defined by place, and *where* one is old matters: "Identities are spatialized, in that where we are says a lot about who we are," Laws comments (93). At the same time, older adults also constitute spaces and places, as she points out (93).

Will Carleton's poem highlights the binary construction of youth and old age by connecting spatial practices to social exclusion. The old woman perceives herself as an inconvenience to her children, no longer belonging, and is thus relegated to the poorhouse—pushed to society's periphery. Carleton's notion of making space for the younger generation aligns with Ralph Waldo Emerson's "Old Age" (1870) in which he observes,

> Youth is everywhere in place. Age, like women, requires fit surroundings. Age is comely in coaches, in churches, in chairs of state and ceremony, in council-chambers, in courts of justice and historical societies. Age is becoming in the country [...]. In short, the creed of the street is, Old Age is not disgraceful, but immensely disadvantageous. Life is well enough, but we shall all be glad to get out of it, and they will all be glad to have us. (285)

Emerson's dire conclusion underscores the social desire to expel older people from shared spaces, a sentiment that echoes the forced displacement dramatized in Carleton's poem. Glenda Laws, who also draws on Emerson's essay, argues that old age is often "peripheralized (its immense disadvantage) into discrete locations" ("Spatiality" 91). She observes that as we age, our place in society, both materially and metaphorically, changes: "The material spaces and places in which we live, work and engage in leisure activities are age-graded and, in turn, age is associated with particular places and spaces" (90). Laws develops the idea of the spatiality of age relations by connecting recent developments in social theory that concern the construction of identities and subjects to an examination of how "aged identities are reflected in and constituted by both materially and discursively constructed built environments" (91). She suggests that "the seeming simultaneous persistence and transformation of these relationships requires gerontologists to pay greater attention to the reciprocal relations between the social and the spatial if they are to understand the (re)construction of aged identities" (91).

My specific objectives in this chapter are to develop an idea of the spatiality of age relations in care home literature and film, demonstrating that the theories developed within the framework of the Spatial Turn can be useful for the construction of subjects and identities. I examine, in the words of Laws, "how aged identities are reflected in and constituted by both materially and discursively constructed built environments" (91). Care homes are not exempt from this observation: the space and place allocated to housing old age contributes to discourses on the aging body and individual. As Gubrium and Holstein put it, the home serves as a "discursive anchor for the aging body [...]. We age bodily, in other words, as much because our bodies are discursively anchored by a particular institution, as because our bodies grow old" ("Nursing" 537). The home shapes its residents' identities by providing a framework of signification and description (533). In this sense, the institutional space of the care home not only reflects societal attitudes toward aging but actively participates in constructing what it means to grow old. As long as aging bodies are spatially and metaphorically relegated to the margins, the exclusion of older adults from dominant cultural narratives will persist. As Sarah Harper aptly observes with regard to frail, aging bodies on the margins of society,

> Only when we are able to accept the changing and declining body as part of the normal experience of humanity, one that is crucial for defining human life and (while recognising the extreme diversity of the human ageing experience), return it spatially and metaphorically to centre-stage within human experience, will the inclusion of all older adults within the mainstream occur. (191)

Recognizing this interconnectedness between space, identity, and cultural perceptions of aging is essential for challenging stereotypes and fostering alternative, more inclusive representations of later life, as well as reimagining spaces and places of care for older adults. This, in fact, needs a conscious rethinking of the metaphorical language used in the narratives we tell about long-term care.

The Spatiality of Care Relations

Like age, care as a social practice must also be understood through the lens of spatiality, as it is deeply embedded in the physical and social environments in which it takes place (Lin et al.). Care, as Joan Tronto and Berenice Fisher famously maintain, is "a species activity that includes everything that we do to maintain, continue, and repair our 'world' so that we can live in it as well as possible. That world includes our bodies, our selves, and our environment, all of which we seek to interweave in a complex, life-sustaining web" (Fisher and Tronto 40). This widely cited definition extends beyond the conventional understanding of care as solely care work, instead emphasizing its broader, relational nature and its connection with space and place.

The built environment of care homes—ranging from their architectural design to their spatial organization—plays a crucial role in shaping the experiences of both caregivers and care recipients. Institutional cultures within these settings evolve in response to broader political and economic shifts, particularly in times of neoliberal privatization presenting us with, in Emma Dowling's words, a "toxic cocktail of recession and austerity" (1) which often leads to cost-cutting measures, staff shortages, and increased workloads. These changes, in turn, have profound effects on the nature and quality of care relationships, influencing how care work is delivered, received, and experienced on an everyday basis. In such challenging conditions, care work becomes reframed as a task-oriented labor, strictly adhering to standardized institutional protocols, guidelines, and regulations. Emma Dowling captures the severity of these shifts by describing them as a "crisis of care," a concept that underscores the widening gap between growing care needs and the diminishing resources allocated to meet them:

> To speak of a crisis of care is to point to the growing gap between care needs and the resources made available to meet them. […] In an unequal world, no crisis affects everyone equally. To speak of crisis is thus to ask the question, a crisis for whom? It means to highlight class and inequality in the way the crisis is experienced, and in the way that care is organised to entrench division and pit us against one another. It means asking: who is cared for and who is not? (Dowling 6)

In her book, Dowling addresses intersectional perspectives and discusses how care and care work are increasingly structured through transnational care arrangements and migration, which are fundamental components of what Arlie Hochschild calls global care chains (Dowling 12). The movement of care workers across borders, often from lower-income to higher-income countries, reflects larger economic disparities, geopolitical inequalities, and moral conflict (von Kutzleben et al.; Dowling; Armstrong and Braedley, "Care;" Owusu et al.). These global care chains—wherein care responsibilities are transferred across different geographic and social spaces—also highlight the spatialized nature of care and care work, as they reshape family structures, labor markets, and social policies.

Within this context, neoliberal policy frameworks have increasingly redefined care not as a shared social responsibility but as a private transaction, a commodity to be purchased in the marketplace. As public infrastructures recede, the care home itself becomes a spatial manifestation of these market logics, reframed through ruling metaphors of the hospital, hotel, and home—and, more darkly, the prison. Such metaphors underscore how institutional spaces are shaped by economic rationalities, where the quality of support, the degree of autonomy, and even the possibility of "aging well" are contingent on financial resources.

The COVID-19 pandemic has further underlined the significance of spatial dimensions in care work. Nursing home residents have been disproportionately affected by COVID-19, experiencing higher rates of infection, hospitalization, and mortality (H. Armstrong 19). Lockdowns, social distancing measures, and restrictions on mobility not only altered the logistics of caregiving but also exacerbated existing vulnerabilities within care systems, as Margaret Gullette discusses in *American Eldercide*. The crisis exposed and intensified the fragility of institutional care structures, the precarious conditions of migrant care workers, and the emotional and physical toll on both caregivers and those receiving care, as well as their families and friends. Care homes were making headlines due to the devastating conditions and became labelled the pandemic's "ground zero" (Barnett and Grabowski 1), which significantly contributed to the nursing home specter.

1.1 From Almshouse to Nursing Home

"Modern long-term care cannot escape its history," Martha Holstein and Thomas R. Cole write in their thorough overview of the evolution of long-term care in America (21). For most of American history, they maintain, caring for older relatives and people with disabilities was predominantly the task of families, primarily women (19). As Joe Gaugler points out, care in old age was primarily ensured either by having multiple children who could provide support for parents experiencing chronic or age-related disabilities, or through accumulated wealth (422). From the founding of the United States until the early nineteenth century, he observes, American society was mostly rural and relatively younger compared to later periods. After the colonial period, beginning with 1820, care began to be institutionalized: the period from 1820 to 1865, Holstein and Cole note, "marked a deliberate turn to institutional poor relief" while medical care, except for the poorest, took place in domestic settings (19). From 1865 onwards, "institutional poor relief became harsher, hospitals increasingly biased toward acute care, and older people the dominant populations of the almshouse" (Holstein and Cole, "Evolution" 20).

In *Disciplining Old Age*, Stephen Katz analyzes the discursive construction of old age from a Foucauldian perspective, and traces the development of caregiving facilities back to its origins with the Elizabethan Poor Law (1601). The contradictory discourse of reform that emerged in the seventeenth century, as well as the complex structures of the almshouse and the poorhouse, contributed to a definition of old people as a separate group that has up until today been framed as burdensome. This is significant, because statistically only a relatively small number of persons have relied on public support (Katz, *Disciplining* 57–58). Since the 1830s, middle-class American culture has responded to the anxieties of growing old with a psychologically primitive strategy of splitting images of a "good" old age of health, virtue, self-reliance, and salvation from a "bad" old age of sickness, sin, dependency, premature death, and damnation (Cole, *Journey* 230). Katz explains this splitting as he writes with reference to Brian Gratton (*Urban Elders*, 123):

> In 1880, 10 out of 1000 persons 65 and over lived in almshouses while in 1923 it was 9 out of 1000. The number of elderly almshouse inmates in relation to the total elderly population was quite small. […] Nevertheless, popular and negative definitions of the elderly as a problem population abounded and were linked to their being left behind in the deteriorating almshouse system. (*Disciplining* 57–58)

Katz goes on to explain how old people became the butt of finger-pointing, emphasizing the belief that an improvident old age was the result of a misspent or dissolute life. "Thus, their care continued to be premised on the almshouse ethos of punitive reform and minimal charity," he writes (*Disciplining* 58). During this period, it became evident that almshouses could not meet the special needs of old people, which led to the enactment of the 1935 Social Security Act and the establishment of the modern long-term care system (Holstein and Cole 20).

The discourse of old age as a problem and the parallel development of institutional eldercare are closely linked to the establishment of geriatric medicine[3] which, as Stephen Katz notes, "was born in the hospitals and hospices of nineteenth-century Europe, especially in France, because confined within their walls were the elderly subjects upon whose bodies clinical researchers tested their ideas about senescence" (*Disciplining* 47). A key figure in this process was the physician Jean-Martin Charcot, whose observations on old age at the *Hôpital de la Salpêtrière* in Paris were compiled in *Clinical Lectures on the Diseases of Old Age* (1881). His work played a pivotal role in shaping the medical discourse on senescence by establishing, as Heike Hartung observes, "a clinical perspective on the aged body as a distinct system of meanings and problems" (*Narrating* 80). These developments contributed to the emergence of a burden narrative of old age, which, according to Katz, can be traced back "to a profound shift in the physiological and cultural conceptions of old age" (*Disciplining* 47). At the same time, the almshouse evolved into one of the "strongest institutional bases for the subjective homogeneity attributed to the elderly in general" (58), further reinforcing the association between aging, dependency, and institutionalization. Katz explains the institutional impact as follows:

> By the late nineteenth century, they [the old] constituted the majority of its residents and justified its continued existence. In return, the institutions made visible the social presence of the elderly as a poor, dependent, infirm, incapacitated, unproductive, unreformable, and differentiated population. The public got to know the elderly through a custodial gaze that uncharitably framed them as a subjected population who had been means-tested and classified as deserving of the state's welfare. Furthermore, [...] advocates for social reform embellished the symbolic significance of the dreaded almshouse in order to highlight the poverty of old age (Haber 1993). Given the dramatic increase in elderly occupants relative to the graduate removal of other groups, almshouses eventually became public old age homes. (*Disciplining* 58)

In the late nineteenth and early twentieth century, similar trends could be observed in Great Britain, the United States, and Canada, although in Canada, the process of transformation from a work house system to a network of old age homes took much longer than it did in the United States (59). Katz reports

3 For a detailed overview of the development of geriatric medicine, see Katz, *Disciplining*, and Cole, *Journey*. Cole also points to Mary Wilkins Freeman's text *A Mistaken Charity* (1887), which illustrates the discourse and conditions (*Journey* 204).

that it was not until 1947, with the passing of the *Homes for the Aged Act* in Ontario, "that the term *house of refuge* was changed to *home for the aged*, and the term *inmate* was replaced by *resident*" (59). People still slept in large dormitories, were separated according to sex, and were not allowed to leave the premises without permission (Blaikie, *Ageing* 49), and "the poorhouse became a symbol of brutality and corruption" (Cole, 1992, qtd. in Holstein and Cole, 28). Almshouses and related institutions of geriatric care, Katz states, "have been considered as a technology of differentiation, however gruesome or humane their conditions may have been. Their practices of relief and ethos of reform eventually became reserved for the elderly, mapping out their differentiated status and unifying their subjective attributes" (59).

Katz's observations are critical when considering the development of discourses about old age and its spatial differentiation. He shows how, in the United States, old age came to be defined as a "social problem," a narrative which is also reflected in the *Social Security Act* that was signed into law by President Franklin D. Roosevelt in 1935, and granted money to "aged needy individuals" (Title I, *Social Security Act*, qtd. in Achenbaum, "Risk" 69). Together, Title I, which inaugurated a federal-state program of old-age assistance, and Title II, an old-age insurance program, helped older Americans gain new rights, but also significantly contributed to the definition of old age as risk, especially for those who were not eligible for the program. This was because the right to old-age insurance was narrowly defined (Achenbaum, "Risk" 69), and offered little help for marginalized groups among the old.

This discourse on old age as a time of impoverishment, helplessness, and dependency is also described in Richard M. Garvin and Robert E. Burger's 1968 much-cited review of American nursing home care, *Where They Go to Die: The Tragedy of America's Aged*. It can be read as a vehement reaction against the commercialization of care homes in the early 1970s, reflecting the protests that arose and the demands for radical reform. Calling nursing homes "pre-funeral homes" or "death traps," Garvin and Burger argue that "[t]he nursing home today holds a terror for the aged that Bedlam once held for the insane, that chain gangs once held for convicts, and that sweatshops once held for children" (22). They emphasize the maltreatment of elders in such institutions and compare terrible situations to those of inmates of jails and asylums, reminding readers of what Erving Goffman calls a "total institution" (xiii). Goffman introduced this concept in his seminal 1961 work, *Asylums: Studies on the Social Condition of Mental Patients and Other Inmates*, in which he examines life within enclosed, regimented spaces such as hospitals, mental asylums, prisons, military barracks, monasteries, and nursing homes: "A total institution may be defined as a place of residence and work where a large number of like-situated individuals, cut off from the wider society for an appreciable period of time, together lead an enclosed, formally administered round of life" (xiii). By situating nursing homes within this framework, Garvin and Burger reinforce the idea that such institutions systematically strip older adults of autonomy and dignity. In their epilogue, they issue a forceful plea for urgent political intervention, concluding their analysis with the call to "save Granny from her dungeon" (186). They contend that their work should not be regarded merely as a social study but as an impassioned appeal to recognize and empathize with the plight of nursing home residents, or rather inmates: "To present the facts about homes for the aged, it is necessary to recreate the feeling of desperation in dilapidated rooms, the terror of fire" (11). *Where They Go to Die* encapsulates the dominant discourse of the late 1960s and early 1970s, which framed nursing homes as punitive and dehumanizing institutions, at a time when care home reform was still in its infancy. In many ways, these critiques of inhumane conditions in nursing homes echoed the earlier twentieth-century protests against the almshouse, underscoring a persistent historical pattern of institutional neglect and marginalization of older adults.

In *Old Age and the Search for Security: An American Social History*, Carole Haber and Brian Gratton describe a simultaneous development—the rise of the nursing home industry: "Between 1960 and 1976, the number of homes increased by 140 percent, the number of nursing beds by 302 percent, and most significantly, the revenues received by the industry by 2.000 [!] percent" (141). While in the 1960s, most of the homes were small, privately run facilities, private investors began to see old age as a new business: Holiday Inn and Sheraton Hotels were among the first to plan nursing home chains (Burger 15). This development indicates a shift in the culture of care-giving, which—as I will elaborate on later—was subsequently reflected in fiction and film. This shift contributed to discourses on changes in eldercare that began to take root in Canada and the US in the 1970s, leading to significant nursing home reform. That nursing home reform was widely discussed is reflected not only by the fact that Simone de Beauvoir added Robert E. Burger's full-length article "Who Cares for the Aged" as an appendix to *The Coming of Age (La Vieillesse)*, but also, and most importantly, through the implementation of Medicare and Medicaid in the framework of the 1965 amendments to the *Social Security Act.*[4] Together with the new quality control mechanisms that were implemented in the early 1970s, Medicare and Medicaid promoted discussions in both the United States and Canada, and facilitated the creation of new facilities that no longer resembled the dreaded Victorian poorhouse.

Canadian institutions also underwent radical changes in the latter half of the twentieth century. Discussions about Canadian eldercare are complicated by the lack of agreement on common language in terms of the names of long-term care facilities. Albert Banerjee observes that long-term care has different developmental histories in each province and territory, and that few pan-Canadian analyses of long-term care exist (3). Institutionalized eldercare, he writes, is "practically invisible at the federal level" (5). Megan Davies maintains in her excellent review of the development of nursing home care in Canada, *Into the House of Old: A History of Residential Care in British Columbia,* that just as in the U.S., institutional care can be traced back to the British legacy of the English Poor Law of 1601, a legacy that was "transmitted from one generation to another and reconfigured in various state and institutional policies and practices" (*Into* 4). The welfare state created in the 1950s and 1960s, Davies argues, "was laid on top of older poor law institutions and programs" (4), and led to developments in the second half of the twentieth century that were shaped by discourses highly similar to those prevailing in the United States, which framed the care home "as a place quite separate from the community, rather than a community institution" (Davies, "Renovating" 175). This development has fueled imaginations of the populace of these countries with images of gloom and horror.

From 1970 onwards, policymakers in the U.S. reacted to inspectors' allegations of poor standards and elder abuse in homes. Beginning in 1971, government regulations were put in place that attempted to ensure quality control, and the newly founded Office of Nursing Home Affairs within the Department for Health, Education, and Welfare provided a structure to reinforce these new measures (D. B. Smith 22). Even though in the nineteenth and early twentieth century the "dread of the poorhouse" had never relied on any statistical probability, because only an average of two percent of old people have lived in institutions, the fact that the poorhouse was considered a forerunner of today's nursing home played a decisive role in the history of American older adults (Haber and Gratton 116). "As part myth and part reality, institutionalization [...]

4 "Congress passed legislation in 1965 establishing the Medicare and Medicaid programs as Title XVIII and Title XIX, respectively, of the *Social Security Act*" (Klees et al. 3).

possessed a symbolic meaning," they contend (117): "The isolation and predominance of the aged in almshouses and private old-age homes became a broadly accepted symbol of the declining status of the old. [...] The elderly's longstanding fear that their days would end in the almshouse has a clear parallel in the contemporary belief that the nursing home might be their fate" (142).

Today, especially after the COVID-19 pandemic, nursing homes still represent a focal point for society's fear of aging. They are commonly described as terminal places from which there is no exit but death. In recent years, however, the question of how and where to live in old age has become more relevant than ever due to changing demographics:

> In 2011, the first of the baby boom generation reached what used to be known as retirement age. And for the next 18 years, boomers will be turning 65 at a rate of about 8,000 a day. As this unique cohort grows older, it will likely transform the institutions of aging—just as it has done to other aspects of American life. Will boomers redefine this life stage, or will it redefine them? (AARP)

As the website of the American Association of Retired Persons (AARP) informs us, new forms of eldercare are emerging, and the image of a hospital- or prison-like institution that focused primarily on the management of the old body in terms of a medical model is gradually being replaced by images of modern and comfortable homes that put personalized care and individual needs first. New housing schemes are being conceptualized where "leisure and consumption play an important symbolic role in affirming personal identities" (Blaikie, *Ageing* 175). As Andrew Blaikie comments, the "land of old age" is being redeveloped in such a way that congregated housing units emulate the appearance of grand-deco hotels and explicitly offer a "hotel lifestyle," while traditional homes for old people serve a population of frail elders who are largely excluded from the new construction of the life course and become "marginalized relics" (176). Which type of care-giving is suitable, affordable, and accessible for an individual depends on a plethora of parameters that are to a large extent related to aspects of the traditional matrix of "race, class, gender, age, and able-bodiedness."[5]

---

5 For an excellent analysis of how the material environments of retirement and assisted living communities "frame" their residents in ways that have deep implications for elder identities, identity management, and cultural citizenship (10) especially with regard to class, see Green Kuhn, *The Eye of Beauty: Creating a Place for Elite and Aging Elders*.

Only slightly more than 5% of the 65+ population in North America live in long-term care facilities, and about 70% of these people are women (Harris-Kojetin et al. 40). Holstein and Cole emphasize that the story of long-term care has mostly been told from the perspective of "white, middle-class [and I should add, male] reformers, providers, and administrators" (20), largely ignoring the care work accomplished by families, mostly women, and their informal networks. They are aware of the need of addressing more diverse stories of long-term care, "refracted through the prisms of gender, race, class, age, ethnicity, and geographical region" (20) but found ways to give voice to ethnic and racial minorities in their article (20).

Invisible Care

The novels, short stories, plays, poems, and films I have analyzed in my research mirror this demographic data not only with regard to gender, but also in terms of race and class[6] because they almost exclusively depict relatively privileged white residents as recipients of care. Changing demographics[7] show that as an increasing proportion of the population ages, an ever-increasing number of persons will be in need of professional care. This will also affect demographics within care-giving institutions, and culturally competent care-giving may become even more important in the coming years than it has been in the past (Kunow, "Aging").

This matter is closely linked to issues of globalization because care of old people, as Kathleen Woodward observes, "increasingly becomes a matter of the global market in our neoliberal economies" (17). Care-giving is perceived

---

6 "Non-Hispanic white persons accounted for at least three-quarters of users in all long-term care services sectors, except adult day services centers" (Harris-Kojetin et al. 34). According to Feng et al., more than 80% of American nursing home residents are White, whereas only ten percent are Black, three percent are Hispanic, and two percent are Asian (Feng et al. 1364). Likewise, Canadian nursing homes are populated by a majority of White, female customers (Mehrotra et al. 227).

7 The United States' National Center for Health Statistics' 2013 report *Long-Term Care Services in the United States* says that "recent projections estimate that over two-thirds of individuals who reach age 65 will need long-term care services during their lifetime. Largely due to aging baby boomers, the population is expected to become much older, with the number of Americans over age 65 projected to more than double, from 40.2 million in 2010 to 88.5 million in 2050. [...] The oldest old [those aged 85 and over] are projected to almost triple, from 6.3 million in 2015 to 17.9 million in 2050, accounting for 4.5% of the total population (U.S. Census Bureau, 2012)" (Harris-Kojetin et al. 3).

to be a relatively low-skilled job, and, as such, is a job usually performed by women. According to Farrell, almost 90 percent of the front-line workers in both institutional and home- and community-based settings are women, 56% of them from minority groups and many of those who work as nursing aides or UAPs (unlicensed assistive personnel) in North American care homes, an under-regulated and underpaid profession, have insufficient training, and need to work more than one job in order to earn a livable wage. Caregiver migration in the framework of the global care chain from the "Global South" to the "Global North" has critical implications for older members of society in the caregiver's countries of origin, leading to a "care crisis" (Calasanti 145; Dowling) in the "Global South" where children and old people are left without a primary caretaker. This dynamic not only exposes deep-seated gender and labor inequalities but also underscores the ethical and social consequences of a globalized care economy that prioritizes profit over the well-being of both caregivers and those they care for.

Kathleen Woodward addresses the invisibility of caregivers in her essay "A Public Secret: Assisted Living, Caregivers, Globalization," arguing that they are "shamefully unacknowledged by our society" (21). She renders this "scandalous public secret" visible by exploring the representation of caregivers and old people together, suggesting that "one of the most effective modes of advocating for changes in public policy is engaging in people's understanding through stories and images" (17). Woodward advocates for a new way of representing care-giving—a way that focuses on both the care-giver and old person: "Isolated and separate, caregivers and elders are vulnerable. Together, caregivers and elders are strong. [...] We need scholars without borders in age studies, scholars who understand that it is important not just to think globally and act locally but also to think locally and act globally—and who will call attention to the public secret of the caregivers of frail elders" (46). By reframing caregiving as a shared experience rather than an isolated burden, Woodward calls for a more inclusive and ethical discourse—one that not only acknowledges the labor of caregivers but also fosters a collective responsibility for aging and care in a globalized world.

The public secret Woodward identifies is, in fact, brought to light in several fictional and filmic accounts, challenging the notion that the caregiver's voice is universally silenced. As my analysis in the following chapters demonstrates, these representations occur more frequently than one might assume, offering multifaceted portrayals of both caregivers and the elders they assist. In the last year, 2024, several films appeared, addressing this topic. Two of them deserve to be mentioned here as they were shown in my hometown Graz's film festival "Diagonale" and won several awards. The first is *Tomorrow I leave* (Mâine Mă Duc), an Austrian/Romanian movie directed by Maria Lisa Pichler and Lukas Schöffel. The film highlights the invisibility of transnational carers through Maria's endless cycle of sacrifice. Every four weeks, she leaves her Romanian village to care for frail, old clients in Austria, while her own aging parents and family manage without her. Her work sustains others, yet she remains in constant transit, dreaming of one day settling down and opening a small bed and breakfast. The second film I would like to mention is the documentary film *24 Stunden* (24 Hours) that reveals the unseen daily reality of caregiving. Harald Friedl's film follows Sadina Lungu, a Romanian live-in caregiver in Lower Austria, uncovering a system of exploitation. Despite these harsh conditions, Sadina emerges as a compassionate, dedicated, and deeply caring individual. She provides Elisabeth, a bedridden woman living with dementia, with dignity and unwavering respect. In an interview, Friedl explains why he needed to address the "public secret:" "The final push to make this documentary came when Romanian caregivers were flown in during the COVID lockdown. The borders were closed, and they were quarantined in Schwechat [Vienna's airport]. That's when I realized how essential they are. And suddenly, everyone else did too. [...] They are never recognized as key contributors—but they are" (Bachmann, my transl.).

I contend that such literary and cinematic depictions, when critically examined alongside the systemic issues Woodward highlights, have the potential to shift societal perceptions of aging and care. By fostering a deeper awareness of both the vulnerabilities of frail elders and the precarious conditions faced by their caregivers, these narratives can serve as catalysts for meaningful change in both public consciousness and care practices.

1.2 Age Studies and the Spatial Turn

In "Of Other Spaces," an essay that is based on a lecture given in 1967 (first translated into English in 1986), Michel Foucault writes that while "the great obsession of the nineteenth century [...] was history [...], [t]he present epoch will perhaps be above all the epoch of space. We are in the epoch of simultaneity" (22). In *Mappings: Feminism and the Cultural Geographies of Encounter*, Susan Stanford Friedman argues that spatial thinking needs to complement temporal analysis (130) and urges us in response to Fredric Jameson's famous "Always historicize!" (9), to "Always spatialize!—that is, always ask how locational and geographical specifics particularize any given phenomenon or interpretation of it" (Friedman 130). The issue of space as an analytical category of the production of meaning and the question what it "does" and how it is "produced" has received increasing amounts of attention from members of various academic disciplines. Cultural geographer Edward Soja, who is said to have coined the term "Spatial Turn" in his book *Postmodern Geographies* (1989) (Döring and Thielmann 33), maintained in 1996 that the scholarly debate about the spatiality of human life "will eventually be considered one of the most important intellectual and political developments of the late 20th century" (*Thirdspace* 2).

Soja's objective is to encourage us "to think differently about the meanings and significance of space and those related concepts that compose and comprise the inherent spatiality of human life: place, location, locality, landscape, environment, home, city, region, territory, and geography" (1). He argues that the Spatial Turn contemporary Critical Studies has experienced since the 1990s signifies a development in which "scholars have begun to interpret space and the spatiality of human life with the same critical insight and emphasis that has traditionally been given to time and history on the one hand, and to social relations and society on the other" (verso).

The works of Doreen Massey, Susan Stanford Friedman, Edward Soja, but also of Mikhail Bakhtin, Michel de Certeau, Michel Foucault, Henri Lefebvre, and John Urry have shaped the Spatial Turn. These works have brought about a critical reevaluation of space and place from a background of primarily two traditions: cultural materialism on the one hand, which is influential primarily in the English-speaking world, and phenomenology on the other, which is influential particularly in German and French speaking contexts (Ganser, *Roads* 61). A strictly phenomenological approach that focuses on the experience of built space was represented most famously by Gaston Bachelard in *The Poetics of Space*, first published in 1958, or the abovementioned Yi-Fu Tuan's *Space and Place*, whereas American Cultural Studies mainly approach discussions of space and place from the perspective of cultural materialism, which is interested in space and place as a site and means of power (61).

In connection with the study of aging, aspects of social relations and space have been brought to the fore, especially by geographical gerontology, a discipline that since the 1970s has significantly influenced the development of critical and cultural gerontology (Andrews and Phillips 8). Although the Spatial Turn has not yet touched the mainstream of Age Studies, critical gerontologists have been interested in aspects of space and place particularly with regard to questions of the body, the home, residential care settings, and more generalized landscapes of aging (Kearns and Andrews 15). Before I develop a working hypothesis for the spatiality of aging in care home narratives, it is important to provide an (admittedly limited) overview of theoretical approaches to space relevant for the analysis to follow.

The terms "space" and "place" have so far been used interchangeably in this book. Scholars from various disciplines have, in the context of the Spatial Turn, elaborated on the difference between the two concepts. Depending on their approaches (phenomenological, social, political, geographical, aesthetic), their explanations highlight different aspects. American geographer and phenomenologist Yi-Fu Tuan in *Space and Place* (1977), for instance, focuses on "The Perspective of Experience," as the subtitle reads. He is interested in exploring the ways in which we feel and think about space, how people develop attachment to specific places such as "home," and how our sense of time affects our sense of space and place. He differentiates the two concepts as follows:

> "Space" is more abstract than "place." What begins as undifferentiated space becomes place as we get to know it better and endow it with value. Architects talk about the spatial qualities of place; they can equally well speak of the locational (place) qualities of space. The ideas "space" and "place" require each other for definition. From the security and stability of place we are aware of the openness, freedom, and threat of space, and vice versa. Furthermore, if we think of space as that which allows movement, then place is pause; each pause in movement makes it possible for location to be transformed into place. (Tuan, *Space* 6)

In *Environmental Gerontology: Making Meaningful Places in Old Age* (2013), editors Graham D. Rowles and Miriam Bernard define spaces similarly as "locations within a Cartesian world that, in and of themselves, have no meaning" (xii) and places as "those same locations transformed through processes of habitation and life experience into sites of great meaning that reinforce individual and group identity" (xii). They assert that space matters, but place matters even more, framing the care home as a place that threatens identity: Place "captures the essence of meaning in life" (20). "To be placeless," they write, "is to be alienated in the world and is a threat to identity. It is a fate that in our contemporary society confronts many people as their residential circumstances change toward the end of life" (20).

Co-Presence and Coerced Immobility

For the concrete analysis of my primary texts, I draw on John Urry's work on mobility which highlights the significance of physical travel in shaping social life, questioning why individuals persist in corporeal movement despite its challenges. He argues that social citizenship entails active participation in society, which requires spatial access and opportunities for co-presence. Restrictions on movement, such as those found in institutional settings like care homes, contribute to social exclusion by limiting both physical and social engagement. Urry envisions a "good society" as one that minimizes "coerced immobility" (270) and maximizes conditions for co-presence, ensuring that all members can participate meaningfully in social life. In this context, escape narratives (see Chapter Four) challenge these spatial constraints, resisting the institutional limitations that confine individuals and restrict their agency.

The Chronotope

Another theorist that is important for my analysis is Mikhail Bakhtin, especially his idea of the "chronotope," which refers to the "intrinsic connectedness of temporal and spatial relationships that are artistically expressed" (Bakhtin, *Dialogic* 84). "What counts for us," he writes, "is the fact that it expresses the inseparability of space and time [...]. In the literary artistic chronotope, spatial and temporal indicators are fused into one carefully thought-out, concrete whole. Time, as it were, thickens, takes on flesh, becomes artistically visible; likewise, space becomes charged and responsive to the movements of time, plot and history" (84). Ganser et al. explain the concept as a "means of measuring how, in a particular age, genre, or text, real historical time and space as well as fictional time and space are articulated in relation to one another. [...] The chronotope operates on two important levels: first, as the means by which a text represents history; and second, as the relation between images of time and space in the text, out of which any representation of history must be constructed" (Ganser et al. 2). Bakhtin exemplifies this by means of the road in adventure narratives: "Of special importance is the close link between the motif of meeting and the chronotope of the road ("the open road"), and of various types of meetings on the road. In the chronotope of the road, the unity of time and space markers is exhibited with exceptional precision and clarity" (Bakhtin, *Dialogic* 98). I will use this concept in Chapter Four, where Bakhtin's "idyllic chronotope" and the chronotope of stagnation will also play a role. I find it also enlightening in other contexts, for instance to explain aging in relation to the body, which, I will argue, can also be read as a chronotope.

The Spatial Triad

While Mikhail Bakhtin explores how the chronotope structures the relationship between time and space in narratives, Henri Lefebvre maintains that space itself is socially produced, shaped by ideological, economic, and political forces that regulate and control human activity. A key figure in spatial theory, Lefebvre's book *The Production of Space* (1974, first English translation in 1991) is considered "the most important book ever written about the social and historical significance of human spatiality and the particular power of the spatial imagination" (Soja, *Thirdspace* 8). Known for "spatialising Marxist theory" (Shields 8083), he observes that "space is never empty: it always embodies a meaning" (Lefebvre 154). He posits space as a product of power struggles writing that "(Social) space is a (social) product. [...] [S]pace has taken on, within the present mode of production, within society as it actually is, a sort of reality of its own. [...] [T]he space thus produced also serves as a tool of thought and of action; [...] in addition to being a means of production it is also a means of control, and hence of domination, of power" (26). He implies that "empty space," in the sense of an absolute space, cannot exist: "Natural space was soon populated by political forces" he notes (48) because once it is appropriated or colonized through social activity, it becomes "relativized and *historical*" (48). In other words, space is "the product of ideological, economic, and political forces (the domain of power) that seek to delimit, regulate and control the activities that occur within and through it" (Zieleniec 61).

Although, as Edward Soja rightly observes, *The Production of Space* is not easily approachable, it was through Lefebvre's work, and especially his "trialectics of spatiality," conceived space, lived space, and perceived space,[8] that a new way of theorizing space has evolved (*Thirdspace* 11). As Stanka Radović argues, "Lefebvre's three-dimensional analysis of space [is] based on the continuous interplay between material production, the production of knowledge, and the production of meaning" (11). I look at care homes as shaped by the interplay of (a) *perceived space* (spatial practice; the material space, social practice, and functional aspects of the institution), (b) *conceived space* (representations of space; the ideological and administrative frameworks that govern care, the knowledge production linked to it), and (c) *lived space* (representational spaces; the personal, affective experiences of those who reside there, i.e., the production of meaning). There is a dynamic interplay between material spatial practice

8 For an excellent overview of Henri Lefebvre's "trialectics of spatiality" (Soja, *Thirdspace* 10), see Elden; Shields; Radović; Soja; Ganser (*Roads*).

and its imaginative appropriations, marked by both interdependence and contradiction (Radović 11). In other words, these frameworks shape not only how care institutions are designed and managed but also how aging individuals are cared for—and, crucially, how their bodies are imagined, categorized, and regulated within cultural narratives of aging. A 2017 study by Christine Buse et al., "Imagined Bodies: Architects and Their Constructions of Later Life," illustrates this point, taking a similar approach and examining how architects conceptualize the aging body when designing residential care homes. The study found that architects' "conceptions of bodies were also permeated by prevailing ideologies of caring: although we found that they sought to resist dominant discourses of ageing, they nevertheless reproduced these discourses" (Buse et al. 1435).

Although Radović develops her theory in the context of Caribbean fiction, her insights, which include caregiving spaces, are equally relevant to this study. I align with her argument that "Lefebvre's *lived space* of daily human experience is reconceived through fiction into new forms of knowledge (*conceived space*), which in turn seek to critique and transform the material social practice (*perceived space*)" (11). Radović further draws on Christian Schmid's observation that, for Lefebvre, materiality in itself or material practice per se has no social existence without the thought that directs and represents it, and without the lived experience—the emotions and meanings invested in it (Schmidt 41, qtd. in Radović 11). Space, therefore, is not a fixed entity but emerges through the continuous interaction of all three dimensions (Radović 11). I also agree with her reasoning that, despite the primary challenge of applying Lefebvre's framework to literary analysis—namely, its foundation in material spatial practice—his approach remains valuable and relevant (12). As she explains, literature's engagement with spatiality is inherently indirect, yet it possesses a unique capacity to influence how space is perceived and understood:

> As an art of representation, literature is already at a remove from this concrete spatial practice. Yet literature's imaginative engagement with daily reality has a transformative potential, and, instead of understanding it as a passive formulation of utopian fantasy or ideological acquiescence, we may also think of its undeniable capacity to reshape the very terms of our engagement with the real. My use of Lefebvre's theory should therefore be understood as a frame of reference for a particular kind of literary reading, which seeks to preserve the continuous dialectical correlation between materiality, its conceptualization, and its symbolic meanings. (Radović 12)

This dialectical relationship between materiality, representation, and meaning is particularly relevant in the context of care homes, which are not just physical spaces but sites where aging is socially, culturally, and discursively constructed. As institutions that mediate the experience of old age, care homes embody both the material constraints of institutional life and the symbolic meanings attached to aging, dependency, and autonomy. Lefebvre's theory will thus be mainly a guiding theory for my understanding of the spatiality of aging in institutions.

Space, Place, and Gender

Doreen Massey adds the perspective of gender to the analysis of space and place. As a Marxist scholar, she has a high degree of awareness of class-based injustice and is certainly right when she contends that factors such as gender and ethnicity significantly shape how individuals engage with and experience space and place. Like Lefebvre, she emphasizes that these identities intersect with broader social and economic forces, influencing one's position within the dynamics of time-space compression: "Social relations always have a spatial form and spatial content. They exist, necessarily, both in space (i.e., in a locational relation to other social phenomena) and across space" (Massey 168). She describes social space as the intricate network of interwoven and dynamic relationships. From this perspective, a place emerges through the unique set of social interactions occurring within it. The distinctiveness of any given place is shaped both by the specific combination of interactions present—one that is not replicated elsewhere—and by the new social dynamics that arise from these converging relationships (168).

Apart from her focus on gender, Massey's work is also crucial to my study because it reveals how care home stories are shaped by social inequalities, often centering white, middle-class residents while marginalizing others. Her insights into intersectional power dynamics demonstrate that these spaces are not neutral but are deeply shaped by historical and social structures. This insight is particularly relevant as a backdrop to my analysis of narratives of colonialism, displacement, and queerness in *Cereus Blooms at Night*, which I analyze in Chapter Two. Massey critiques the dominant narratives of globalization, suggesting that fears of instability and uprootedness characterizing different kinds of postmodern identities often reflect the perspectives of a relatively privileged elite. She argues that feelings of disorientation and loss of control stem from a prior sense of stability and dominance—one that is not universally shared. She questions whose experiences of displacement and placelessness are being centered in these debates, asking, "To what extent, for instance, is this a predominantly white/First World take on things?" (165). Massey suggests that analyses of globalization have often, perhaps paradoxically, been shaped by a Western, white, and globalized perspective, overlooking the historical and ongoing displacements experienced by marginalized communities (166). She references bell hooks, who argues that "the very meaning of the term 'home', in terms of a sense of place, has been very different for those who have been colonized, and that it can change with the experiences of decolonization and of radicalization" (165). She also includes Toni Morrison's work, particularly *Beloved*, that challenges the romanticized notion that everyone once had a stable, unquestioned home—a place of belonging and ownership where identity could be securely rooted. "Yet some 'Others' of the dominant definers in First World society have always been there – women," she writes (Massey 166). For my work, it is Massey's focus on the spatial aspects of gender that helps me explore the role of female protagonists in shaping and navigating the care home spaces they inhabit—and escape from—as I will show in Chapter Four. If women have long been marginalized in these narratives, what happens when we turn our attention to older women?

Power Relations: Heterotopias and the Panopticon

A key shift in spatial thinking emerged through the work of Michel Foucault. Edward Soja observes that the reimagining of spatiality, as developed by Foucault and Henri Lefebvre, challenges and deconstructs all conventional modes of spatial thinking" (*Thirdspace* 163). Foucault's approach to spatiality, particularly his analyses of power, discipline, and institutions, redefines space as an active force in shaping social relations, making his work central to contemporary spatial theory. Like Lefebvre and Massey, although not from a Marxist point of view, and without a particular focus on gender, Foucault also argues that space is a "historico-political problem," linking issues of space to questions of power and knowledge:

> A whole history remains to be written of *spaces*—which would at the same time be the history of *powers* (both these terms in the plural)—from the great strategies of geo-politics to the little tactics of the habitat, institutional architecture from the classroom to the design of hospitals, passing via economic and political installations. It is surprising how long the problem of space took to emerge as a historico-political problem. (*Power* 149)

Here, Foucault stresses modern reconfigurations of knowledge and the organization of new institutions such as asylums, clinics, and hospitals in the eighteenth and nineteenth century. Already in his texts *Madness and Civilization* (1973), *The Birth of the Clinic* (1975), and *Discipline and Punish* (1979), the spatiality of power and knowledge played a role for Foucault who, although never explicitly mentioning old age, illustrated how "vagabond and 'unproductive' people were identified as political problems in seventeenth and eighteenth century European societies" (Katz, *Disciplining* 19). Divided by the state into mad, poor, or delinquent, these people were disciplined in institutions: asylums, hospitals, prisons, and schools (19), places Foucault calls "heterotopias" ("Of" 24). Every society, Foucault notes, needs and creates such spaces of "otherness" to deal with crisis and deviation so as to maintain its structured, rational order.

My analysis of the spatiality of old age is guided by the concept of "heterotopia," which—even though Edward Soja dismisses it as "[f]rustratingly incomplete, inconsistent, incoherent" (162)—serves as a useful concept to open up a discussion on the marginalization of old age. Foucault briefly mentions "heterotopia" in the preface to *Les Mots et Les Choses* (1966, Engl. *The Order of Things*) and develops it further in "Of Other Spaces." He focuses on the spatiality of power relations, and on the way cultural norms and social practices are revealed through space. In this brief text, he talks about those spaces "which have the curious property of being in relation with all the other sites, but in such a way as to suspect, neutralize, or invert the set of relations that they happen to designate, mirror, or reflect" (24). These spaces, he observes, "are linked with all the others," but at the same time "contradict all the other sites" (24). They are, he argues, utopias, imagined perfections or inversions of society *without* real space, or heterotopias (literally: "the other space"), spaces that in a way simulate reality. Heterotopic spaces are defined in dependence on and in contrast to utopias. While utopias are emplacements that have no real spatial existence, heterotopias are real places, "effectively enacted utopia[s]" (24)—or, in the case of involuntary confinement as in prisons or nursing homes, dystopias:

> There are also, probably in every culture, in every civilization, real places—places that do exist and that are formed in the very founding of society—which are something like counter-sites, a kind of effectively enacted utopia in which the real sites, all the other real sites that can be found within the culture, are simultaneously represented, contested, and inverted. Places of this kind are outside of all places, even though it may be possible to indi-

> cate their location in reality. Because these places are absolutely different from all the sites that they reflect and speak about, I shall call them, by way of contrast to utopias, heterotopias. ("Of Other Spaces" 24)

Foucault begins his essay by historicizing heterotopia, arguing that every society constitutes its own heterotopic sites that can take various forms. Like Soja and Lefebvre, he also observes that space is not neutral: "We do not live in a kind of void, inside of which we could place individuals and things. We do not live inside a void that could be colored with diverse shades of light, we live inside a set of relations that delineates sites which are irreducible to one another and absolutely not superimposable on one another" (23). As one central example, he determines the "crisis heterotopias" of "so-called primitive societies," sites which are "privileged or sacred or forbidden places, reserved for individuals who are, in relation to society and to the human environment in which they live, in a state of crisis: adolescents, menstruating women, pregnant women, the elderly [...]" (24). In modern societies, crisis heterotopias have increasingly been replaced by heterotopias of deviation (25). Such places can be brothels, colonies, or cemeteries, but also psychiatric wards, prisons, hospitals, or rest homes (25). With regard to the latter, Foucault writes that these are places where "individuals whose behavior is deviant in relation to the required mean or norm are placed" (25). He notes that old age is a deviant "since in our society where leisure is the rule, idleness is a sort of deviation" (25). This assumption and juxtaposition of leisure and idleness already emphasizes a particular image of old age, which is very often one of decline and physical decrepitude. The nursing home specter gains its potency precisely through such ageist discursive practices of marginalization and objectification in a dystopic space. Admitting, however, that in his earlier work he had overemphasized "technologies of domination," which render the body "docile" (135), Foucault corrected his own theory in later writings, ascribing agency and self-determination to the subject according to the subject positions that are obtainable. Such "technologies of the self" ("Technologies") are employed by individuals as power strategies through their recognition and instrumentalization of the subject positions available, thereby allowing them to actively participate in the creation of discursive formations. This agency not only opens up possibilities of resistance and subversion, but also enables individuals "to change history" (Olssen 32). With regard to the nursing home, this could mean that resisting and subverting everyday practices may eventually trigger change in institutional routines

(Harnett; Ryvicker). Stanka Radović sees the potential to challenge as inscribed even in heterotopia:

> Nevertheless, although heterotopias function by exclusion and serve to order and segment social space, they also hold the opposite potential: challenging the order they have helped establish, providing, as Foucault puts it, "a kind of contestation, both mythical and real, of the space in which we live" ("DS," 179). In other words, as soon as a space is created to uphold imaginary social barriers and keep the deviant at the margins of social life, that same space also offers a vantage point from which centrality and order can themselves be perceived and challenged. (196–97)

Even as institutions like care homes function to segregate aging bodies from the rest of society, they also provide a vantage point from which dominant norms about aging, dependency, and institutionalization can be questioned and reimagined. This means that care homes, often viewed as sites of confinement, can also become spaces of subversion—whether through small acts of resistance, communal bonds that defy institutional expectations, or narratives that reframe aging beyond the limitations imposed by institutional structures.

Another way of thinking the spatiality of institutional control is illustrated by Foucault in his examination of "Bentham's Panopticon" (*Discipline* 205). According to Foucault, power is exercised through institutions which facilitate self-regulation through the internalization of norms ("normalization," *Security* 56). The panoptical structure, consisting of a tower surrounded by a circular structure of light-flooded cells in which the inmates can easily be watched and controlled, is an "important mechanism, for it automatizes and disindividualizes power" (202). It makes inmates feel as if they are being observed all the time without knowing whether they are being watched or not, which creates paranoia—they are "caught up in a power situation of which they are themselves the bearers" (Foucault, *Discipline* 201). This system of internalized control held by wielding invisible modes of power is, according to Foucault, inherent in institutions like hospitals, infirmaries, the military, universities, or schools (*Discipline* 159):

> The Panopticon [...] is a type of location of bodies in space, of distribution of individuals in relation to one another, of hierarchical organization, of disposition of centres and channels of power, of definition of the instruments and modes of intervention of power, which can be implemented in hospitals, workshops, schools, prisons. Whenever one is dealing with a multiplic-

> ity of individuals on whom a task or a particular form of behavior must be imposed, the panoptic schema may be used. (*Discipline* 205)

Although many nursing homes have adapted their floor plans during the last decades and are, therefore, usually no longer structured like a panopticon, there is a notable exception that is worth mentioning in this context because it illustrates the abovementioned ideas by means of a Foucauldian work of art. When the German-Dutch artist Hartmut Wilkening was asked to design a sculpture for a newly built nursing home called *De Burcht* ("fortress") in Hoogezand, Netherlands in 2009, its floor plans inspired the artist to create a sculpture of Michel Foucault's head. In an article describing the design process of his project entitled *Vrij Geestig* ("Quite Witty," see fig. 1), he explains:

> The building of the De Burcht residential nursing home has the form of a panopticon. From the open well on the first floor there is an all-round view of the galleries on the upper floors where the entrance doors of the apartments are located. Inspired by the idea of a central point in the building from which everything can be seen in a single glance, and which can itself be seen from all angles, Hartmut Wilkening proposed to make a large sculpture depicting the head of Michel Foucault, the theoretician of panopticism. The concrete portrait of the French philosopher sports a broad smile, his arm emerges from the floor and his hand is resting on his bald head. (Wilkening, "Foucault")

Michel Foucault, Wilkening notes, was supposed to be the first inhabitant of the new building: "Before the placing of the roof, the sculpture was hoisted in with a crane, under the watchful eyes of the future residents and other invited guests" (*Foucault*). The head with its weight of seven tons cannot be removed anymore without destroying it. The artist's interpretation clearly links the care home's floorplans to Foucault's theory of the panopticon (Wilkening, "Michel" 83–88). Wilkening states that the head has received attention and popularity in artists' circles mainly because of the fact it has been moved into the home like a Trojan horse. He never meant this to be a cynical comment on residential care in any way, Wilkening says, and continues, "But the true potential for subversion lies not—neither in my view nor in Foucault's—in a possible uprising of the panopticon's inmates breaking free from their confinement. Rather, it emerges when the institution's content overflows, dissipating into endless details, ultimately rendering all forms of registration, measurement, treatment, and surveillance insignificant"[9] (Wilkening, "Frage" 1). In this sense, the sculpture not only invokes Foucault's panoptic gaze but also gestures toward the possibility that institutional control, when stretched to its limits, may unravel under the weight of its own rigidity, leaving space for new and unpredictable forms of agency to emerge.

Fig. 1: Hartmut Wilkening, "Vrij Geestig" ("Quite Witty").

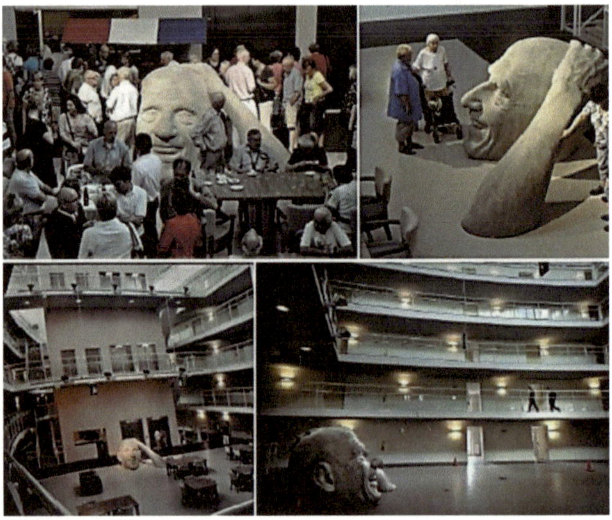

Photo credit: John Stoel. Photo collage assembled by the author from material obtained from the artist.

The Spatiality of the Care Home

While I agree with Hartmut Wilkening's interpretation of Foucauldian subversion in the context of care homes, I also find Glenda Laws's perspective compelling. She notes that the physical environment of a care home shapes

9 In the original text, Wilkening writes, "Aber das eigentliche Potential der Subversion liegt nicht – nach meiner Meinung und auch nicht nach der Überlegung von Foucault – in einem möglichen Aufstand der Insassen des Panopticons, die ihre Einschliessung durchbrechen, sondern eher darin, dass der Inhalt der Anstalt ausufert, sich in unendlichen Details verliert und so jede Form von Registration, Vermessung, Behandlung und Überwachung unbedeutend werden lässt" (Frage 1).

identity and social dynamics, noting that space "might place limits on the type of community that can develop in a particular place and thereby limit potential social interactions" ("Spatiality" 92). Once nursing homes were established, she explains, perceptions of where certain individuals should receive care shifted. "The webs of social relations in which we are enmeshed are constituted by space," she writes, reinforcing the idea that social relations are deeply tied to spatial structures (92). At the same time, she emphasizes that space not only shapes but also constrains these relationships (92). If we view social relations as influencing personal life narratives, then institutional settings can both enable and constrain individual identity development.

One of the most important readings of the panopticon in the context of theorizing the nursing home that focuses on the limits of identity development has been presented by the critical gerontologists Jaber Gubrium and James Holstein, who argue that "[o]rganizations establish general parameters for how narratives may be produced and who is authorized to produce them" (*Analyzing* 174). In their article "The Nursing Home as a Discursive Anchor for the Ageing Body," they maintain that "as populations age, the nursing home becomes a kind of 'panopticon' for discursive embodiment (Foucault 1979). While the nursing home applies healing, palliative, and custodial technologies, it also provides a framework for signification and description" (533). The nursing home does so as a physical entity, but unfolds its potency at a distance through the medical gaze:

> Staff, residents, and family members inspect and, in turn, are incited to describe bodies served and cared for in accordance with institutional categories, in the language of decay, decrepitude, or surprising fitness. [...] The panopticon even works in the opposite direction, providing the scrutiny and discourse of the healthy body with a source of comparison and the resulting gratitude that "it hasn't come to this", meaning the need to be placed in a nursing home because of frailty. ("Nursing" 533)

The fear of becoming frail, a "bag of bones," or a "vegetable" (522) after undergoing institutionalization is rooted in the discursive anchoring of the care home that focuses only on the body. This fear plays a constitutive role with regard to the decline narrative inherent in the cultural construction of old age—the fourth age, because it guides body talk relevant to disease, care-giving, and death. Together with the term "nursing home," it discursively encourages the appropriation of aging characteristics while talking about the body rather than about other matters (521). While the "third age" is commonly thought of as a time of independence, the "fourth age" is "marked by the arrival of major health problems" (Twigg, *Body* 50). Twigg notes that the distinction made between the third and fourth ages is not chronological, but qualitative: "In this the body is key, for it is the onset of serious infirmity that marks the point of transition. As a result, the fourth age can seem to be not just about the body, but nothing but the body. It dominates subjective experience, to the extent that it swamps all other factors in determining matters like morale or wellbeing" (*Body* 64). The fourth age, defined by its focus on bodily decline, is often equated with disease and deterioration—standing in stark contrast to the ideals of "successful" or "active" aging. Chris Gilleard and Paul Higgs further explore this divide and the marginalization of the oldest old:

> The fourth age emerges from the institutionalization of the infirmities of old age set against the appearance of a third-age culture that negates past representations of old age. [...] The fourth age is important as a cultural and structural component of aging but it is not constructed around the same coordinates as those of the third age. It is not simply the terminus of the third age, nor some kind of third-age anti-matter—the unsuccessful but necessary counterpart to successful aging. One way of approaching this issue is to consider the fourth age as a kind of social or cultural "black hole" that exercises a powerful gravitational pull upon the surrounding field of aging. ("Aging" 121–22)

Gilleard and Higgs address the difficulty of representing oldest old age by explaining it as a "black hole," a metaphor that signifies a place, or rather a space-time, where gravity is so intense that nothing can escape. This powerful metaphor evokes a sense of existential erasure and the end of signification, and those who enter risk vanishing from cultural recognition altogether. This concept, sociologist Amanda Grenier explains, "confronts the invisibility of the fourth age and the void of cultural space allocated to this group" (174). The use of the metaphor of a black hole, interpreted as a place of atemporality, highlights the sense of threat emanating from this phenomenon and seeks to explain the cultural "othering," reinforcing the ways in which society pushes the oldest old into the margins, rendering them almost untouchable, both literally and figuratively.

As a final example in my discussion of the Spatial Turn and critical gerontology, I include Haim Hazan's theory of the fourth age as "a-temporal territory of the fourth space" ("Beyond" 91). Like Gilleard and Higgs as well as Grenier, Hazan interprets the fourth age as a space/place beyond dialogue, a realm without language. He highlights the difficulty of representing this stage through language or any other form of cultural expression. Building on this idea, Heike Hartung contends that, unlike the "third space," the fourth age is defined by "a refusal of narrative continuity and closure" and becomes a space of "incommunicable oldest age" (21). It is beyond common cultural codes, as Hazan puts it: "[T]here exists no common experiential ground" ("Beyond" 94) in this "twilight zone of another human existence, a buffer separating the living from the dead" (96). In his essay "The Home Over the Hill: Towards a Modern Cosmology of Institutionalization," Hazan notes that the othering of old age "reflects the fundamental discord between human mortality and modernity. In a society where death is conceived of as being ahead of a person rather than alongside him, terminality is culturally unaccounted for, death becomes a taboo area, and the dying are rendered untouchable" (327). He sees the care home in modern societies as a holding space for the transition between life and death, shaped by modernity. As secularization and social fragmentation weaken traditional beliefs in an afterlife, what remains is the stark contrast between life and an "inconceivable nonlife." In this context, care homes step in to symbolize the blurred boundary between the two (328). Hazan echoes Gilleard and Higgs in maintaining, as Hartung summarizes, that the "third age," shaped by midlife norms, has taken control of the oldest age through management and surveillance (Hartung, *Ageing* 17).

As Gilleard and Higgs note, "[p]art of the definition of the third age is its active exclusion of 'old age' and 'agedness'. In that sense the cultural and structural boundaries of the third age may provide, through a process of antagonistic reciprocity, the structural boundaries for the 'fourth age'" ("Aging" 122). The "fourth age," they assert, does not so much represent a particular age cohort or stage of life as it "functions as a social imaginary" because it represents "a kind of terminal destination—a location stripped of the social and cultural capital that is most valued and which allows for the articulation of choice, autonomy, self-expression, and pleasure in later life" (123). Once in a care home, older individuals are refused any kind of futurity as they are not expected to develop in terms of a progress narrative anymore. It is commonly understood that any change signifies decline in the "waiting room for death." Hazan describes old age metaphorically in spatial terms: "The separation of the aged from society, the identification of ageing with ugliness, evil, and horror, and the reluctance to engage in physical contact with the aged all indicate that ageing is perceived as a dangerous area located, as it were, between life and death" (Old 68).

To further explore how the fourth age is shaped through spatial and cultural exclusion, it is useful to consider Gilleard and Higgs's argument on the structural boundaries between the third and fourth ages. Their perspective aligns with Hazan's notion of the fourth age as a realm beyond cultural representation, reinforcing the idea that old age is not only marginalized but fundamentally othered through spatial, social, and narrative separation. This interplay between exclusion, representation, and identity formation leads directly to a discussion of how cultural texts—particularly film and fiction—shape and challenge dominant portrayals of long-term care and aging. Concerning questions that address old age, identity, and long-term care, I argue that the Spatial Turn has put space and place on the agenda of researchers engaged in the interdisciplinary field of cultural gerontology. While many of them position the care home as a place "over the hill" where the old, as W.H. Auden writes, are "stowed out of conscience / as unpopular luggage," I will describe in the next section that the question of cultural representation of long-term care is also a central theme. In the next section, I will explore how film and fiction actively construct and deconstruct old age as "other," shaping societal perceptions and challenging dominant narratives.

1.3 The Care Home in Film and Fiction

In literature and film, the care home often serves as a symbol, a spatial metaphor for the experience, fears, and uncertainties associated with old age. Used as a setting or spatial frame, the care home illustrates the marginalized social position of old age ("over the hill" being one such position). The threat of ending up as inmates of the "'halfway houses' between society as we know it and the cemetery" (Garvin and Burger 11) has been mirrored in literary texts since the late 1960s and has become increasingly common up until today. Since then, the number of novels, plays, short stories, and films grappling with the complexities of housing the oldest old has grown significantly and shape our cultural understanding of long-term care. As Grist and Jennings write in their analysis of care and caregiving, "When care homes are visible in screen and in print their depictions as, at best, a badly run hotel staffed by ineffectual fools or, at worst, a ruthlessly run prison camp staffed by sadistic caretakers fuels the popular cultural imagination. These depictions undermine and undervalue the work done by real carers in real homes" (Grist and Jennings 2–3). I largely agree with their assessment—fiction and film frequently reinforce negative stereotypes of long-term care, emphasizing neglect, loss of agency, and institutional confinement. While such sensationalized and dystopian portrayals remain dominant, there has been a gradual shift toward more nuanced representations. Some recent narratives acknowledge the varied realities of eldercare, depicting settings that range from restrictive and infantilizing institutions to supportive, well-run communities with compassionate caregivers and even high-end amenities. Nonetheless, the "horrible home" trope—often drawing on Gothic elements and the sublime—continues to prevail. Although more balanced portrayals have started to emerge, they remain in the minority. The dominant cultural narrative still positions care homes as spaces of confinement and decline, reinforcing long-standing anxieties about aging and institutionalization. This ongoing tension between entrenched stereotypes and evolving representations underscores the complexity of how eldercare is imagined in contemporary literature and film.

Since the emergence of public old age homes in the early 20th century, both theories of aging and concepts of caregiving have evolved. Yet, the "nursing home specter" continues to loom large in the collective memory of aging societies on both sides of the Atlantic. This lingering fear has been both reinforced and challenged through a growing body of literature and film. One of the earliest literary explorations of the care home as a fraught space is *The Hearing Trumpet* (1974).[10] Written by Leonora Carrington, a British-born surrealist writer and artist who fled to Mexico during World War Two, this surreal and darkly humorous novel critiques institutionalization and the treatment of older women. Blending elements of detective fiction, the prison narrative, and the escape story, it also engages with climate change, caregiving, utopian feminism, queerness, and even anticipates posthumanism. As Helen Byatt observes in her excellent introduction to the 1996 edition, "It spans past, present, and future" (Carrington, *Hearing 1996* vi), while Ali Smith, in her introduction

10 Although this book focuses on North American novels, *The Hearing Trumpet* deserves a mention because of its significant influence on the genre. If one considers Leonora Carrington a British author, the novel does not strictly fit within the scope of this study. However, its pioneering depiction of the care home, along with its exploration of themes that later became central to North American narratives on aging and institutional care, makes it too important to ignore. While not part of the North American canon, its impact extends beyond national boundaries, making it a key reference in discussions of care home fiction.

to the 2003 edition, describes it as a "post-war, post nuclear vision, and one with ramifications in the global-warming era. Its reprint could not be more timely (Carrington, *Hearing 2003* x). The novel's fantastic and visionary narrative, centered on the empowerment of an old woman with a hearing disability, aligns with Mariana Cruz's characterization of it as a "geriatric and ecofeminist utopia" (Cruz 1) rich in social critique. In many ways, I argue, *The Hearing Trumpet* not only encompasses, but also anticipates many of the key themes that would come to define care home narratives over the following fifty years.

The category comprises a large variety of texts including comedy, drama, crime stories, slap stick "geezer lit mystery"/"geezer noir" stories, and novels that Barbara Frey Waxman calls *Reifungsromane*, novels of ripening, in which the authors portray their heroes and heroines "as forging new identities or reintegrating fragmented old ones and as acquiring the self-confidence, self-respect, and courage to live the remainder of their lives fully and joyously" ("From" 320). Recently, a wave of graphic novels has emerged, often focusing on adult children navigating the emotional and logistical challenges of caring for their aging parents and debating moving them into long-term care (Dalmer and Cedeira Serantes; Venema; DeFalco). A prime example is Roz Chast's *Can't We Talk About Something More Pleasant?*, whose title itself captures the discomfort and avoidance surrounding the topic.

In *Figurenmodelle des Alters in der deutschsprachigen Gegenwartsliteratur* (2010), Miriam Seidler asks whether the nursing home novel[11] ("Pflegeheimroman"), a type of novel which is primarily associated with places of physical and mental decline, would ever spark any interest in readers (316). Today, the answer is clear: authors who use the care home as a setting or theme have struck a chord. Fiction and films about long-term care institutions have grown increasingly popular, reflecting the public's rising interest in aging and old age. In Germany, Miriam Seidler was the first to explicitly define the care home novel as a distinct and emerging genre. While her classification of "closed" and "open" care home novels—those set entirely within care facilities versus those that only partially take place in them—offers a helpful framework, it provides only a limited perspective on how these narratives construct old age. Her work still delivers a valuable overview of the genre in German literature, and the questions she raises are equally relevant for analyzing North American literature. Why is

11 Peter Simonsen refers to the genre of the care home novel in the context of Scandinavian literature in his book *Livslange liv: Plejehjemsromaner og pensionsfortællinger fra velfærdsstaten* (2014).

this new genre gaining traction so rapidly? What discourses shape these narratives?

In the North American context, Sally Chivers was among the first to analyze literary representations of care homes. In *From Old Woman to Older Women* (2003), she explores this theme in her chapter "'Here, Every Minute Is Ninety Seconds': Fictional Perspectives on Nursing Home Care," where she implicitly identifies the emergence of the care home novel as a distinct genre (59). By juxtaposing multiple North American novels set in long-term care institutions, her work laid the foundation for further studies in this field. Chivers later expanded on these insights through her involvement in a Canadian research project led by Pat Armstrong and funded by the Social Sciences and Humanities Research Council Canada (SSHRC), which deepened her understanding of aging, caregiving, and institutional care. Her contributions have been invaluable to the field, and I am deeply indebted to her analysis.

In her PhD thesis from 2015 entitled *Long-Term Caring: Canadian Literary Narratives of Personal Agency and Identity in Late Life*, Patricia Life also argues that the genre has recently been emerging in anglophone Canadian literature (4). Analyzing several Canadian twenty-first century texts, Life, too, acknowledges that nursing-home narratives have become "a recognizable genre, under the general umbrella of age narratives" (4):

> [It is a genre] that begins with realism flavoured by the gothic, evolves into mystery edged by black humour, and finally transforms into fantasy with an undercurrent of grim awareness. I compare the image of the dreaded nursing home of mid-twentieth-century texts to its metamorphosed images in late twentieth- and early twenty-first-century texts, and I argue that authors are now beginning to combine narratives of fear of the nursing home, aging, and death with narratives of positive-aging and late-life agency. This mixture has culminated in the birth of new fantasy stories featuring successful escape from nursing homes and aging, although awareness of reality's grim truths also still lurks within them. (Life 4)

In my analysis of the genre's development, which I began in 2011, I have reached similar conclusions but diverge slightly from Patricia Life regarding the chronological shifts she outlines. Life rightly observes that earlier novels—particularly those from the mid-20th century—often depicted care homes as dreadful places, a pattern evident in both Canadian and U.S. literature, as seen in Margaret Laurence's *The Stone Angel* (1964) and May Sarton's

As We Are Now (1973) as respective examples, but I am not entirely convinced that this portrayal has disappeared in more recent works. John Mighton's 2005 play *Half Life*, for instance, still presents a care home setting that evokes confinement and loss rather than comfort or agency. Life argues that the shift in representation—from hospital- or prison-like institutions to more hotel-like facilities—mirrors a broader narrative transformation: from stories of decline to those emphasizing late-life agency:

> While in the past nursing-care institutions epitomised decline, I will argue that now they are often presented as sites where late-life individuals exert agency over their surroundings, further enrich and expand their personal identities, and avoid application of the decline narrative to their own lives. I will also show that early twenty-first-century texts have begun to add a surprising new narrative where residents have acquired so much agency that they are able to walk away from the nursing home and even from old age itself. (Life 4)

While this trend is certainly visible in some texts, I question whether it fully encapsulates contemporary representations of care homes. It is certainly true that care-giving institutions have traditionally been linked to a cultural imaginary of old age as a state of decline, but Life's claim rests upon the assumption that novels which present the care home as a prison-like institution do not allow for or transport narratives of late-life agency. As the following analysis shows, this assumption cannot be confirmed. Whereas on the surface, narratives set in homes that are presented as "total institutions," to use Goffman's term (14), may at first seem to symbolize decline, they often subvert and challenge ageist stereotypes and decline narratives fervently. They do so by offering striking individual narratives of self-determination and agency, representing escape stories or novels set in luxurious retirement lodges. Read as *Reifungsromane* (Waxman, *From* 2) or *Vollendungsromane* (Rooke 244–245), they narrate resistance, and sometimes even progress, despite adverse conditions.

Care Home Story Typologies

When characters walk away from the care home—the escape narrative being a recently emerged sub-genre, as Life rightly observes—this can definitely be interpreted as a sign of self-determination and agency. While newspaper reports sometimes cover incidents of residents who live with dementia and walk away unintentionally and accidentally, the escapes narrated in such literary texts are always well planned. Examples of such escape narratives are Gail Radley's *The Golden Days* (1991), Clyde Edgerton's *Lunch at the Piccadilly* (2004), Sara Gruen's *Water for Elephants* (2007), as well as two novels which will be discussed in Chapter Four, Oscar Casares's *Amigoland* (2009) and Janet Hepburn's *Flee, Fly, Flown* (2013). Interestingly, the specific nature of the institution—whether it is depicted as a humiliating prison, a deindividualizing hospital, or a luxurious, hotel-like facility—matters little to those who seek to escape. What truly drives their desire to run away is the feeling that they do not belong, that they do not feel "at home" in their respective institutions, or that they have one final mission to fulfill. The reasons behind this impulse vary. Genre conventions, such as the prison narrative, escape story, or quest, significantly shape the level of agency and self-determination afforded to the protagonists. The common thread in all these works is the implicit belief that somewhere beyond the institution, there exists a place where they truly belong—a space they can call *home*.

The care home novel borrows elements and themes from several other genres. The previously mentioned escape narratives, for instance, are often modeled after road movies. Comedy and romance offer other templates, for instance in Joyce Magnin's *Blame It on the Mistletoe* (2011). Another popular genre is detective fiction, in which older residents often slip into the role of the investigator. A prime example is the "geezer-lit mystery"[12] series invented by Mike Befeler, the author of six books featuring "Paul Jacobson, a crotchety octogenarian amateur sleuth" (*Retirement Homes Are Murder*) three of which involve long term care institutions, *Retirement Homes Are Murder* (2007), *Care Homes Are Murder* (2013), and *Nursing Homes Are Murder* (2014). Resident-detectives also play a central role in M. Scott Peck's *A Bed by the Window: A Novel Of Mystery And Redemption* (1991), James Moore's *They Should Live So Long* (2001) and Al Stevens's *Nursing Home Ninjas* (2013), suspense stories in which a band of vigorous seniors take it upon themselves to find out who is behind the sudden and unusually high death rate in patients and employees.

12 The "geezer-lit mystery" series includes Mike Befeler's books *Retirement Homes Are Murder* (2007), *Living With Your Kids Is Murder* (2009), *Senior Moments Are Murder* (2011), *Cruising In Your Eighties Is Murder* (2012), *Care Homes Are Murder* (2013) and *Nursing Homes Are Murder* (2014). Furthermore, he is the author of *The Back Wing* (2013), another novel set in a care home that is the "first book in a new paranormal geezer-lit mystery series" (http://www.mikebefeler.com/index.html).

Horror narratives are almost as popular as "care-home whodunits." The fourth age as an expression of the uncanny is presented in stories where the oldest old are featured as the "living dead," existing as zombies in a timeless limbo state. This horror setting corresponds to the realm Hazan terms the "twilight zone of human existence" ("Beyond" 96) when he talks about the final stages of life in old age. In such horror novels, the "fourth age" is represented as a time of suffering, and is the true horror that haunts newly arrived inmates, who have not yet been initiated into the terrors of the nursing home. The mysteries driving the plot in such novels are usually resolved with recourse to slapstick and comic relief, as in Joe R. Lansdale's short story and movie "Bubba Ho-Tep" in which Elvis Presley meets John F. Kennedy in a nursing home where they have to defeat a "redneck mummy" (Lansdale 7). Other novels containing horror elements are *The Tides* by Melanie Tem (1999), winner of the Bram Stoker Award, or *The Nursing Home* by James J. Murphy III. (2009), books whose covers feature creepy images of haunted castles, the grim reaper, and the undead. Here, the "nursing home specter" looms large as an expression of the threatening forces associated with old age that need to be kept at bay. Eudora Welty's short story "A Visit of Charity" (1941/1992) is an early example that "borrows repeatedly from the arsenal of the gothic," as Rüdiger Kunow argues ("Coming" 300), representing the aged "as alien, as totally *Other*" (301).

One of the predominating themes in the care home novel is that of the home as a prison. In general, it can be said that care home narratives tackle questions of life-course identity and old age, and that a movement to or within the space of the care home is often used to signify transition, change, or crisis. As in the boarding school novel, a character's loneliness and their difficulty to cope with a new phase of life away from "home" is placed in the foreground. The care home, like the boarding school, is often depicted as a microcosm of society—a disciplinary institution that is often run by overbearing and despotic administrators who rule what is often depicted as a panoptical institution by using discipline and punishment. In addition to being subject to the institution's regulations, the inmate is also subject to the dynamics of a small social group whose rules have yet to be understood by the newcomer.

The care home, positioned at the intersection of public and private life, rarely provides genuine privacy. For characters who feel lonely and powerless, carving out counter-spaces—places of agency where they can assert self-determination or cultivate a sense of home—is particularly difficult. Many care home narratives engage with this dilemma, centering on one fundamental question: what does it mean to be "at home"? The care home is often portrayed as a trivialized simulacrum of home, a professionally constructed environment that mimics domesticity but rarely fulfills the deeper emotional and existential dimensions of being at home. This tension highlights the complexity of defining what *home* truly means, especially in later life. Since moving into a care home is frequently depicted as a character's final relocation, these narratives foreground the existential weight of this transition, exploring the loss, adaptation, and redefinition of home in institutionalized settings.

Against this backdrop, older protagonists have to challenge and fight against, sometimes subvert, institutional constraints in order to maintain or renegotiate their sense of self, and regain their independence and agency. In some novels, this struggle may go hand in hand with the need to transgress borders and defy rules and regulations in order to resist becoming a "patient." Tim Sandlin's *Jimi Hendrix Turns Eighty* (2007), or Paul Quarrington's *King Leary* (1987) are excellent examples of such narratives. As opposed to boarding school novels where the transitional age of adolescence is highlighted, an age that leads to maturity and adulthood, care home narratives often deal with protagonists' struggle against the transition from adulthood into the culturally constructed state of senescence, and highlight the difficulty of remaining "adult" in the sense of maintaining self-determination and independence. Residents are often victimized and infantilized in such narratives, and the grade of senescence is very often expressed through space; moving to the next floor in a care home often signifies moving further away from adult life, and eventually into oblivion. The space of the home can be experienced as limiting and confining, but also serves as a space of protection and redefinition of a protagonist's self, such as in Todd Johnson's *The Sweet By and By* (2005), Lola Lemire Tostevin's *The Other Sister* (2008), Joan Barfoot's *Exit Lines* (2008), or Shani Mootoo's *Cereus Blooms at Night* (1996).

Whereas the previously mentioned texts center around protagonists who are themselves residents/patients in care homes, the last decades have also witnessed the production of texts written from the perspective of adult children or other care-givers, who struggle with decisions of putting loved ones into nursing homes. Some of them are fictional, such as Michael Ignatieff's *Scar Tissue* (1993), and some are autofictional or autobiographical, such as Dudley Clendinen's *A Place Called Canterbury* (2008). Autobiographical/creative non-fiction accounts also include those of nurses' aides and nurses, for instance *Harvest Moon* by Sallie Tisdale (1987) or *Endnotes* (2008) by Ruth Ray. In addition, a vast number of advice columns, manuals, how-to-guides and self-help books such as *Planning Long-Term Care for Dummies* (Levine), and specialist reports, as well as a large number of care home ethnographies, are available.

During the past three decades, and especially the last few years, movies have also begun to play an important role, adding to the genre of the care home narrative.[13] Most of them have been based on novels, plays, or short stories, such as Kari Skogland's *The Stone Angel* (2007), which is based on Margaret Laurence's 1964 novel of the same title; Sarah Polley's film *Away From Her* (Canada/USA/UK 2007), which is adapted from Alice Munro's famous short story "The Bear Came Over The Mountain" (1999/2003); or Nicholas Sparks's novel *The Notebook* (1996), which was made into a movie by the same name by Nick Cassavetes (2003). *Away From Her* and *The Notebook* are dementia narratives that deal with the meaning of true love in old age while *The Stone Angel*, a family saga, portrays the struggle of a woman at the end of her life to reconcile herself to her past. It tells the life story of 90-year-old Hagar Shipley who runs away when her son wants to assign her to a nursing home. Other movies that center on efforts to keep characters out of long-term care include *Iris*,[14] *Cloudburst*,[15] *Up*,[16] *Robot and Frank*,[17] and *The Savages*.[18]

Two recent and very popular British movies that address the question of where to spend the last years of one's life are John Madden's *The Best Exotic*

13 Two notable European examples of animated films are Paco Roca's *Arrugas* ("Wrinkles," Spain 2012), which is based on the graphic novel with the same title (2007, the English version was published in 2015), and the Flemish short film *Memee* by Evelyn Verschoore (2010).

14 Richard Eyre's movie *Iris* is based on John Bayley's memoires of his wife, *Iris: A Memoir of Iris Murdoch* (1998) and *Elegy for Iris: A Memoir* (1999).

15 *Cloudburst* premiered as a stage play in 2010 and was adapted by its author, Thom Fitzgerald, for the screen in 2011.

16 "Shady Oaks Retirement Village" is the care home featured in the animation films *Up* and *George & A.J.*, the bonus film narrating what happens to the two retirement home workers after witnessing Carl Fredricksen's house flying off in *Up*.

17 *Robot and Frank* (2012) tells the story of an ex-jewel thief whose increasing dementia causes his children to buy him a care robot that becomes his friend—and partner in crime. In the end, Frank moves to a nursing home in which all care-givers are robots.

18 *The Savages* (2008) is a film by Tamara Jenkins in which the central characters are a brother and sister who have to take care of their old father after his girlfriend passes away in Sun City, Arizona. They decide to relocate him to a care home in Buffalo, where he dies.

Marigold Hotel,[19] based on Debora Moggach's novel *These Foolish Things* (2004), and *Quartet*[20] based on a play with the same title by Ronald Harwood (1999). A variety of short films (*Rhonda's Party; The Greyed Escape*) also deal with the topic of long-term residential care. Furthermore, a number of "cinema verité" documentaries have come out that portray life in the care home, including the award-winning movie *Room 335* (2006) by Andrew Jenks, who decides as a young college student to move to a Florida senior residence for one summer; Brad Lichtenstein and Lisa Gildehaus's *Almost Home* (2006), which chronicles the daily lives of staff and residents at Saint John's On The Lake, a retirement community in Milwaukee, Wisconsin, documenting the "Culture Change" movement that strives to improve quality of life for residents and staff; Jared Scheib's award-winning film *The Mayor* (2011), which tells the stories of several octogenarian long-term care facility residents in Texas; and *Gen Silent* (2010) by Stu Maddux, a documentary that focuses on LGBT elders in care homes.[21] The 2014 film *Penelope: The Documentary* deserves special mention because it is the capstone of the groundbreaking "Penelope Project," (Basting et al.) with an aim to "dramatically raise the bar on activities in long term care." The film shows how residents, some with severe dementia or who are wheel-chair bound, collaborate with playwright Anne Basting and the Sojourn Theater to create "Finding Penelope," a play reinterpreting Homer's Odyssey to recount it from Penelope's point of view (371 Productions).

Who and What is (Not) Represented?

An additional analytical aspect of my research is the question of who gains visibility in cultural representations of care homes, and who does not. The set-

19 *The Best Exotic Marigold Hotel* (2012) tells the story of a group of British retirees who move to India, lured by promises of luxury at the Marigold Hotel. As Sally Chivers writes about the "The Best Exotic Marigold Hotel cinema franchise (2011 and 2015, UK)," "These star-studded comedies – *The Best Exotic Marigold Hotel* and *The Second Best Exotic Marigold Hotel* – feature a set of white British seniors not quite able to finance their mature years while living in the UK, who decide to outsource their retirement to India, thereby transforming from excess into consumers and even producers yet again" ("What" 85–86).

20 The 2012 movie *Quartet*, Dustin Hoffman's debut as director, is set in a luxurious retirement residence for talented musicians where four singers plan to raise funds for the home by putting on a revival concert.

21 A comprehensive overview of further documentaries and other films can be found on the website programforelderly.org which has a special section on "nursing films."

tings of care-home films and novels range from retirement lodges and assisted living facilities to nursing homes (a true categorization is difficult due to the lack of standardized terminology), and also include places where around-the-clock care is standard. While "illness narratives," including dementia narratives, have gained popularity as a genre in the second half of the twentieth century (Hartung, *Narrating* 282), and include pathographies that end with the death of the narrator, the sick and dying oldest old are, interestingly, rarely represented in nursing home narratives. Although a few exceptions exist, such as in Canadian writer Edna Alford's short story cycle *A Sleep Full of Dreams*, protagonists who are frail, sick, in pain, or bedridden rarely are given a voice or position from which the action is narrated. Unlike in illness narratives, such characters are often only referred to as "the other" living in the "black hole" of an inaccessible closed ward, such as on the "second floor" in Alice Munro's short story "The Bear Came Over the Mountain" (309), or the "Advanced Living" wing in Margaret Atwood's tale "Torching the Dusties" where, the narrator assumes, "things are different. She hasn't wished to imagine exactly how different" (232).

Although statistics indicate that many care-home residents require full-time care due to dementia, frailty, or illness, literary and filmic representations of care homes often focus on older characters who are relatively healthy. This discrepancy raises the question of why such protagonists are depicted as living in long-term care facilities at all. In some cases—particularly in care home detective stories—the residents are still firmly in the third age, portrayed as pensioners without significant physical or cognitive impairments.

While several dementia narratives have actually been written from an agent position, which aims to represent what is going on in the brain as memory slowly disintegrates (e.g., Lisa Genova's *Still Alice*, 2009), the "representational dilemma" (Hartung, *Narrating* 15) of depicting the frail and sick oldest old living in nursing homes has so far barely been tackled, and the oldest old are usually not developed into full-fledged characters. Heike Hartung approaches the difficulties related to representing frail old age from a narratological perspective and points to the "problem of narrating the unnarratable" (Rimmon-Kenan qtd. in Hartung, *Narrating*, 15) in dementia and illness narratives.

The absence of the oldest old in care home narratives may reflect the taboo of death, an unspoken presence that lingers in the background. Margaret Atwood's protagonist in "Alphinland" refers to it as the "D-word," an unavoidable truth that looms like "a huge advertising blimp, but to mention it would have been like breaking a spell" (15). Julia Twigg offers a possible explanation for this omission: she argues that old age itself is a cultural taboo because of its proximity to death. She asserts that since death empties old age of meaning, the stage that precedes it—extreme old age—becomes something society prefers to ignore: "It is hard to invest the body in old age with a stronger sense of subjectivity, when old age itself is avoided as a topic, seen as having no meaning, or at least no meaning other than decay, decline and final absence" (Twigg, *Body* 50). The reluctance to confront oldest age, decline, and ultimately death is evident in most care home narratives, despite the fact that the space of the care home itself inevitably evokes such associations. Drawing on Ernesto Laclau and Teresa de Lauretis, Rüdiger Kunow explains: "To call age an impossible object means that it is something which established discourses or hegemonic representational practices promise to describe, yet cannot do so" (306). In this sense, oldest age remains a gap in cultural representation, a presence that is both acknowledged and erased at the same time.

As a literary studies scholar working in the field of Age Studies, I fully agree with Anne Wyatt-Brown who describes it as "a daunting task" for scholars to "study gerontological issues and theories, master an unfamiliar social science vocabulary, and attract an interdisciplinary audience capable of responding intelligently and critically to their insights" (299–300). Wyatt-Brown admires those "pioneers" among literature scholars who have, since the mid-1980s, "mastered gerontological theory, thereby bridging the gap between the two fields and creating a legitimate sub-specialty in literary studies" (300). At the same time, it is crucial to recognize that literary gerontology must also remain rooted in a deep understanding of literature itself; rather than relying solely on traditional gerontological methods, this field benefits from examining what literature is and how it works as a mode of inquiry ("American" 256).

In this context, Hannah Zeilig raises two essential questions: "Is it feasible to extrapolate from literature in order to gain insight into other fields of inquiry? If so, what can be gained from literature, what is the type of information which it can yield?" (40). A response to Zeilig's questions can be found in Barbara Frey-Waxman's book when she argues that literature "can take us out of ourselves and our usual settings, making us more conscious of our unexamined beliefs and assumptions and giving us new food for thought" (83). The power of fiction lies in its ability to render the inner worlds of older individuals and "affirm the contradictions, complexity, and uncertainty that lie at the heart of the experience of aging" (Yahnke 86). Expanding on this idea, Sally Chivers emphasizes that "a humanities-based approach to aging can consistently maintain the crucial complexity of growing old because works of art, such as literature, can comfortably encompass contradictions and even gain their aesthetic strength from doing so" (*From*, x). In this way, literature not only represents aging but also reflects its paradoxes and ambiguities, offering a depth of understanding that more rigid scientific approaches might struggle to capture. While striving to understand fictional characters, we acknowledge them as being different from, but also similar to, ourselves at the same time; we recognize ourselves in them through a personal and a political act of understanding, as literary philosopher Martha Nussbaum asserts:

> It is for this reason that literature is so urgently important for the citizen, as an expansion of sympathies that real life cannot cultivate sufficiently. It is the political promise of literature that it can transport us, while remaining ourselves, into the life of another, revealing similarities but also profound differences between the life and thought if that other and myself and making them comprehensible, or at least more nearly comprehensible. (111)

This is what the texts analyzed in this book accomplish, as is shown in the following chapters. They all draw, in one way or another, readers into the world of the care home, permitting them to identify with their protagonists in their struggles against institutionalization, or in their attempts to redefine themselves in a way that makes sense for them in a new environment. While it is clearly not the task nor the focus of sociological, gerontological, or medical texts to facilitate identification on the reader's part, understanding the "visceral prose" (Waxman, *From* 18) and aesthetics of literary texts can enable readers to identify with a literary character, and experience aging by proxy. This argument resonates with Nussbaum's claim that we as readers gain a better understanding of the world by "learning both to see the world, for a time, through their eyes and then reflecting as spectators on the meaning of what we have seen" (*Poetic* 93). As literary gerontologists, we can take the matter one step further, as Waxman observes. Literary texts, she maintains,

> can affect whole societies and do important work for social betterment, even when they are presenting sexist or ageist notions in their characters and plots, precisely because resisting literary critics will interrogate and undermine these sexist or ageist notions in the texts and raise general readers' awareness of how these damaging notions operate both in texts and in society. (Waxman, "Literary" 88)

Here, Waxman refers to the concept of the "resisting reader" that has been developed by Judith Fetterley in her book *The Resisting Reader: A Feminist Approach to American Fiction* (1978). Fetterley's concept is very useful when applied as an approach to challenge and deconstruct patriarchal hegemonic and colonial power structures, and has also already been applied by Maierhofer:

> Readers who resist the imposition of traditional interpretations, question the overt meaning of the text, and challenge the codification of meaning and received opinions about specific texts, perform political acts that transcend the realm of literary studies. When, for example, the subject of aging in literary texts is merely treated as a point of reference for the young protagonists or when older people are portrayed as playing inspirational or redemptive roles by rescuing young protagonists from indecision or desperation, this calls for a resisting reader who claims aging characters in their own rights as portrayals of human existence incorporating all stages of life. ("Desperately" 130)

In recent decades, not only the different types of care facilities have been increasing in North America, which are also mirrored in fictional works, but also the representation of old characters in film and fiction has significantly changed, as Anne Wyatt-Brown points out:

> In 1992, Canadian gerontologist Constance Rooke pointed out that 'fiction concerned with old age' was growing "for both literary and sociological reasons" (1992, 242). As the aging population increased, writers and readers, she argued, were eager to explore what it felt like to be old. As a result, elderly characters were less likely to be what the English novelist E.M. Forster (1927) called "flat characters" and instead became fully round. (57)

Cultural representations have the capacity, as Wyatt-Brown claims, "to create a picture of aging, one that most readers can easily understand and appreciate. Without literary gerontology, however, the representation might be one-sided, the view of the author and few others. Only by combining research with novels and memoirs can we begin to comprehend the varieties of aging experience in our time" (57). In a similar fashion, Mike Hepworth emphasizes the importance of literature when he states:

> Fiction evidently adds a further dimension to our understanding of the quality of the ageing experience. Because fiction is a creative mental activity re-

> quiring author and reader to extend her or himself imaginatively into the minds of other characters, novels are in the advantageous position of admitting readers to a variety of different perspectives on the situation of an ageing individual. (5)

Now, at the onset of the twenty-first century, the nursing home seems to have been firmly established as a setting, and its residents have been developed into central characters. These developments add weight to the argument that narratives that represent older protagonists living in long-term care institutions need to be addressed from the perspective of literary studies and Age Studies. One notable exception mentioned earlier is Sally Chivers's insightful book *From Old Woman to Older Women* in which she refers to novels depicting institutional care:

> These depictions of institutional care, more than commenting on the possibilities of such facilities to provide improved care, demonstrate the complicated process of forming attitudes toward the frail old and help to counter the impetus to think of age as either positive or negative. They provide examples of how narrative fiction can offer a perspective on the individuality of elderly residents that differs from clinical interaction. (Chivers, *From* xlvi)

As Chivers shows, it is important to re-imagine old age in order to reimagine structures of institutional care. In order to develop convincing arguments for such a paradigm change, however, it is also important to analyze why the nursing home specter still looms so large in our minds. Where does the deep-rooted cultural fear of care homes for old people come from, and why is it so deeply engrained in our minds? Defining old age as an uncanny and dangerous space inherently frames the care home as an uncanny site as well. To counteract ageism, it is essential to reimagine care homes as spaces that support meaningful identity development in later life. Literary representations play a key role in this process, as they encourage readers to engage in alternative narratives of aging. Many texts depict protagonists who undergo transformative experiences in the final stages of their lives—experiences that allow them to re-narrate their pasts and arrive at meaningful conclusions, despite, or perhaps even because of, their physical frailty. By offering new ways of conceptualizing eldercare, film and fiction have the potential to challenge and ultimately dismantle the "nursing home specter," shifting cultural perceptions of long-term care. "[T]he figure of the 'nursing home,' typically as a symbol of cultural failure and a fate worse than death, haunts representations of older adults across the popular culture spectrum, in television, magazines, cinema and newspaper coverage," (Chivers, "Blind" 134). Care home novels and films add to these kinds of cultural representations of old age, and in most cases fuel rather than calm the fears of ending up in such an institution.

In contrast to ethnographic research on residential care facilities in which old people can easily be objectified and unintentionally rendered passive (Kearns and Andrews 20), I claim that especially through the mediums of art, literature, and film as well as the criticism thereof, this passivity can be counteracted, and a voice can be given to all—care-givers, family members, and old people. Fiction has already been functionalized as a resource that can be used by researchers from disciplines ranging from sociology to anthropology, from geography to critical gerontology to better understand aging and old age. The methods and approaches of literary criticism, however, have not been incorporated into the analysis of spatial aspects of institutional care as represented in care-home novels or films. The focus of my analysis, therefore, is on the fictional representation of the space of such institutions, and the way in which it determines or contributes to the cultural "othering" of old age, as well as to the definition of the self-identity of "patients," "residents," or "clients."

American novelist May Sarton also offers an explanation for difficulties encountered when writing about old age, and employs a spatial metaphor to emphasize the binary opposition of young and old when she writes, "[t]he trouble is that old age is not interesting until one gets there, a foreign country with an unknown language to the young, and even to the middle-aged" (23). The strangeness of the other country, which is of no importance until one enters it, is additionally reinforced by the fact that the old are not intelligible to the young. Sarton describes the problem of the binary construction of young and old in her novel, set in the Twin Elms nursing home, a space that houses those who are perceived as "other." The journal Caro Spencer, an old resident, keeps is, as Barbara Frey-Waxman puts it, "a vehicle that transports us to the foreign country of dependent senescence and translates its language into terms that adult readers, regardless of age, can comprehend" (140). In *As We Are Now*, Sarton expresses the inability to communicate the experience of old age to those who have not yet reached the "fourth age," an "era of final dependence, decrepitude, and death" (Laslett 4). The experience of old age, she implies, cannot be passed on via a common language. Sarton uses a spatial metaphor, the "foreign country," to describe this wordless realm.

The metaphorical language employed when speaking about aging and old age has been investigated by numerous scholars from various disciplines (Cole, *Journey;* Blaikie, *Ageing;* Blaikie, "Imagined"; Dekkers; Krasner, "Accumulated"; Krasner, *Home;* Kunow, "Chronologically"; Vincent). The metaphors, particularly in terms of cultural representations of institutional long-term care still need to be examined in more detail though. Sarton uses the prison as a *pars pro toto* to express what it means for her to live in the foreign country of old age: "Old age, they say, is a gradual giving up, [...] a real test of character, a kind of solitary confinement," as she puts it (14). As one of the first books in the history of the genre of the care home novel, *As We Are Now* invites, or rather urges, readers of all ages to enter and explore this "uncharted terrain," and contest its boundaries and borders. With this book, I accept Sarton's invitation.

2 Hospital, Hotel, or Home?
Renegotiating Identity at the Nexus of Public and Private

"See the number on your door, the big 14 here?
That's how you'll know this is your room when you're coming back."
From meals. Games. TV movies. All the promised fun.

— Joan Barfoot, *Exit Lines*

The ache for home lives in all of us. The safe place where we can go as we are and not bequestioned.

— Maya Angelou, *"All God's Children Need Traveling Shoes"*

Home is a place that offers security, familiarity and nurture.

— Yi-Fu Tuan, "Home"

A liminal space at the intersection of private and public, the care home has been compared to the hospital, hotel, prison, concentration camp,[1] or heterotopic spaces such as the luxury hotel, the cruise ship,[2] and even the airplane: "Airplanes are flying nursing homes," Dorothy Pringle states, emphasizing that both of these places are heavily managed in terms of time and space, restrict

1 As Margot O'Neill writes on ABC NewMail, "Mistreated nursing home residents 'better off in a concentration camp'" (M. O'Neill). May Sarton in *As We Are Now* (9) uses the same comparison in a disturbingly inappropriate manner.

2 See Lerner et al., as well as Lindquist and Golub.

and allow certain behaviors, and involve routine and ritual (Andrews et al. 110). Pringle's comparison of airplanes to nursing homes highlights the drawbacks of residential life by depicting the restrictive and often uncomfortable nature of both environments:

> Not having a choice of whom one sits besides and risking that this seatmate may smell, slurp food, chatter endlessly or refuse to participate in even occasional exchange of pleasantries; [...] eating on the schedule imposed by the airline not when one is hungry and, moreover, having little choice over what one eats; having to use and wait for communal facilities, such as bathrooms and not being able to get to the toilet when needed [...] having television sets turned on regardless of one's interest in watching them; having to wear a restraint to protect against the rare possibility of injury; and having nothing to do and nowhere to go. Arguably, relationships with staff can vary considerably and can either dramatically improve or detract from the overall experience. Notably, the quality of service can also depend on one's ability to pay. (Andrews et al. 110)

Just as air travel confines passengers in a tightly regulated space for the duration of their journey, care homes structure the daily lives of residents within a framework that prioritizes efficiency, safety, and institutional control. A crucial distinction between the two settings, she maintains, is "that passengers are allowed to leave airplanes at the end of their journeys, whilst residents of nursing homes often live out the rest of their lives in these settings" (110). Andrews et al. use the image of the airplane to evoke empathy: while many can relate to the frustrations of air travel, far fewer can truly imagine the experience of long-term institutional living. Regardless of whether one agrees with the analogy, it undoubtedly invites deeper reflection on the nature of institutional environments and the limitations they impose (110).

As the comparison of a nursing home with an airplane or a hospital shows, it seems difficult to think the institution as "itself," without resorting to familiar concepts such as a hotel, holiday resort or—as shown in Chapter Three—a prison. Susan Braedley reflects on this issue in her article "Reinventing the Nursing Home: Metaphors that Design Care," thinking about these concepts as "ruling metaphors" that "have come to dominate the everyday life of many nursing homes, bringing in the material realities and social relations of private households, hotels as commercial enterprises and hospitals as places of medical practice" (57). These metaphors, she states, shape not only physical design but also social relations, care practices, and institutional policies. However, she argues that

> the resulting environments are often disappointing when assessed for conditions of equity, dignity and respect for residents and for those who care for them, yet also have some benefits. They produce Baudrillardian environments, approaching but never realising fantasies that dependence, frailty and dying can be cured in a hospital, evaded by luxurious hotel living or escaped through the familiarity of something "like home." (Braedley 57)

These metaphors, she notes, reinforce existing social inequalities, rather than creating genuinely new and equitable care models. Even if we managed to break out of these guiding frameworks, it is difficult to come up with models that do not operate within capitalist structures that undervalue care work and reinforce gendered expectations: "In industrialised countries, few people have extended experiences of collective living that could offer a prefigurative metaphor for collective caring" (57). In this chapter, I will investigate these metaphors that shape the care home as a synecdochical space.

Hospital, Hotel, Holiday Resort, or Home?

The care home, it is often stated, is an institution that lies at the intersection of hospital and hotel. Due to its history of long-term care, its architectural plans with double-loaded corridors and linoleum floors, and its focus on caregiving, the association of the care home with a hospital is probably the most obvious one. Yet there is one fundamental difference: like tourists, who will leave the airplane, hospital patients will eventually be discharged. As Kearns and Andrews claim, "even against the odds, people are expected to graduate from hospital into greater independence, but the reverse prevails in the nursing home: it would be counter-intuitive to graduate into anything but greater dependence (e.g. a geriatric ward)" (15). In other words, hospitals are supposed to enable people to live independently after being discharged, whereas care homes are usually seen as a final destination.

To downplay the institutional character, architectural firms, designers, funders, researchers, advocates, and operators "have been reimagining the nursing home, working to escape its poor reputation through design. They have adapted the architecture, furnishings, décor, spatial and social arrangements of familiar environments with positive associations, such as 'home', 'hotel', 'village' and 'hospital,' to produce new forms of nursing home care"

(Braedley 45). They increasingly emphasize the hotel-like aspects of care homes, designing them as spaces of relaxation, entertainment, and comfort. Sterile, cold hallways are now softened with carpeting and warm lighting, shifting the focus away from the facility's institutional nature and toward aesthetic appeal. Care homes designed under the "hospitality" model feature light-filled corridors, courtyards with lush, green gardens, gyms, cafés, hair and nail salons, bars, and shops, all intended to emulate a hotel lifestyle "suggesting places of consumption and active leisure" (Buse et al. 1446). Such amenities with their emphasis on "luxury" and "elegance" insinuate that care homes can be places of enjoyment, presenting "a vision of life that is implicitly classed and remote from institutional models associated with welfare and need" (1446). As intended, the impermanence suggested by such "non-places" (Augé 110) may, as architect Annmarie Adams and Age Studies scholar Sally Chivers maintain, "make the transition to care easier for many residents" (Adams and Chivers, "Architecture" 144). Yet, these design choices shaping the expectations of future residents frame the facility as a temporary place. "It is always understood [...] that even those residents who are 'permanent' will only last so long" (144). No matter how carefully curated the aesthetics, the reality of institutionalization can hardly be masked.

In another article, "Home Pages: Domesticity and Duplicity in Images of Architecture for Ageing," Adams and Chivers critique the unoriginal hospitality approach often taken in care home design:

> In North America, long-term care (LTC) architecture has traditionally been the work of mediocre architectural firms. Highly constrained by governmental regulations, the design of the places where most of us will age and die is far from inspired, and marked by a remarkable conservatism. Many LTC buildings look like hotel chains and are sited like strip malls, forming undistinguished backdrops to unremarkable thoroughfares, designed more for cars than for people. Rarely do the top students in architecture schools take on long-term care buildings for their thesis projects, perhaps because of this reputation for design constraints rather than innovation. ("Home" 82)

The traditional nursing home, as Peter Uhlenberg describes it, is constructed as the opposite of what is commonly understood as "home," a notion that is based on the ideal of the family model.[3] He writes, "No one who lives in a nursing home could possibly confuse it with a home. Sharing a bedroom with a sick stranger, being served institutional food on a fixed schedule, having no control over the design and furnishing of your room, and being cared for by indifferent aides contradicts the idea of home" (73). Most care home ethnographies and analyses by gerontologists who study place attachment among old people seem to perpetuate, for a variety of economic and ideological reasons, the idea that the domestic, familial space is the ideal place where old people wish to remain, or where they wish to return to at the end of their lives. It "symbolizes all the positive associations we have with hearth and home," Jennifer A. Parks explains in her critical feminist study of home health care. "Whether or not patients are *actually* better off in their own homes, [...] home care symbolizes a 'kinder, gentler' form of health care delivery where patients can remain in the bosoms of their families" (Parks 11).

Aging in place is not always the ideal solution it is often portrayed to be. Websites offering advice to adult children caring for aging parents frequently present it as a blessing to all involved, but the reality is often far more complex. Parks' research on the home health care industry highlights its highly exploitative nature, affecting not only workers but also families and patients, while raising significant ethical concerns (9). Although a majority of individuals, she writes, "invariably prefer home-based to institution-based care" (3), this preference is often rooted in an idealized vision of "home" rather than the actual ability of family members to provide adequate care. A recent Gallup and Robinson poll in the United States reflects this contradiction: when adults aged 35 to 64 were asked whether they would take in an aging parent, 53 percent answered yes. But when older adults (65+) were asked whether they would want to live with their children if they could no longer live independently, only 25% said they would (Span n.p.). These findings suggest that while aging in place may seem desirable in theory, the practical and emotional realities for both older adults and their families often tell a different story.

The juxtaposition between idealized conceptions of home and the true reality in the context of long-term care institutions has been reviewed in detail

3 For an extensive overview of the symbolic meaning of "home," see Linda McDowell, who theorizes the notion of "home" and "domesticity" from a gendered perspective, drawing upon the works of David Harvey, Martin Heidegger, Gaston Bachelard, and Pierre Bourdieu, to develop a feminist reading of home, place, and identity (71–95).

by Roger Fay and Ceridwen Owen in their article "'Home' in the Aged Care Institution: Authentic or Ersatz," in which they observe that "one of the strongest criticisms of aged care homes is the tendency towards romantic and stereotyped meaning of home for elderly people" (35). This ideal of familial domesticity seems to be trivializing and sentimentalizing the notion of "home" vis-à-vis the institution which, due to its developmental history, has always been portrayed as its opposite. Although personal relationships are central to a person's "feeling at home," the concept of "home" is highly complex and multilayered. "Home," as Elaine Caouette states, is related to control over one's own environment, and assures a sense of security: "It offers freedom of action and expresses its resident's ideas and personal values. The experience of home establishes a state of permanence and continuity, which provides a sense of belonging. Home permits us to develop and secure our relationships with family and friends. […] Home is an indicator of social status" (Caouette 254).

In traditional institutions of long-term care, "homelikeness" is usually not placed in the foreground—on the contrary. Many of aforementioned ethnographic or sociological accounts of life in residential care institutions portray the care home, which is usually based on a medical model, as an anti-domestic, homogenizing space in which all the qualities that are stereotypically ascribed to the family home, such as continuity, relationships, control, or social status, are overturned (Börjesson and Torgé; Fleming et al.). Environmental gerontologists Graham Rowles and Habib Chaudhury describe this opposition between home and institution as a dialectic, and contend that nowadays, "long-term care facilities strive to create a homelike physical and social environment within an organizational/institutional framework" (15). A trend to design modern long-term care institutions with the home aesthetic in mind has begun in the past decades, creating spaces that can be adapted and personalized. The "homelikeness" is often fostered by allowing residents to bring their own furniture and personal objects, acknowledging that the transition from home to institutional care can pose a threat to personhood for many older adults (Rubinstein and Medeiros 59). These familiar belongings are intended to minimize the ruptures and discontinuities such a move might introduce, helping residents maintain a coherent life-course narrative, preserving autobiographical continuity, and reinforcing a sense of belonging even in institutional settings. They still remain Baudrillardian hyper-realities, "approaching but never realizing fantasies that dependence, frailty, and dying can be cured in a hospital, evaded by luxurious hotel living or escaped through something 'like home'" (Braedley 57).

As James Krasner observes, "The elderly home is more like a fictional world than most spaces, because every path and every object is likely to be 'storied'" (*Home* 50). This highlights the interconnection between home and memory, suggesting that personal spaces are not just physical environments but also repositories of identity, history, and selfhood, making empty space into place. This link between memory and home is represented in Margaret Laurence's *The Stone Angel*. As has also been observed by Kathleen Woodward (*Aging* 146), the novel highlights how a person's sense of self can be connected to the place they inhabit, and how care homes can be of "debilitating sterility" (Woodward, *Aging* 142).[4] Hagar Shipley, the ninety year old protagonist who is struggling against being moved into a care facility, resists the sale of her house. She experiences her home as an extension of her identity, with each object anchoring her to her past: "My shreds and remnants of years are scattered through it [the house] visibly in lamps and vases. [...] If I'm not contained in them and in this house, something of all change caught and fixed here, eternal enough for my purposes, then I do not know where I am to be found at all." Hagar's memories are stored in each object, in the house itself. This passage aligns with Gaston Bachelard's concept of "topoanalysis," which he defines as "the systematic psychological study of the sites of our intimate lives" (8). Bachelard describes this phenomenon as a "memory of the body," emphasizing that "the house we were born in is physically inscribed in us. It is a group of organic habits" (14). In other words, our homes shape not just our memories but also our embodied experiences, becoming an integral part of our identity.

One example that illustrates the garage-like "unhomeliness" of the nursing home appears in Thomas Edward Gass's report, *Nobody's Home: Candid Reflections of a Nursing Home Aide*, which begins by Gass describing the setting of the care home as a storage unit for the old: "Let me walk you through this little world that thrives within our sealed people-container. The economy of the building, with its flat metal roof and concrete block walls spread out low and

4 In *Aging and its Discontents*, Woodward uses *The Stone Angel* as a "counter text" illustrating her point, but not interpreting it separately. As one of the first Age Studies scholars, she reminds us in a footnote that "In the last two decades several novels have appeared in the United States which portray the life of the elderly in nursing homes as debilitating, of which I mention four: May Sarton's *As We Are Now* (New York: Norton, 1973), Ellen Douglas's *Apostles of Light* (Boston: Houghton, 1973), John Updike's *The Poorhouse Fair* (New York: Knopf, 1969), and Hilda Wolitzer's In the *Palomar Arms* (New York: Farrar, 1983)" (222).

long, is void of ambition or pretense. Like an industrial complex or self-storage unit, it is clean, efficient, and functional" (Gass and Vladeck 1). In the foreword, Bruce Vladek describes how the institution Gass works for resembles a "mini-hospital" (xii) governed by "rules and regulations meant to preclude the worst sorts of abuse or disaster or embarrassment, not by an effort to create especially sensitive or responsive environments for lonely, frightened, frail old people" (xii). The care home, he writes, is "managed clinically by nurses" and "operated predominantly by entrepreneurs who can survive economically only by squeezing nickels and speculating in real estate" (xii). Gass describes how the residents he cares for are "in a continual state of identity loss and reclamation, due to dementia and to the nature of institutional life" (Krasner 130). The title of Gass's memoir, *Nobody's Home*, expresses the "distortions of identity for both patient and caregiver," as James Krasner observes:

> The phrase seems to be a truncated version of "the lights are on, but nobody's home," which would apply to many of the nursing home residents. But it also reminds us that the facility is no kind of home; nobody would ever choose to live there, as it cannot sustain any sort of authentic domestic life. As a result, it becomes the home to a sequence of nobodies—both residents and aides exist in a twilight world of social marginalization and indeterminate identity. (Krasner, *Home* 130)

Krasner's analysis highlights the problems of isolation and the loss of identity experienced in nursing homes. The bleak environment is not only unpleasant for residents, but also for everyone working and visiting. This "aesthetic deprivation" (Moss and O'Neill) can have effects on the quality of life. As Moss and O'Neill note,

> Of course, health-care professionals also suffer from aesthetic deprivation. If the health-care settings in which they practise are poorly designed, aesthetically barren, and polluted by noise it is not surprising that such an environment may have a negative influence. Aesthetic enrichment is likely to have an impact on staff wellbeing and empowerment, and might also promote a clinical framework that rises above task and technique-oriented health care. (1033)

What is often overlooked in analyses such as Krasner's is the fact that long-term care institutions in fact have multiple functions, including a medical one; most residents live there because they can no longer cope by themselves, or have special care needs that cannot be taken care of in their own homes. Californian health care designer and architect Gregg Maedo points out the pitfalls of dysfunctionality such design concepts can create when translated into reality:

> Making a Nursing Home more like a hotel and mimicking the aesthetics does theoretically create a more inviting atmosphere. Unfortunately, this approach is a mistake. Even though conceptually, a Nursing Home and a hotel may have similarities in terms of balance between public vs. private space, the hospitality design lacks the underlying medical support that composes the actual function of a Nursing Home" (Maedo n.p.).

Just as the notion of home is multi-dimensional and complex, as Fay and Owen pragmatically state (41), so is that of the institution. "Contemporary well-designed nursing homes do provide aspects of home while at the same time providing the resources required of an institution that cares for people in a state of physical and cognitive decline," they assert (41). The design concept of a "home-like" environment may differ from good institutional design:

> This acknowledges the true purpose of these facilities—the support and wellbeing of people experiencing the ageing process not only through the design of the physical landscape of the building and exterior spaces, but also through the relational everyday practices and social connections—and may more readily support the privacy, autonomy and selfhood that are fundamental to making home. Furthermore, many aspects of these facilities will necessarily respond, through design, to the practical necessity of addressing the very real needs of people who are frail and ill—not all of which are compatible to the idea of being "homelike". The provision of a home is only one aspect of that purpose. (Fay and Owen 41)

Fay and Owen note that increasing care needs may necessitate adopting a more medical model in nursing homes, since, unlike retirement communities or assisted living settings—which prioritize a homelike atmosphere—nursing care may require additional space and higher hygienic standards to effectively manage residents' complex health conditions. In a more medicalized environment, residents may have complex health conditions requiring specialized equipment, treatment spaces, and rigorous infection control protocols. For instance, rooms might need extra clearance for mobility aids, beds must accommodate medical equipment, and areas need to be designed for efficient sanitation.

Culture Change: Can We Find New Models?

Despite these arguments that support the medicalized model, long-term care began to change towards more homelike atmospheres beginning with the Culture Change Movement in the 1980s (Gaugler 430). Recent innovative long-term care models, Gaugler explains, are the Butterfly Approach, the Eden Alternative, the Green House Project, the Wellspring model, or the Hogeweyk Village, a long-term care residence in the Netherlands designed for individuals with dementia but, "comprehensive culture change in nursing homes has proceeded slowly" (431).

Among those who challenge conventional approaches is Peter Whitehouse, who explores future models of care in his article "Long-Term Care for the Future: Just What is Real Anyway?" featured in our edited collection *Care Home Stories*. In his piece, Whitehouse offers a critical perspective on his visit to the Hogeweyk Dementia Village, which he found less impressive than anticipated. Drawing on his firsthand research in both Canada and the Netherlands, he calls for a fundamental reimagining of long-term care. He maintains that intergenerational learning should be at the heart of this transformation, fostering resilient communities capable of addressing the complex social, economic, and ecological challenges ahead.

One more recent example I would like to mention here is the *Dagmarsminde Method* that was popularized in 2021 through a documentary movie, *It Is Not Over Yet* (Denmark 2021, dir. Louise Detlefsen). It refers to a small Danish nursing home, Dagmarsminde, which is a "'Care Oasis' for people with severe dementia," as the website[5] states. It was established in 2016 through the private initiative of nurse May Bjerre Eiby who, after witnessing her own father's lonely death in a nursing home, wanted to create a new way of caring that actually resembles and modernizes Florence Nightingale's initial ideas of holistic care and the importance of the environment. Eiby describes her concept and tells the success story of her home in her book *Living Normally With Dementia: One Care Home's Story and How to Make It Yours* (2022) (Eiby and Kyhn). Most importantly, the "Dagmarsminde Method" consists of de-medication: "Dementia changes the way we are human. That's why the solution is human, not medical," she states (Eiby). In addition, she believes in person-centered care and

5 https://www.dagmarsminde.dk

home-like, pleasant surroundings: Dagmarsminde, the home's website reads, "is designed in every detail as a 'care oasis', prioritizing a sense of nature, well-being, closeness, and equality." With regard to the aesthetics of the home, the website mentions that "art, lighting, furniture, acoustics, temperature, green plants and fresh flowers, pets, fine table settings, essential oils, music, tone of voice and the food we serve are some of the important components to create the right atmosphere" ("Interior Design"). Dagmarsminde provides a caring environment for twelve residents experiencing varying stages of dementia and frailty, with staffing actually being equal or even lower than in other Danish nursing homes. This care model does not distinguish between different care levels and is accessible to anyone in need; but as demand is high, there are extensive waiting lists.

In this chapter, I engage in a discussion of the "production of space," as Lefebvre calls it, in textual representations of care-giving institutions. I do so to explore and deconstruct the binary opposition of "home" and "institution." As will be shown in my analysis, "feeling at home" is not necessarily linked to careful design, but can take various shapes. It can, for instance, be linked to a place that offers the possibility of rewriting one's life-course narrative in a potentially different, but meaningful way. Such a place, as the texts analyzed will show, can also be found in the care home, regardless of its design. These texts illustrate the difficulty of renegotiating identities in institutions of long-term care, not only for patients/residents, but for all individuals involved. Most importantly, this difference points to the function of the care home as a metaphorical and metonymical space when used as setting.

Renegotiating the Self: Fictional Representations of the Nexus of Hospital, Hotel, and Home

In Edna Alford's *A Sleep Full of Dreams*, the first text analyzed in this chapter, readers encounter Calgary's Pine Mountain Lodge primarily through the focalization of Arla Pederson, a young nurse struggling to reconcile herself with the demands of her challenging profession. The narrative problematizes the tension between Arla's tendency to perceive the old women as "other" and her simultaneous identification with them. This conflict is expressed on a spatial level; the homogenizing power of the care home is embodied by both the institution and Arla, and is especially at work in the institution's public areas. It is counterbalanced by her acknowledgement of her charges' individuality, which is expressed through Arla's caring relationship with them in their private rooms.

The second book discussed is Caribbean-Canadian author Shani Mootoo's novel *Cereus Blooms at Night*, which tells the turbulent life-story of Miss Mala Ramchandin through the narrative of Tyler, a homosexual male nurse at Paradise Alms House. In the secure place of the nursing home, Tyler and Mala develop a friendship that changes both their life-course identities, and allows them to find new meaning in their lives. The story tells a progress narrative of old age that is only made possible through good and nurturing institutional care.

While the first two texts emphasize the role of the care-givers, the third text, Joan Barfoot's novel *Exit Lines*, focuses on the alliance of four residents living in the Idyll Inn, a luxurious hotel-like retirement lodge. One resident, Greta, sets her suicide plans aside after realizing that friendship and solidarity have made her life meaningful. Finally, the short film *Rhonda's Party* introduces the character of Rhonda, a care-home resident who has spent months planning her best friend's Margaret's 100th birthday party, much to the dismay of the institution's administrator. When Margaret dies on the eve of the celebration, Rhonda must overcome her loneliness in the care home and decide whether the party will go on. What unites the narratives discussed in this chapter is that they all represent long-term care institutions as a place where characters (both nurses and residents) renegotiate their sense of self.

2.1 Care, Concern, (Dis-)Connection: Edna Alford's *A Sleep Full of Dreams*

In her 1981 short story cycle *A Sleep Full of Dreams*, Edna Alford depicts everyday life in a Canadian nursing home by introducing eleven old women and presenting their individual relationships with Nurse Arla Pederson. While John Keats in his poem "Endymion" talks about "a sleep / Full of sweet dreams, and health, and quiet breathing" (Keats 65), Alford's elision of the word "sweet" in the title "leav[es] readers to question the nightmare that 'a sleep full of dreams' may involve" (Chivers, *From* 72). In fact, unlike Keats's poem, the ten vignettes in the book are not set in joyful, paradisiac Elysian fields, but walk readers from room to room in Pine Mountain Lodge, a nursing home in Calgary, Canada.

In an interview with Alan Twigg, Edna Alford states, "I see *A Sleep Full of Dreams* as being a book about compartmentalization. It's there in the form. You will go into another room and into another room. It was suggested at some points that I might want to write a novel out of the stories. But I was absolutely determined that it be presented in this form" (A. Twigg 3). The cycle's compartmentalization not only reflects the reality of the architecture of many nursing homes, but also underlines the individuality of each of the women Nurse Arla deals with. Sally Chivers notes, "[o]verall there is a stark disjunction, reflected architecturally, within the nursing home. The contrast between the individual stories of the characters as located in their personal rooms and their uniformity in the dining room and common areas crystallizes the conflict between homogeneity and individuality that inhabits the institutional settings of any nursing home" (*From* 69). The very same conflict burdens Arla, who oscillates between perceiving the old characters as a homogeneous mass of bodies ("old women who lined the porch walls like assorted house plants on window sills," 57), and seeing them as individuals each with their own life story, women with whom she develops personal relationships and a certain level or trust.

The stories are linked through a single narrator's perspective, mostly Arla's, which is refracted in an indirect, sometimes omniscient third-person narrative. *A Sleep Full of Dreams* traces Arla's personal development and her difficulties finding a voice of her own, while coming to terms with her ambivalent feelings towards her exhausting job as a nurse and the stigma that caring for the dying involves. She feels that "just by working with these old women, she carried some kind of curse, some contagion, some odour" (19). Like her charges, Arla is part of institutional regimes, rules, and discourses. The narrative successfully portrays her struggle to find an answer to her boyfriend's question "[i]f you're so upset about it, Arla, why don't you leave?" (21). As is typical of the genre of the short story cycle, "the emphasis in most of them is on transition and the experience of change," as Maria Löschnigg points out (260). She observes that the short story cycle is "episodic in nature, allowing for glimpses of significant moments in the lives of the protagonists" (258–59). In fact, the book centers on Arla's development at a particular stage in her life. The narrator's perspective changes in only two stories that are set outside of the nursing home to that of an old woman resident, Tessie Bishop ("Half-Past Eight") and Harold Simpson, an old man in the bingo hall ("Under the I"). Löschnigg describes this narrative organization as a "Munrovian pattern"—a monovocal homodiegetic structure, "i.e. the narrative voice remains more or less constant throughout the whole cycle" (257). Although each vignette can be read as a separate story, the space of the nursing home and its effects on the individuals living and working there creates a certain sense of unity.

Pine Mountain Lodge is represented as a threatening place to the old women's individual identities, but it also challenges Arla's sense of self. She is conscious of the processes and power games at work in the institution, and through her encounters and relationships with the individual old women, she begins to critically reflect on her own life. Through her growing engagement with the women, she finds it increasingly difficult to deal with the central aspects of a nursing home: old age, dependency, and death. Arla's identification with her patients leads her to the painful discovery that she, too, is aging and might one day end up in a similar situation. She questions her own norms and values, both in her capacity as a nurse as in her private life, especially her relationship with her boyfriend, David. As readers, we follow Arla's inner conflicts and personal development until one day, at the end of the book, she decides to quit her job.

Despite Arla's personal development, Jeremy Lalonde cautions against reading *A Sleep Full of Dreams* as Arla's *Bildungsroman* as "one would expect Arla to be a more fully developed character" (87). Although Arla is the prime focalizer, and does undergo personal development, I agree with Lalonde's argument that the book is not a Bildungsroman in the classical sense. This supposition is supported by Edna Alford when she states in an interview that "[t]he vignettes are not narrated to portray a story of Arla's development and progress, [...] but to depict life in an institution" (A. Twigg 2). Maria Löschnigg emphasizes the difference in genre between short story cycle and *Bildungsroman* when she writes, "I would be careful about labels which again imply the conventional concept of a totalizing form which these authors have tried to undermine or escape" (258). *A Sleep Full of Dreams* corresponds to Löschnigg's description of the short story cycle:

> [t]he meaning of the incidents which are recalled by the narrator and around which the stories are built often lies in the fact that they signify processes of transition and transformation with regard to the protagonist. The narrative process appears as disjointed, as it offers a series of segments which—even if put together—resists the pattern of the linear and coherent life story which is typical of the *Bildungsroman*. (259)

As readers, we only share a small portion of Arla's life. The cycle, beginning in spring and ending after Christmas, comprises merely about one year of her work at the Pine Mountain Lodge. The book does not offer a happy or romantic ending that leaves readers satisfied with the insights Arla has gained. Rather, it contains a series of snapshots of Arla's life. Understanding and interpreting

Arla's development happens through the creative acts of reading and synthesizing the individual stories and their ambivalences. Sally Chivers observes:

> Although Alford writes in the third person, Arla's continued presence encourages the reader to evaluate and relate to her constantly changing and developing perceptions of the older adults she attends. Arla's assumptions are continually undermined, whether she begins a story with a negative opinion that some new knowledge thwarts or starts out full of optimism that is debunked. Accordingly, readers can accompany Arla through this third-person, partially omniscient narration in her continual reevaluation of her job, Pine Mountain Lodge's residents, and her own thoughts on aging. Alford subtly and gradually alters the seeming neutrality that the third person sets up by introducing various Pine Mountain residents. (*From* 69)

In the following interpretation of the individual vignettes, I focus on the spatial context of the nursing home as an institution located at the intersection of public and private, hospital, and home. As a bearer of meaning in its own right, the setting impacts the development of the protagonists' identities and interpellates them into their individual roles; Edna Alford's relatively unknown text represents one of the rare examples of care home narratives that grant visibility to the "fourth age." It provokes existential questions by portraying the challenges of coming to terms with death and dying—and indeed life itself. I deliberately decided to exclude three vignettes, "The Visitor," "Poll 101," and "Under the I" because they do not significantly engage with spatial dynamics or add any new perspectives.

Read in Bakhtinian terms, Pine Mountain Lodge can be seen as operating as a chronotope of stagnation, representing temporal suspension within institutionalized aging. Residents' pasts remain inaccessible or misunderstood, trapping them in perpetual present isolation. The vignettes' spatial-temporal dimensions reveal how personal histories and identities are disregarded or suppressed by institutional routines. The Lodge emerges as a chronotopic space where time is static, defined by repetitive routines, surveillance, and gradual erasure of individuality, further intensified by institutional control and neglect.

In terms of the spatiality of aging, Lefebvre's idea of contradictory and contested spaces comes into play. His argument that space is socially constructed, encompassing power relations that shape and are shaped by social interactions is rendered visible in the care home described by Alford. Pine Mountain

Lodge is a perceived space through its spatial practices; its dimly lit corridors and regimented routines symbolize the confinement and isolation. It is also a conceived space as its institutional logic constructs the home as a controlled, panoptical environment. Finally, in Lefebvre's terms, it is a lived space or space of representation where dominant discourses of aging, vulnerability, and dependency are materially and symbolically inscribed.

The Hoyer

In the first vignette, "The Hoyer," Arla Pederson is introduced to the reader as a hard-working young nurse in Pine Mountain Lodge, who is just about to take Miss Bole to the bathing room with the help of the eponymous hoyer. Miss Bole fears this apparatus because she feels it dehumanizes her by making her absolutely defenseless: "Miss Bole glared suspiciously at the apparatus. [...] [She] hated the hoyer, regarded it as a sinister and contemptible contraption. Most of all, she was afraid of it. It was unsafe, she maintained, dangerous, and sooner or later it would grab her and, like a madman, mangle her limbs" (Alford, *Sleep* 9). Arla, however, cannot move the heavy woman without the device. She is disgusted by the naked body, which "fat and distorted, lay open to the curious eyes of anyone passing her doorway and to the three old women who also occupied this room" (10). There is no privacy in this degrading procedure, and Miss Bole's dignity and her status as a person, as a prolific painter in high demand, which becomes clear later in the story, is absolutely irrelevant in this situation. She is reduced to her sheer physicality, a body exuding "the unmistakable stench of rotting flesh" (10) due to a "festering bed sore, angry and red at the centre, blue and mud-yellow and running around the outside" on her club foot. An object of disgust without any agency or personal control, Miss Bole's old body is publicly displayed in the aisle of the nursing home on its way to the bath. Arla quickly covers it with a sheet in order not to upset anybody they encounter. Miss Bole's body is, in Julia Kristeva's words, rendered "abject." Kristeva explains the abject as "something rejected from which one does not part, from which one does not protect oneself as from an object. Imaginary uncanniness and real threat, it beckons to us and ends up engulfing us. It is thus not lack of cleanliness or health that causes abjection but what disturbs identity, system, order" (4). The abject threatens Arla's sense of self through its dissolution of proper boundaries, and position at the borderline between life and death. Abjection disrupts the identity and order integral to Lefebvre's idea of the conceived space. Miss Bole's body destabilizes the neatly arranged social order symbolized by institutional spaces. Her body becomes a site of contestation, a lived space where boundaries of self and other, life and death blur.

The hallway and bathing room exemplify spaces where private and public domains collapse, enhancing the visibility of abjection. The hoyer, described as a monstrous contraption, embodies Kristeva's idea of the uncanny boundary violation, simultaneously medicalizing, objectifying, and threatening Miss Bole's identity and autonomy. Thus, the spatial arrangement itself becomes complicit in the production and reinforcement of abjection. The institution as both home and hospital creates inherent contradictions, as personal dignity conflicts with institutional efficiency. Miss Bole's forced visibility—her public exposure—demonstrates how institutional space prioritizes perceived efficiency over lived experiences.

In "The Hoyer," bathing is not a matter of pleasure, stress relief, or even luxury, but is explicitly located within a medical discourse. The "medical gaze" is dominant in the institutional context where authority is exercised over the individual, as Julia Twigg points out in her studies of bathing ("Deconstructing" 221; "Bathing;" *Bathing*). She observes that "[e]quipment both distances the person from direct human contact, putting a barrier between them and the operator, and acts to objectify them by providing the means whereby they are trapped, caged, made subject to the machine" (*Bathing* 25). The story highlights this objectification: Miss Bole is extremely terrified that the machine will not hold her weight, her eyes "black with the fear of what seemed to the old woman uncontrolled and sinister levitation" (*Sleep* 12). Julia Twigg's observation that "sanitary machinery and equipment often have a slightly bizarre and surrealist quality to them" (*Bathing* 25) is confirmed in the story: "Once in the hallway, the machine looked for all the world like a large bird of prey, a vulture or a hawk with a hapless body victim tangled up in its claws. It looked as if it had just swooped off a Bosch nightmare and snatched the fat old woman with the full intent of pecking her to death" (*Sleep* 13). The hoyer is depicted as a fantastic and alienating creature, such as those created by 15th century Dutch painter Hieronymus Bosch, and is experienced as threatening by both Miss Bole and Arla, who is this passage's focalizer. Although both women dread the machine, the institutional context does not allow them to change their daily routines; Arla puts Miss Bole into the contraption, reinforcing the asymmetry of power through the "gaze of youth," as Julia Twigg explains:

> Clients are naked, dependent, and below; workers are clothed, powerful, and above. Bathing subjugates the person in a second sense also. We are accus-

> tomed from Foucauldian and feminist writings to the notions of the professional gaze or the phallic gaze, but there is also a gaze of youth. [...] Recipients of help with bathing are literally subject to the gaze of youth in that their old bodies are exposed to the surveillance and view of younger workers. Many older people [...] internalize a sense of their bodies as no longer attractive, something that might be distasteful to see or handle; and this contributes to the unsettling experience of body care and to the asymmetrical nature of the exchange. ("Body" 65)

Arla, aware of Miss Bole's shame, observes the old woman in the bathtub, and contributes to the power imbalance by commenting on the process:

> [Miss Bole] absently lifted her sagging, mottling breasts, each in turn. She swiped beneath each with the cloth. Then she swiped at the white, curly pubic hair above her vagina. "You better do that thoroughly, Miss Bole," Arla said sharply, under the guise of efficiency. "You won't be having another bath till next week." That was one way of getting back at her. Ruthless, Arla was aware, but one way. The remark was double-barreled, with the humiliation of having to wash even the most private parts of her body in the presence of another person as well as the threat of next week's bath. (*Sleep* 17)

The asymmetry of power created by this procedure is increased by the juxtaposition of young Arla's crisp white uniform and Miss Bole's naked, old body, a "great mass of white flesh" (11) that is helplessly dangling from the contraption. In these scenes, the focalization shifts between Miss Bole and Arla, so that both perspectives become available to the reader, a narrative technique that also illustrates the power-struggle between the two women. Both of them, each acutely aware of the other's reaction, wish that the routine should come to an end as quickly as possible (Chivers, *From* 69).

Alford challenges the stereotype of the of old woman as helpless by presenting the bathing scene as a power struggle. While Arla takes control over Miss Bole's body via the machine, Miss Bole takes control of Arla's mind through the telling of horror stories during the bathing procedure. In these cruel stories that involve farming accidents and other disasters with people being killed or mutilated by contraptions such as threshing machines, Ferris wheels, or a rope going down into a deep well, Miss Bole's own fears are mirrored while she dangles from the hoyer's arm. The stories do not miss their aim—that of invoking similarly unpleasant feelings in Arla, who "despised this feeling of terror which crept over her every time she bathed the old woman" (*Sleep* 14–15). For instance, when the hoyer slowly dips Miss Bole's body into the water, she is terrified and recounts a tragic story in a strange and deep-throated, eerie voice. In this story, which took place decades ago, she recounts watching her niece drown after going down into a well with a rope, describing the drowned and accidentally strangled little body in minute and disgusting detail—to create the desired effect: "Arla winced. It was a direct hit" (16). In addition to Miss Bole's festering club foot, the morbid imagery she uses in her violent stories causes a feeling of abjection in Arla: "She despised this feeling of terror which crept over her every time she bathed the old woman. It always rooted itself in her stomach..." (14–15). Looking at Miss Bole's body, and listening to her horrible stories, Arla is painfully confronted with her own fears of aging and dying. These visual and auditory stimuli signify the abject "other" that confronts Arla with thoughts about her own death. She feels disgusted and alienated, and has difficulty concentrating on the machine that could so easily hurt Miss Bole. Arla can hardly control herself, which makes Miss Bole smile, settling the power imbalance in her favor: "Miss Bole knew she had the girl, again" (15). Bathing Miss Bole becomes a dehumanizing procedure for both of them. The hoyer comes to symbolize contested terrain, with Miss Bole reclaiming her power position while dangling in it, but she is aware that she must not go too far with Arla, whom she disindividualizes by calling her "the girl:"

> [S]he always tested only as far as she safely could, never far enough to push the girl over the edge into anger because that was very dangerous. She had observed that when angered, the girl ignored the ladies, prodded and pushed them like lumps of breaddough. The bath could become even more hazardous and painful if the girl became reckless with the machine, raising it too high, lowering it too fast. (11)

When Miss Bole is finally wheeled back to her room, a representative from the Department of Cultural Affairs is waiting for her in the corridor, and she is "obviously embarrassed to be presented to company in such a humiliating fashion" (23). Lyanda Weatherby has come to inquire about Miss Bole's artwork, which she would like to purchase for a permanent collection in the new provincial gallery. The "well-dressed, middle-aged woman" is also uncomfortable when confronted with "the apparition of this sheeted old woman who hung somehow from a sinister metallic machine" (23). In this scene, the liminality of the nursing home's private-public space and the lack of privacy are again highlighted.

While Ms. Weatherby is asked to wait outside until Miss Bole is dressed, Arla begins to feel excited for Miss Bole. Ms. Weatherby's respect for Miss Bole's artwork changes Arla's attitude towards her. Now, back in her own room, Miss Bole is no longer defined as an abject body, but as a person in demand, an individual with whom Arla can relate on a new and different level, thereby also reevaluating her mixed feelings of superiority and guilt: "The young woman felt somehow better about Miss Bole, somehow not so guilty for being young and whole and mobile" (24). The gaze of youth is relativized, and Arla is able to see Miss Bole as more of an equal, a precondition for identification, which is suggested in the story when Arla "looked at her with what felt like different eyes" (25). Here, the feeling of abjection seems to give way to a genuine interest in Miss Bole as an artist. Arla realizes that Miss Bole has a different voice, too, as she has started singing happily, sounding "like a trilling bird, eerie [...] completely different from the deep-throated purring voice Miss Bole used to tell her stories. Whoever knows anybody, Arla thought. Everybody is full of secrets" (25). A new image of Miss Bole, now queen-like, is presented:

> Arla could feel the warmth, the happiness. [...] She saw Miss Bole nestled comfortably in her wheelchair, resplendent in her quilted autumn robe which covered her club foot, now slippered anyway. She folded her hands in her lap, her whole hand completely hiding the clawed hand. Her eyes appeared to have red sparks at the centres. She looked like a queen prepared to hold court. Arla was proud of her. (25)

This reevaluation, however, is only of very short duration. When Arla leaves the room with the wet towels, Miss Bole reassumes her deep voice, telling yet another horror story about a person's arm being caught and burnt in Pine Mountain Lodge's laundry mangle, this time referring to a recent event, which Arla has been trying hard to forget. Here, the third category established by Lefebvre, lived space, can be employed to analyze how Miss Bole contests her abjection by reclaiming agency through the horror stories she tells Arla. Miss Bole resists and reclaims her dignity as an act of subverting the dominant spatial narrative, despite adverse institutional conditions. Miss Bole succeeds in bringing the terrible accident back to life in Arla's mind. In the last scene, the nurse, pulling herself together, pushes the hoyer out the door and into the hallway.

Sally Chivers concludes her interpretation of the story by stating, "[h]aving followed Arla as an exemplary interpreter of old people and sensed her error in failing to comprehend the significance of Miss Bole's ruthless replication, readers reevaluate both the stories of the old and the interpretations Arla offers" (*From* 70). As readers, we witness Arla's difficulties to understand Miss Bole's behavior. Arla is shown as ultimately failing to make sense of Miss Bole's stories. She does not understand them to be an expression of the old woman's fear, vulnerability, and discomfort. While identification and understanding on Arla's part seems to be briefly possible while they are in Miss Bole's room, Miss Bole is reduced to her physicality in the public areas of the care home.

For this vignette, Lefebvre's "spatial triad,"—perceived space, conceived space, and lived space, is a helpful analytical tool that elicits how spatial arrangements influence experiences of aging. The perceived space, read as spatial practice, becomes evident on the routines and practices of the care home, such as bathing and the use of the hoyer, that govern the daily rhythms and interactions. Arla's and Miss Bole's interactions with the hoyer exemplify how perceived space disciplines bodies, regulates privacy, and manifests social attitudes towards aging, abject bodies as "problems" that need to be contained and controlled. Lefebvre's second category, conceived space, refers to the conception of the care home as a medicalized space with a high level of efficiency. It is a "care" space, but prioritizes functionality and hygiene, which contributes to Miss Bole's humiliation and objectification. The medical gaze creates a sense of clinical detachment and exerts institutional control, reinforcing power asymmetries based on age, mobility, and authority. The third category established by Lefebvre, lived space, can be employed to analyze how Miss Bole contests her abjection by reclaiming agency through the horror stories she tells Arla. Miss Bole resists and reclaims her dignity as an act of subverting the dominant spatial narrative, despite adverse institutional conditions. Despite institutional constraints, Miss Bole's storytelling creates an alternative space of representation where power is renegotiated. Her narratives disrupt the dominant spatial practice by foregrounding personal histories and fears, at least temporarily challenging the spatial power dynamics of Pine Mountain Lodge.

Mid-May's Eldest Child

In the second vignette, "Mid-May's Eldest Child," Arla's youthful zest for life is contrasted with old Miss Moss's decline. The contrast is reinforced by the setting: Alford juxtaposes the grey, sinister world of the care home to a lush, green park, and a shopping mall, places which are represented in the story as "fit surroundings" for youth, not for old age (Laws, Spatiality 90). The vignette's title again stems from a famous poem by John Keats, "Ode to a Nightingale," that Miss Moss, a former high school teacher, had taught Arla. The intertextual reference hints at the central theme of the story: the finiteness of human existence.

The story opens with Arla walking to work, reminiscing how she and David had made love in the spring sun on their balcony the day before. Arla compares the balcony to Miss Moss's "silly bowers," contrasting her romance with David to Miss Moss's imagination of the romance in Keats's work. Keats's poem is also referenced when Arla, crossing a park, basks in the morning sun and enjoys nature with all her senses:

> When she reached the park gates she threw away her sweater, her vinyl purse and her lunch bag on the infant grass and, like a child, raced toward the naked white flag pole. Grabbing hold of it with one arm, the other swinging up and outward like a wing, she flew around and around. [...] Quickly dizzy, she let go of the pole and spun outward between a clump of lilacs and a bed of tulips and daffodils, running till she fell, then rolling over and over on the grass, her arms stretched upward, reaching toward the clear young sun. [...] Right then it seemed to Arla that anything was possible, probable even—that her future was as brilliant and certain as the leaves. (Alford, *Sleep* 28)

Arla happily immerses herself in nature, displaying a hunger for life and love, lying down in the grass, "her eyes closed, her face relaxed, her lips parted to receive the mythical 'man-of-the-morning' kiss" (28). Nature and sexuality merge metaphorically as she smells "lilacs and daffodils, tulips and columbine all warm between the labia of the earth" (28). When she gets up, she notices a grass stain on her uniform, describing it guiltily as if it came from making love on the lawn. The sunny, lush green park and Arla's youthful vigor are contrasted with the "dim corridor of the lodge" (30) and its inhabitants that await her. The contrasting spaces of the park and the nursing home are distinct, yet connected spaces representing different meanings and practices related to aging and youthfulness. Arla's spontaneous and sensual interaction with the park contrasts with the regulated space of the care home, exemplifying Lefebvre's spatial practice as the enactment of social rhythms and power relations on the physical plane.

On this particular day, she is expected to take Miss Moss, whom the matrons call "an irascible, uncompromising old witch" (29), to the hairdresser's. Arla looks forward to the trip, and slightly bends the institution's rules by planning to take Miss Moss to lunch and for a walk through the park where she "could see the new flowers and they could share this remarkable spring day. And they could talk" (30). Arla, thinking she understands Miss Moss's love for romantic poetry, hopes to please the old woman by bringing her in contact with nature. She sees this shared "quality time" as an expression of thankfulness on her part for the recognition Miss Moss gives her as a nurse, establishing a bond which allows them to subvert the rigid authority of the matrons. Arla sees something special in Miss Moss, not least of all because she showed appreciation for Arla's poetry recitals.

The story is told in retrospect through Arla's focalization, and Arla's mental listing of what she could have done wrong during the outing indicates that some disagreement must have occurred between the two women. While the narration does not reveal any feeling of guilt on Arla's part, it seems to slow down in pace when Arla—still in third person narration—remembers how she flirted with both the taxi driver and the hairdresser, enjoying their lustful looks at her body. Arla, in hindsight, draws a connection between these situations and Miss Moss's sudden anger and disintegration. Already a few moments after leaving the home, Miss Moss starts to change. When getting out of the taxi, in which Arla had been flirting with the driver, Miss Moss grows dizzy and falters a little, which surprises Arla "who had hitherto thought of Miss Moss as a kind of lady metronome, her gait confident and measured, self-assured along the smooth brown linoleum of the lodge" (35). Outside of the care home, Arla notices that Miss Moss "became progressively more confused and she began to wheeze" (35). At the hairdresser's, both the barber and Arla treat Miss Moss in an ageist way, Arla by speaking for her (noticing in retrospect that it was something "she had never had to do with Miss Moss," 36), and the hairdresser by asking her, "And how will you have it cut, little lady?" (36). The hairdresser "glanced at Miss Moss, then winked at Arla and Arla smiled weakly, knew that he and she were somehow, sadly, on the same side. She felt like a traitor" (37). Miss Moss now seems to break down entirely, with her sudden deterioration also affecting her speech:

> Arla couldn't understand it—this woman who had perfect command of the English language, whom Arla regarded as if she were the high-priestess of poetry, of beautiful, well-formed syllables, all of a sudden could not manage to say anything that made sense. Her speech was splintered, like the speech Arla remembered from the burnt-out old schizophrenics at the government hospital. (36)

The only intelligible words Miss Moss utters after a period of muttering incoherently are an attempt to offend the hairdresser. Taking into account Doreen Massey's insight that public space is highly structured by masculine forms of visibility, power and autonomy, it becomes clear why Miss Moss feels vulnerable in these public interactions. Her difficulty speaking and her embarrassment stem from societal expectations that devalue the aged female body and voice, relegating her to dismissive treatment in public interactions. But she fights back: When he is finished cutting her hair, and hands her a mirror, "She riveted her needle eyes on the mirror and snapped, 'Sir, you are incompetent—but what can you expect—nowadays'" (37). Arla is embarrassed and offended at the same time by Miss Moss's unkind comments, because they also include criticism of her own abilities. She is disappointed by the realization "how important it was for [Miss Moss] to believe the best was in the past, *her* past, that everything was slip-shod now, derelict, renegade, worthless" (37). Her idealized image of Miss Moss gives way to a strong sense of disappointment, and Arla begins to think that her feeling of connectedness with the old woman has been an illusion. Arla can no longer see any common ground, an insight that is expressed on the level of space through the juxtaposition of Miss Moss's behavior in the home and in public.

While in "The Hoyer," Arla developed a sense of connection with Miss Bole, bridging a generation gap that had previously seemed insurmountable, this feeling is completely reversed in "Mid-May's Eldest Child." Arla tries hard to appease Miss Moss, but to no avail. Feeling powerless and sad, Arla still does not give up, hoping that a short walk through the park with its daffodils and tulips would cheer Miss Moss up, "that the new spring growth would revive her, that she might still give a spring recitation" (38). It is now, Arla notices, "more glorious, more opulent, more fragrant" than in the morning, but Miss Moss only "focused her eyes on the dull grey boulders lining the walkway" (38) and does not bother to look up.

Again, Arla's perception of the space around them contrasts with that of Miss Moss's. Arla's last resort is to lead Miss Moss to a circle of moss roses blooming close to the ground. They were "pink and red and purple [...] they all looked soft and open-mouthed and Arla felt an urge to touch them, to run her finger round their inner lips. She was delighted" (38). This very sensual description and its imagery parallels the first scene of the story in which Arla recalls David caressing her on the floor of their balcony. Arla tries to interest the old woman, "Look Miss Moss,' she said, 'roses!' "Mid-May's eldest child, the coming musk rose"– Keats, right?' No answer, 'Miss Moss?' Still no answer. 'Let's go have a look'" (38). Arla recites from "Ode to a Nightingale" to reassure Miss Moss that Arla remembered what she had been taught. Miss Moss's sudden reply comes as a shock: "'You may go yourself, Miss Pederson,' Miss Moss growled, 'but if you think this conduct is acceptable during working hours, I disagree and I'll have no part of it. I will not serve as an excuse for your irresponsible behavior'" (38). Arla feels betrayed as Miss Moss seems to side with the institution, and threatens to report her.

Walking back towards the nursing home, the lodge seems to crumble just as Arla's recognition and esteem for Miss Moss does: "From the distance, the lodge looked benign to Arla, though she knew better [...] It sat like an aristocratic old woman, [...] But age had levied a heavy tax and if you really looked at it, you could see that the fine old three-storey building was approaching dilapidation" (39). From this moment on, Arla dismisses Miss Moss as being no different than the other old women in the residence. Her former appreciation for Miss Moss's kindliness changes to disdain for the old woman's insensitivity when she watches her poke "at a tulip or daffodil along the side of the path with her cane as she might have poked at the carcass of a dead cat" (39). When Miss Moss finally, instead of reciting poetry inspired by nature as Arla had happily expected, breathes heavily, heaves, and vomits on the lodge's steps, Arla's disappointment causes a physical reaction: "Now she felt welling up with her a different kind of emesis, not only the disappointing turn of the day, but disillusionment, a disenchantment so deep it seemed to turn her inside out—a dry heave" (40). Like her reaction with Miss Bole, she again experiences a feeling of abjection when her identification with Miss Moss and ego-boundaries are challenged. As Arla witnesses Miss Moss's disintegration in public, the abject becomes tangible, representing the fragility and unpredictability of aging. She experiences discomfort as her idealized perception of Miss Moss falls apart, triggering her own fears and a visceral reaction of disgust, a physical and emotional embodiment of abjection. Now, she uses the poem Miss Moss had taught her cynically against the old woman: "'A thing of beauty is a joy forever,' she recited to herself, her voice mocking the old woman's, her mouth twisted, her eyes glazed with anger—'its loveliness increases; it will never / Pass into nothingness; but still will keep / A bower quiet for us and a sleep / Full of sweet dreams and health and quiet breathing'" (40). In an interpretation of this scene, Lalonde maintains,

> Arla rejects the argument of Keats's *Endymion* — that things of beauty are immortal since they live in the memory. There is, however, no reason to suppose

> that the consolatory power that Miss Moss ascribes to reading and reciting poetry will be in any way diminished by this temporary loss of her faculties. If we read Arla as the central figure in this story, the message is profoundly negative: she rejects the consolatory power or art in a world where death and dying are never distant, and she loses the compassion she initially showed toward Miss Moss. (92)

While in "The Hoyer" Arla came to realize Miss Bole's uniqueness, "Mid-May's Eldest Child" shows Arla, even if only to protect herself, making a sweeping, ageist statement about old women: she "began to feel not so much hurt any longer, but anger toward the old woman. She felt herself withdraw, felt the old woman's power over her diminish, was relieved to find herself objective. Miss Moss was just an old woman. That was all she was" (39). Arla oscillates between individualizing and homogenizing the nursing home residents, which can be read as "as a metaphor for a cultural necessity to interpret the elderly as complete entities" (Chivers, *From* 71). Arla calls Miss Moss "just an old woman," meaning that she is no different from all the other lodgers who, as she mentions earlier, get on her nerves. As Chivers points out, this conclusion is "insufficient because it has been proven in the previous story to have no inherent meaning; there is no such thing as 'just an old woman' any more than feminists at the very last would agree that there is no such thing as "just a woman" (*From* 71). Arla finds it difficult, even impossible, to find a professional yet empathic way of caring for the lodge's residents. The reference to Keats's poem reveals her difficulty of accepting life's finiteness. While the nightingale is "immortal" through its song, humans are not. The care home symbolically reminds Arla of this fact.

The institutional rules, embodied in Arla's nursing uniform and the restrictive policies she slightly transgresses by taking Miss Moss for an outing, represent Lefebvre's conceived space defined by institutional authority and medical rationality. Arla's bending of these rules—attempting to humanize the institutional experience by introducing leisure and outdoor enjoyment—reveals tensions between institutional expectations and individual autonomy. The spaces outside the institution (the taxi, the park, the hairdresser) unexpectedly become sites where institutional ageist dynamics follow Miss Moss, suggesting the institutional discourse's pervasive influence even beyond its physical boundaries.

Lefebvre's notion of spatial contradictions becomes especially relevant as the spatial distinctions between the park, the public, and the nursing home blur. The transition from the home to public space becomes a source of vulnerability rather than liberation for Miss Moss. Outside the nursing home, she loses her institutionalized protection and authority (as an educated former teacher) and becomes vulnerable to ageist stereotypes from strangers and Arla's inadvertent infantilization. Read through a Foucauldian spatial lens, Miss Moss's increasing loss of agency symbolizes how institutional disciplinary power extends beyond physical spaces, shaping interpersonal dynamics and perceptions of self-worth. The juxtaposition of Arla's youthfulness and Miss Moss's diminishing vitality underscores how social perceptions shape these contrasting spatial experiences, reflecting the assertion that spatiality actively participates in constructing identities and power relations.

Communion

The next story, "Communion," problematizes Arla's troubled sense of self by juxtaposing her "private 'communion,'" as Lalonde calls it (93), with "the public rites that Reverend Paul performs for Mrs. Pritchard" (93). Arla is the focalizer of the third person narration that presents a detailed account of her sexual arousal and masturbation in the nursing home's toilet, while the Reverend administers communion to Mrs. Pritchard in her room. While Mrs. Pritchard's soul "longed for the body and blood of the Lord" (58) Arla also gets "hungry" (59). She notices the priest's voice jumping "without warning to a higher pitch" (61), then again drifting "down into low throat tones," (61), perceiving the ritual next door as if it were a sexual act. The nursing home's structured, controlled environment sharply contrasts Arla's private space within the bathroom, where institutional surveillance temporarily breaks down, allowing intimate acts typically repressed by institutional norms. The institutionalized religious ritual conducted by Reverend Paul reflects the nursing home's role as a morally regulated space, reinforcing ideals of propriety, sanctity, and discipline. Arla's personal sexuality, in stark opposition to these institutional values, highlights the conflicting spatial ideologies around purity, discipline, and bodily control.

At the same time, Arla observes two dogs repeatedly mating on the hill outside the kitchen window. Arla, agitated by the tone of the Reverend's voice and looking at the "hard pointed flesh" (62) of the "Shepherd" (the term, even more semantically ambiguous because it is capitalized, is only used for the dog), runs down to the washroom in the basement and masturbates in the dark. "The end was convulsive, almost doubled her, she knowing where they were—the dogs, the Reverend Paul and Mrs. Pritchard" (63). Immediately afterwards, she feels guilty, repeating "quietly, mechanically, 'have mercy upon us, have mercy upon us...'" (64).

Her guilt and shame suggest the fragility of lived space, showing how institutional controls (both of the care home and the church) influence her internalization of moral judgment, even outside direct surveillance. While the institutional space epitomizes Foucault's notion of discipline, control, and normalized surveillance, Arla temporarily escapes this surveillance within the private confines of the restroom. Nonetheless, her immediate guilt afterward demonstrates the deep internalization of disciplinary power—reflecting Foucault's concept of panopticism, where institutional surveillance shapes individual self-perception and behavior even when direct observation is absent. The juxtaposition of Arla's personal, intimate space (the bathroom) against the public religious ritual further highlights gendered spatial tensions. The Reverend, performing a sanctioned public act, symbolizes masculine authority in contrast to Arla's marginalized, concealed feminine desire, which is inherently stigmatized by institutional and religious norms.

When she passes Mrs. Pritchard's door on her way back, she overhears the Reverend whispering, "take and drink this" (64). Arla, "startled by the fact that the service was not yet over" (64), makes herself a cup of tea. As if also attending communion, she drinks it and eats "the one remaining cookie on the tea plate" (64). When she takes a bite, she smells "a faint, sick sweet odor" that stems from the "dark blood on her fingers," remembering "that part of the service which said she wasn't worthy" (63–64). Without completing her chores for the day, Arla decides to go home. She reads "The Prayer of Humble Approach" from a booklet: "We cannot yet praise God as the Angels do. While we are here, the remembrance of our sins and unworthiness must ever mingle, like a dark shadow, with our brightest praises" (65). Upon finishing the prayer, she throws herself on the bed, weeping, "not knowing or remembering in the darkness who or where or even what she was" (65). Unlike Mrs. Pritchard, she cannot find consolation in her feelings of loneliness, shame, guilt, and unworthiness. She has been unable to come to terms with her own self, which she must protect against the threatening, abject image of old age. As in a coming-of-age narrative, she grapples with the difficulty of finding a point of orientation in her life—a point that Mrs. Pritchard has found through her spirituality. As the final sentence reveals, she herself is abject, neither knowing where or who she is, nor even "what"—a question that blind Mrs. Pritchard seems to have found the answer to long ago.

Half Past Eight

The vignette "Half Past Eight" is radically different from the other stories in the collection, not only because it includes Arla only as an absence, and takes place primarily outside of the institution's walls, but also because it challenges the stereotypical notions of how nursing home residents ought to behave. Residents Tessie Bishop and Flora Henderson dress up, as Tessie says, "to see the parade and eat and kick up our heels for a change" (69). Arla is present only in the two rebellious women's cathartic rant: "Goddamn stupid nurse. [...] No more of a nurse than a pig's foot. [...] She hasn't got the brains she was born with. [...] I wouldn't hire her if ya paid me [...] She ain't fit for that kinda work!" (70). The story is linked only through its imagery to the previous one, "Communion," when Tessie puts red lipstick on herself that has a "sickly sweet smell" (66), reminding the reader of Arla's "dark blood on her fingers," (63) and her smelling "a faint, sick sweet odor" (64), which redirects, as Jeremy Lalonde puts it, "the narrative focus away from Arla" (94). He argues that Alford "increases the importance of imagistic links between the stories [...] [which] work to simultaneously bind the stories and the women of the stories together" (86).

In this vignette, the hoyer also reappears in front of Ms. Bole's room. While Tessie "edged her way around it as if she were afraid it were alive, as if it might reach out and grab her" (*Sleep* 70), Flora "stuck out her foot and gave the hoyer a shove and sent it rolling into the wall, clanking when it hit the baseboard, its canvas straps swinging foolishly. 'You'll never get me inta that goddamn thing,' she bellered at the metal hoist" (70). Flora's rowdy behavior at age 86 is juxtaposed to Tessie's attempts to look seductive. Her make-up routine is described extensively in a third-person narration that oscillates between a judgmental, ageist gaze and Tessie's self-perception: "The rouge was pink and had the same sweet sickening odour as the lipstick, like rosewater and glycerin gone rancid in sun and age. The bright pink cheeks clashed violently with her 'Scarlet Fire' lips and together with white, heavily powdered skin in wrinkles, made her look like a clown" (67). This description of a grotesque masquerade contrasts with Tessie's self-perception: "When she had finished, she smiled with satisfaction at the mirror. She began to hum to herself. [...] A very classy number, she thought. [...] Admiring herself in the wavy mirror, she remembered that she had been a very beautiful young woman" (67–68). This play with perspective challenges the readers' possible preconceptions. Whereas parts of the narrative portray Tessie as a poor old lady who even had to "cut down on wool for crocheting" (68) to afford the Stampede Parade where she hopes to see Prince Charles on his horse, her self-appreciation, vitality, and strength are also emphasized throughout the story. Her friend Flora is described as a good companion for Tessie: "Nothing could keep her down. [...] Age meant nothing to her, which was probably why they chummed around together, not because of the drinking" (68). Together they set out to enjoy the day, "a peculiar and somewhat amusing couple" (71). In contrast to Tessie, a little old lady who loves crocheting and the Royal Family, Flora is described as a tall, rebellious, manly kind of woman who swears and curses, drinks whiskey, and spits in the street. In one of the story's key scenes, Flora makes a pass at Tessie:

> Hank had just come back from the washroom and had poured himself another glass of beer when Tessie felt the hand on her stocking, moving up her thigh. She leaned toward Hank, then straightened abruptly. Both of Hank's hands were occupied—a half-full glass of beer in one and a Player's cigarette in the other. She had just watched him light it. She turned on Flora. (79)

With reference to this scene, Lalonde writes, "Alford takes the stereotype of the sexless old woman, turns it on its head, and sets it spinning. [...] Alford manages to reinscribe the sexuality of the elderly without casting heterosexuality as the normative role" (95). First, Tessie is upset, but when the two women return to the lodge, she no longer holds a grudge. Flora attempts to wake up the other residents, banging on each door and roaring obscenities. Tessie has difficulties stopping her, whereupon Flora argues, "What's a matter with ya, Tess? [...] I'd rather be fuckin' drunk than this. [...] [M]ost of the old dames don't even make it to seven-thirty let alone half-past eight—and the worst of it is they wouldn't know what to do with it even if they could get holda some" (*Sleep* 82). Flora expresses her dissatisfaction here with the obedient women who succumb to the homogenizing stereotypes that render old women sexless. She voices her anger about how unquestioningly they have come to endorse the binary opposition between youth and age (Waxman, *From* 127), and feels trapped in a heteronormative environment.

Both Tess and Flora undercut the "sweet old lady" image that does not allow for any kind of diversity, challenging the traditional images of sexless old women in nursing homes. They feel liberated and see themselves as independent subjects who undermine the institution's rules by "breaking out," drinking, and flirting. They position themselves as not belonging to the community of the old age home. For a moment they even jokingly consider opening a brothel in Pine Mountain Lodge—a business Flora used to run unofficially when she was younger—and feel both unshackled and subversive, using the absurdity of the idea as comic relief. This spasm of relief helps them come to terms with the strict institutional regimes imposed by the matrons, with which they know they must comply. They do not see Arla as any different from the matrons. While readers get to know Arla's moral dilemmas with regard to the quality of the Pine Mountain Lodge's care-giving ethics, she is, according to Flora's judgment, part of the institutional authoritarian regime, and not even good at her job (70).

Although the story has been criticized for disrupting the volume's coherence because it takes place outside of the institution, and lacks Arla's focalization (Osachoff 165), Edna Alford argued that she put it into the volume deliberately:

> When Tessie Bishop and Flora Henderson slip the traces and bolt for the Stampede Parade and the Palliser Hotel, their story bolts the form, goes AWOL as well. I had initially intended this story to be told from within the Lodge with more emphasis/dramatization on the consequences of their escapade, but they escaped. I let them. Worse than that, I went with them. And I'd do it again, regardless of the formal, aesthetic consequences. (Alford, "Fear" 177, qtd. in Lalonde 94)

As mentioned earlier, Lalonde suggests reading the collection as a "narrative of community" that is organized according to the compartmentalized structure Alford mentions. Not only are old people compartmentalized as "other," and stored away in a home, but further compartmentalization occurs as a result of the spatial and social structures in the nursing home itself. Therefore, the vignette "Half-Past Eight" does not disturb the unity and coherence of the volume, but instead adds another perspective to the collection, rendering it more diverse (as well as criticizing the lack of diversity in the institution). Alford lets Tessie and Flora escape, and establishes an additional viewpoint by using Tessie as a focalizer to complement Arla's perspective, a technique she applies to challenge and criticize the ageist "othering" gaze in contemporary society (A. Twigg 3).

Fall Cleaning

In "Fall Cleaning," readers are taken into another "compartment" in the Pine Mountain Lodge. This time, the reader is introduced to Mrs. Tweedsmuir, who lives in a cluttered room that Arla and Matron Benstone attempt to clean. To Arla, Mrs. Tweedsmuir is a disgusting hoarder who collects everything from "dry bread crusts and mouldy oranges" (83) to "reeking curdled milk" (84) and "bundles of string, a set of insoles, corn-plasters by the dozen, ribbons of all colours and fabrics, old calendars and ancient, yellowed copies of *The War Cry*" (83). Mrs. Tweedsmuir is upset by the fact that Arla and the matron do not respect her privacy, and begin to clean out her room without requesting her permission: "'These are my *things*, my personal belongings,' began the old woman. 'I want to see what you're taking. I don't want my things thrown out as if they were trash. I have important papers in my room.' Why couldn't she understand that all these things *were* trash, Arla wondered—garbage and nothing more" (84). The institution's medical discourse treats Mrs. Tweedsmuir's belongings purely as "garbage," erasing their emotional significance and personal history. The matron forces her to sit outside her door until the "fall cleaning" has been completed, not allowing her any agency. Both Foucault's and Lefebvre's idea of spatial practices is easy to note here. Cleaning routines designed for efficiency, hygiene, and discipline, reinforce institutional order and norms. Arla's intrusion into Mrs. Tweedsmuir's room exemplifies spatial practices reinforcing the institution's dominance over individual autonomy through surveillance and regulation.

In this story, Arla is again the focalizer, but by now readers are aware of her shortcomings as a nurse, and realize that the perspective presented is biased. Even though Arla reveals a hint of self-criticism by saying that "she could find nothing in Mrs. Tweedsmuir to love" and that this was maybe "the worst thing she could say about herself" (93), she story underlines her lack of empathy for the old woman. For instance, Arla mentions her own passion for collecting "the Royal Albert 'Wild Rose' pattern" (88), but fails to see its similarity with Mrs. Tweedsmuir's hoarding behavior.

To the old woman, the things she keeps in her room are intrinsically connected with her former habit of "fall canning," but, as Lalonde observes, "Arla does not draw the connection between the pioneer spirit that she frequently ascribes to the women of the Lodge and Mrs. Tweedsmuir's refusal to throw anything away. Significantly, all of the food that Mrs. Tweedsmuir hoards away is kept in half-pint sealers; in an exercise that mirrors fall canning, she turns her closet into a pantry for her 'preserves'" (96). The narrative presents the "fall cleaning" as an ambivalent act: while it is necessary to keep the rooms clean to satisfy the institutional hygiene regulations, Mrs. Tweedsmuir's sense of self is endangered by the lack of empathy. The nurses do not display any understanding for the fact that everyone has some level of attachment to their belongings.

When Mrs. Tweedsmuir talks to Tessie Bishop, the narrative reveals how she experiences the cleaning. She fears that she is being cleaned out along with her stuff, and that the room is already being prepared for a new lodger: "'They anticipate my death. […] They are cleaning it out for someone else. […] It won't be my room any more. My room will be in the ground,' she said," (84–85), fearing that her belongings and, thus, her identity will disappear. The radical cleaning of her room has a devastating effect on her.

The next scene meticulously describes Arla helping Mrs. Tweedsmuir get up and walk to the next room, after she had fallen asleep during mealtime and, therefore, not eaten a bite. The excruciatingly slow pace of the narration mirrors the duration of the process. Arla, impatient and bored, does not care that the old lady is hungry, and forces her to leave the dining room. Her dinner tray is taken away, and when Mrs. Tweedsmuir tries to keep a piece of bread with her, Arla demands she hand it over, reminding her that "the matrons don't like you to carry food back to your room. We wouldn't have to shovel it all out so often like we did today" (87). Mrs. Tweedsmuir, slightly jerking, responds, "You ought not have a key to my room. You ought not barge in and root around when I'm not there" (87–88). "'I'm paid to do my job,' said Arla. 'So are pro-sti-tutes, my dear Miss Pederson,'" Mrs. Tweedsmuir counters (88). She is very frail and tired, and her asthma makes it hard for her to walk. Arla prods her to move on, losing what is left of her patience: "If you think that [the asthma] makes you special, Mrs. Tweedsmuir, you're wrong. There's not a woman here who doesn't have something wrong with her but most of them handle it far better than you.' Arla knew she was stretching the truth a little but Mrs. Tweedsmuir was getting on her nerves" (88).

While Arla continues to prod the old woman towards the next room, her associations and thoughts are shaped by the stereotypical ageism, which she usually "tries to counter in her personal life and that her professional experience should help her to avoid" (Chivers, *From* 72). To escape the pressures of her job and avoid acknowledging the threatening idea that she could one day be just like Mrs. Tweedsmuir, she resorts to "othering" her as a monster, a witch, "an old packrat" (88): Mrs. Tweedsmuir "reminded Arla of one of those reptile monsters in old technicolor movies" (87), she observes. "She had whiskers growing out of the many moles on her face, like the witches Arla remembered from fairy tales" (89–90). Arla questions whether there is any meaning to Mrs. Tweedsmuir's life: "There had to be more to a person at the end of her life than a heap of old things. Otherwise, what was the point" (88). Arla's bored description of the dining room underlines the meaninglessness she ascribes to old age and the simulacrum of life in the care home: "Last month, she remembered, there were plastic orchids and at Christmas, large red plastic poinsettias, one at each setting for four in the dingy dining room. So this was what was at the end of the rainbow, thought Arla. The Land of Promise delivered. The gleam in the eyes of the immigrant women—plastic roses. Hardly worth the effort when you stopped to think about it" (89).

When Arla wakes Mrs. Tweedsmuir the next day to get her ready for breakfast, she states that she feels too weak to get up. Arla, despite noticing the feverish look in Mrs. Tweedsmuir's eyes, and realizing that the woman draws her breath "through networks of phlegm growing in her lungs like thick patches of weed on the bottom of a lake" (91), still adamantly demands that she get dressed. A little while later, she finds Mrs. Tweedsmuir lying in a large pool of her own blood, having obviously fallen on her head. However, Arla does not feel any pity: "'Oh God,' Arla muttered. 'Here we go again. This job is just like riding around on a bloody ferris wheel'" (92).

Mrs. Tweedsmuir passes away during the night, and readers are left to wonder whether the "fall cleaning" (the double meaning of the title perhaps intended), including Arla's removal of the board Mrs. Tweedsmuir had used to seal the window against the cold, had weakened her so much that she could not get up by herself anymore. Although the narration encourages the readers to blame Arla for her carelessness, no mention is made of a care-giving mistake, and Arla, as usual, cleans up the room to prepare it for the new lodger, a Mrs. Brockmann, who is already waiting.

Arla's indifference to Mrs. Tweedsmuir's death is stunning. The cleaning, she notes, was "relatively easy for a change. After all, they had thrown out most of the garbage" (93) the day before. However, Arla's negligence regarding the cold air coming in through the window is hinted at, as Lalonde writes, and "the narrator makes plain connections to the reader to which Arla is not privy" (96): "The room she left behind was clean and quiet. Sunlight flickered through the green and red and white blotched curtains. A cold fall breeze fluttered them, lapping them in and out against the screen" (Sleep 93). This description, with which the story ends, is exactly the same as Arla's description of the room after cleaning it the first time, with the exception of the final sentence, "Mrs. Tweedsmuir slept on her freshly plaited bed" (86), which is now missing. Like a hotel room, number 18 waits for a new resident. While readers are presented with both the patient's and nurse's perspectives at the same time, no signs that Arla identifies with her charges appear in this or the following vignette.

Tuesday, Wednesday, Thursday

While Arla has so far found it very difficult, if not impossible, to identify with her charges, she manages to adopt the perspective of Mrs. Langland in "Tuesday, Wednesday, Thursday." Mrs. Langland, a very frail and thin old woman, slips and falls in her own excrement because Arla is too busy and impatient to stay with her during the painfully slow process of getting dressed. The description in this vignette is very detailed and exact, and evokes a strong, nearly abject feeling in the reader, as Chivers contends: "Alford once again imparts to readers a disgust that exceeds the stereotypical disgust of older bodies that younger people often associate with the elderly" (*From* 73). Arla portrays Mrs. Langland as looking "like a ghost" (111) with "[h]er eyes [which] appeared to have grown permanently monstrous, shone silver with horror" (109). The description establishes a stark contrast between herself and the old woman: "Her breasts were empty, flat and wrinkled like crushed tin foil. They disgusted Arla who was young and well-endowed with tight resilient skin enveloping her own breasts" (111). Arla's young body in its "clean white uniform" is further juxtaposed to Mrs. Langland's half-naked and old body, as "a large brown-yellow stain begun to spread over the back of Mrs. Langland's white cotton underpants. Soon it hung heavy inside the cloth and then it escaped through the bottom of her bloomers and ran straight down her right leg, crossing over the maze of cold blue veins till it reached her ankle" (112). Arla scolds her, "Of all mornings to come up with a stunt like this" (113), starts undressing her again and leaves with the dirty laundry. While Arla is away, Mrs. Langland's "old body would jerk into a new set of shivers" (114)—she slips and falls:

> The old woman lay naked, rigid with fear, and again she began to shiver. [...] The yellow mass oozed beneath her and found its way to the edges of her body where some escaped around her boney hips and some just above her armpits, near her shoulders. She held her legs straight out before her, suspended a little above the floor, which gave the body the appearance that it was about to levitate, had already begun to rise. (114)

Mrs. Langland is presented here as close to death, and at the same time lying in her excrement as helpless as a baby. This infantilizing analogy, stereotypical as it is, links the beginning with the end of life, and is frequently applied in nursing home narratives (e.g., *Half Life* by John Mighton). When Arla enters the room, she is shocked to see Mrs. Langland lying there:

> Her face looked like a blank sheet of paper, her eyes large, almost silver, mirroring the eyes of the old woman lying on the floor. The longer Arla stared obliquely at the body, the more she recognized or remembered something familiar in the old woman's frozen face, something unholy in the humiliating posture of the crooked old bone body, framed in the yellow ooze of its own feces. (114)

The beginning of this description merges Arla's face with that of Mrs. Langland. Readers might first think of "her face" as the old woman's, but it soon becomes clear that Arla's face is being described here. The abject is threatening Arla's ego boundaries—she is horrified. Arla suddenly recognizes herself in the old woman:

> Arla couldn't say exactly what it was she recognized there, but she knew it was somehow part of herself. And although she would never really know why, it tore like a ragged fish-knife through the flesh of her indifference, her only ally at times like this, left her with a deeper repugnance, a more palpable fear and disgust than she had ever felt before, even at Pine Mountain Lodge. There was something she saw here, something she smelled in the sulphuric acrid air that made her think of hell, the long-forgotten Sunday School hell of a four year old girl. (114–15)

Here, a process of identification with the old woman begins for Arla. She recognizes that Mrs. Langland is intimately related to her as an individual in her present, her future, and also in her past. The narrator alludes to Arla's indifference, which had been a protective shield ("her only ally"), and indicates that it now slowly gives way to a sense of recognition. Arla is horrified because she realizes Mrs. Langland's lack of personal agency. Chris Gilleard and Paul Higgs argue:

> The deeper abjection of old age lies not so much in the leaking of bodily products nor in the physical stigma of an ageing appearance nor the demonstrable performance handicaps of a disabled person. What constitutes abjection in old age is the evidence of absence, absence of self-consciousness, of self-control, of corporeal ownership—the abjection of the orphaned body. ("Ageing" 139)

Using both George Bataille's and Julia Kristeva's concepts of abjection, Gilleard and Higgs redefine abjection as the cultural and symbolic process by which the aged body becomes emblematic of a deeper existential and social exclusion, where the body is stripped of subjectivity and reduced to an object of care or even horror. Abjection here is not just about the physical signs of aging but about the perceived loss of social and individual agency. Arla's difficulties stem from the breakdown between her personal boundaries and the "orphaned body," the old body's failure—its near-death.

In what is nearly a moment of epiphany, she overcomes this abjection, and feels a deep sense of connection with Mrs. Langland: "The two women stared at each other silently, as if they were in a play and had been directed to 'freeze,' motionless, suspended in time. And although neither spoke or moved, this was the first honest communication between them, the only time Arla had ever been able to imagine the old woman as an ordinary human being" (115). Recognizing herself in Mrs. Langland, almost as if seeing to the bottom of her soul through her eyes, "A red streak slid over Mrs. Langland's face, lit upon the bulbous silver eyes, and only for a moment Arla thought she saw the old lady's eyes on fire, thought she saw flames licking out from her eyelids, then consumed and rekindled in the grey-white irises and finally smothered in the blackness of her tiny, precise pupils" (115). In this moment of epiphany, abjection takes hold of Arla:

> The light reflected on the old woman's body rekindled Arla's memory, haunted her with infernal childish notions she couldn't seem to shake this time. She almost took leave of her senses, screamed and dropped the basin, ran out of the room, out of the lodge, out of the city. Yet, somewhere within her she knew there was nowhere far enough to run, no escape from what she had learned. And so she began to move toward Mrs. Langland, very slowly at first, as if she were a robot or hypnotized. She felt her flesh soften, release her, allow her back into herself. (116)

She then heaves Mrs. Langland onto her bed, cleans and disinfects her and the room, and asks the old woman, this time gently and respectfully, to stand up. She helps her with her food on the sun porch, and Mrs. Langland, although still staring absentmindedly, begins to eat. A few moments later, Arla learns from Mrs. Mackenzie, another old woman, that Mrs. Langland had come to Pine Mountain "from the asylum" (117), after she had "watched her house afire, burned to the ground and her children in it at the time" (117–18). Arla is shocked by this bit of information that gives "the experience an unearthly kind of aura" (119), and starts to shake. She realizes that "more terrifying than anything else, had been the vague, still undefined recognition of some part of herself in the disintegrating mind and body of the old woman, a recognition so deep it seemed to shake her from within" (119). Arla cannot help thinking of this incident again and again, feeling guilty for not treating Mrs. Langland as a human being. As the narrator notes, "her own incompetence and thoughtlessness converged on her. She could have done better. She should have known she couldn't leave the old woman standing by herself" (119). Readers might assume that this revelation would change Arla's perception more deeply, and consequently alter the way she works in the nursing home. In the course of the next few days, however, Mrs. Langland, whom Arla had been treating very patiently and sympathetically as atonement for her harsh behavior, does not react to any of her efforts, "remembering [what Mrs. Langland had been through] became progressively more difficult" (121), and Arla's patience wears thin, increasingly leading her to give way to aggression. When kneeling on the floor, trying to put shoes on Mrs. Langland's feet, Arla "became brutal, grew determined to force the rebellious toes into their proper places" (121). Any connection Arla had felt with Mrs. Langland is now severed, as Lalonde also remarks (97). "Angry now, forgetting grew easy for her, understanding impossible—both finally of the same thing—that these could be her feet, her toes, her somewhere, some other distant time" (121). I agree with Jeremy Lalonde who observes, "Arla appears as compassionless as she was in the opening story, making it difficult to argue that she has undergone any real emotional development" (97). Looking back at the story's beginning, its epigraph, "cold and in the winter weather / comfort is denied / doors are fast but still the weather / rages inside" (108) now makes sense in reference to both the home and Mrs. Langland's inner struggle.

Companion

"Companion," the last and, I would argue, the most complex story of the collection, begins with Arla looking at "the snowflakes intact" (140) on her coat, picking up from where "Under the I" (a vignette not included in my analysis) ends, providing a link between the stories via the cold winter weather through which Harold drives home, focusing on "the spray and hiss of flakes against the glass" (139). The snow during the post-Christmas season not only creates a link, but it establishes a cyclic structure, which connects the ending of the book to its beginning. Ending it with a story set in winter emphasizes the cyclical yet static nature of residents' lives, symbolizing a temporal loop without meaningful change or progression. In this sense, it can be read as a Bakhtinian chronotope of stagnation. Arla reflects on the year that had passed: "Every year she looked forward to Christmas and Easter and summer and always she found herself melancholy afterward, had trouble believing they had come and gone, slipped into her uneventful past with everything else" (140). She is aware of how quickly time is passing, of how she, too, is aging without feeling as though much happening in her life, like the old women in the lodge. The passage of time and, as the natural consequence of its passage, death, is one of the story's central themes. Even when pulling up a blind, Arla cannot help noticing that "it rolled up rapidly, disappearing with a flap flap into wherever it is that blinds go, into nowhere, it had always seemed to Arla, like time, like life" (149).

The diamond ring—another cyclic structure—that David gives Arla can also be seen as a symbol of the natural cycle of life and death. The ring also connects this story back to a previous vignette, "Tuesday, Wednesday, Thursday." In contrast to the yellow and red fiery flames Arla saw in Mrs. Langland's eyes, the ring in this story "glittered and flashed stellate patterns like fractured glass on the smooth white plaster of the wall" (140). Even though it is an engagement ring, it fills her "with doubt and apprehension" (148), and fails to touch her heart. She realizes that "although the ring still glittered in the artificial lights still on in the lodge, [...] the diamond made her sad, was cold as ice, had lost its fire" (140).

The metaphoric connection established between the dark, cold winter and the uneasiness Arla experiences as she enters the lodge on that particular day seem to foreshadow the death of Mrs. Dawson, the story's resident protagonist, who is just a few days away from her 100th birthday. Arla has developed a special connection to this woman, not least of all because she feels that Mrs. Dawson, unlike the other residents, has always shown a genuine interest in her life and respects her. When she received her ring, Mrs. Dawson was the only woman who did not tell her that she was too young to "throw life away" (146). On the contrary, "she knew of the light which danced inside Arla" (147) and "really looked at her as if she was important" (147). Arla gains recognition and respect for what she does from Mrs. Dawson that she does not receive from David or her own family, let alone from the other women or matrons, who show no appreciation for Arla's work. When Arla shows her parents the Christmas card and doily Mrs. Dawson has made for her, she wishes "that they would read the card where it said 'Thank you to a good helper—' that they would know she was of some use to someone, had done something honorable with herself" (147). Her parents, however, are more impressed by the size of the diamond than with an old woman's snowflake-shaped doily. "Biggest chunk of ice I ever saw," her mother had said. 'You're a lucky little lady. Looks like you're gonna be pretty well fixed'" (148). Instead of giving their daughter the recognition and encouragement she craves, they adhere to traditional values that dictate the importance of catching a decent husband who is, they assume, well off. Mrs. Dawson, on the other hand, verbalizes what Arla longs for:

> "Yes, I had a companion once. We were together for forty years, and they were good years, good years." Companion. That was the word Arla lifted out and turned over and over in her mind, studying it from every angle like the ring. That was a good word. Sane and gentle and reassuring. She found herself taking it out whenever she started to worry about David and their future together. Companion. It was all a matter of perspective, she thought. Some comfort here. (147)

Arla is relieved to find a different definition for their relationship, one that is based on understanding and respect, trust and comfort, and equality. "'She didn't want to be 'fixed,' well or any other way," Arla thinks (148). Jeremy Lalonde states, "The perspective embodied by the word [companion] is, along with the snowflake doily, Mrs. Dawson's gift to Arla; together, the word and the snowflake displace the weighty 'chunk of ice' and the threatened loss of self that it implies" (99).

Arla also admires Mrs. Dawson for her "stories full of secrets, clues to longevity, her innocent happiness, the source of her calm and optimism and self-reliance" (146). Their special connection is also visualized in the dance they perform while preparing for the birthday party. Mrs. Dawson "extended one of her withered hands toward Arla. […] Without speaking, they had begun to wheel around the room in a strange, but in its own way, graceful, shuffle-rhythmed waltz" (142). It comes as a special shock to Arla to find Mrs. Dawson in very bad shape when she arrives at work the next day. The old woman has fallen and hit her head; she is confused and suffers a gaping wound on her forehead. The negligent wound treatment administered by the night nurse, an unreliable, confused older woman, adds to the critical nature of the situation, but as Arla knows from experience, "incidents such as Mrs. Dawson's fall were like the top of a toboggan run for these old women. Once the toboggan slipped off the top, there was nowhere to go except down and swiftly" (144). The toboggan run represents another spatial metaphor that symbolizes decline. Still, Arla cannot let Mrs. Dawson go, and resolves "that she wouldn't let her die" (146). She is "furious with Mrs. Dawson who lay motionless, though in pain. She would not fight. Now she was giving up, after all those years, all those hard times she had come through and told stories about. Arla [...] had believed in the old woman, put her faith in her. What was she now but a quitter, a traitor" (149)?

At the same time, Arla feels guilty, and doubts whether she is any good at her job. Although Arla tries hard remain professionally neutral, she can no longer maintain this façade, and hopes for a closer connection with Mrs. Dawson, who seems to be in an "uncommunicable space" far away: "By now, Arla was stooped over the bed, her hands softly cupping the old woman's face, looking hard at the eyes, desperately trying to reach into that space which housed the fight. [...] The woman's eyes glittered like blue ice in the sun" (151). As in previous vignettes, a feeling of "quiet horror" strikes Arla when she realizes that the old woman wants to die, "desired death like a lover, like a friend. Like Arla desired David" (152). Death has now become Mrs. Dawson's companion. Arla cannot deal directly with the situation, but reacts through deferral and avoidance, escaping into her everyday routine by expertly changing Mrs. Dawson's sheets, which gives her a sense of security. But she cannot stand being close to the dying woman, and escapes: "A person had to go to the bathroom regardless of what was going on, she reasoned" (152). When Arla decides to go back after a while, she passes the empty lounge, "but a curious, chill feeling came over her. For a moment she thought she saw Mrs. Dawson dancing with someone" (152). She then re-enters Mrs. Dawson's room, and is struck with sadness. She realizes that Mrs. Dawson is truly dying. She holds her tight, "humming and rocking," until "she felt as if she and the old woman had changed partners" (153).

After Mrs. Dawson has passed away, Arla closes her eyelids, and covers her with a sheet. She then tells Matron Oliver what has happened. "'I quit,' she said, quite without warning to herself" (154). Arla's realization of stagnation—mirrored in her final decision to leave—is pivotal in breaking the chronotopic cycle, symbolizing her personal rejection of the repetitive temporal and spatial confinement institutional spaces enforce on residents and caregivers alike. She leaves the lodge, thinks of moving in with David, and of selling the ring back to afford "a decent bed" (155). She decides that "she might as well face the fact that she didn't give a damn about it" (155). The independence expressed through her thoughts, her deviation from her previously unquestioned adherence to the social norms and values exemplified by the diamond ring, and her newly acquired freedom in making her own decisions render her happy, and mark the beginning of a development that "is projected beyond the close of the sequence," as Lalonde notes (99). Most importantly, Arla realizes that "needing someone didn't make you weak. It made you human" (155). When she finally walks away from the lodge, "she felt she was not alone, because she felt the presence of someone or something walking with her" (155).

The collection ends with an almost supernatural scene that hints at what Arla has gained from her experiences, not only from Mrs. Dawson, but also from the other ladies in the lodge and, perhaps, from her contact with the aging and dying processes in general. The caregiving responsibilities and emotional labor Arla undertakes, as well as the emotional toll this takes, reflect the gendered expectation placed upon women within institutional contexts, reinforcing broader societal power imbalances related to gender and caregiving roles.

A Sleep Full of Dreams—even if not a *Bildungsroman* in the narrowest sense—portrays Arla's struggle to find her own voice, while gaining an understanding of what it means to grow old. While she has difficulties seeing herself reflected in the old women in the earliest stories, such as "The Hoyer" or "Midmay's Eldest Child," the breakup of the binary opposition between young and old, herself and the "other," is already foreshadowed. During the course of the book, and although Arla sometimes seems to move "two steps forward, one step back," she develops an understanding for her own self as a "self-in-relation" (Surrey 51). Roberta Maierhofer emphasizes the importance of such bonds:

> When talking about personal bonding in spite and in acceptance of difference, texts depicting inter-generational relationships can be helpful. The aging individual and the conflicts, passions, and joys, exemplify more than any other stage of life the interplay between the private and the public, the individual and the communal, and stresses the importance of relationships and connections. ("Crossing" 251)

Arla's assertion that "needing someone doesn't make you weak. It makes you human" (155), which appears on the final page of the book, reflects her recognition of the necessary interrelatedness of self and other. Roberta Maierhofer claims with reference to Jacques Derrida's essay "Structure, Sign and Play in the Discourse of the Human Sciences" that an understanding of the self is only made possible when the binary construction of self and other has been replaced by a self-in-relation, by the recognition of difference. She argues, drawing on deconstruction, that the other is not separate from the self, but implicitly imagined as part of the self-understanding because it preconditions the self. The binary opposition described here is deconstructed as arbitrary through an integration of opposites (*Salty* 123–24). The young self, she maintains, can only overcome the binary opposition between young and old by recognizing that the aging self is *not* other, *not* independent from the young, but is its correlate, its completion.[6] This is also exemplified in the case of Arla, for whom Mrs. Langland and Mrs. Dawson are essential reminders of what she is, was, and might become. Arla's identification with the individual old women and her understanding that they are "somehow part of herself" (115) are prefigured in all vignettes presented in the collection that include her.

2.2 Finding Home in a Liminal Space: Shani Mootoo's *Cereus Blooms at Night*

> What is theoretically innovative, and politically crucial, is the need to think beyond narratives of originary and initial subjectivities and to focus on those moments or processes that are produced in the articulation of cultural differences. These "in-between" spaces provide the terrain for elaborating strategies of selfhood—singular or communal—that initiate new signs of identity, and innovative sites of collaboration, and contestation, in the act of defining the idea of society itself.
>
> — Edward Soja, *Thirdspace*

In referencing Homi Bhabha's concept of the "Third Space of enunciation" (Bhabha 37), Edward Soja underlines the importance of moving beyond binary oppositions to embrace the creative potential found within "in-betweenness." The articulation of cultural difference, and the deconstruction of binary oppositions, is central to Shani Mootoo's novel *Cereus Blooms at Night*. I discuss in

6 "Wenn die Vorstellung der Binarität von Selbst und dem radikal anderen durch ein In-Beziehung-Setzen des Selbst zum anderen abgelöst wird, bedeutet das, dass ein Verstehen des Selbst nur dann möglich ist, wenn es in Relation zu dem, was es umgibt, bindet und definiert und durch sein grundsätzliches Anderssein abgrenzt, gesetzt wird. Das andere ist somit nicht vom Selbst getrennt, ist in dem Verständnis des Ich selbst impliziert: Das Selbst ist das, was nicht das andere ist. Anderssein ist somit eine Ergänzung zum Selbst, ohne das das Selbst unvollständig und sogar unvorstellbar ist. In diesem Sinne kann das jugendliche Ich nur durch die Erkenntnis, dass das alternde Ich nicht unabhängig, sondern als Ergänzung zu ihm besteht, zu einer Überwindung des Gegensatzes von Selbst und anderem gelangen." (*Salty* 123–24.)

the following how the nursing home portrayed in the novel operates as such an "in-between" site that facilitates the elaboration of strategies of selfhood, both singular and communal, reflecting and advancing Soja's and Bhabha's insights.

Irish-born Trinidadian-Canadian writer Shani Mootoo sets large parts of her 1996 novel in a care home on a fictive Caribbean island called Lantanacamara. Focusing on the immigrant author's cultural affiliations, most critics have so far concentrated on discussing the novel's place within the postcolonial tradition of Caribbean writers (Warnock 270), and the "shared queerness" (Mootoo 48), which is also at the center of the narrative (May, "Trauma"; May, "Dislocation"; Ashworth; Fox). As Carol Anne Howell states, "Mootoo writes about liminal identities positioned on the margins or between worlds. Such issues relate not only to the immigrant condition but also to sexual and racial politics and the legacy of colonialism" (7).

I argue that *Cereus Blooms at Night* is a text that not only addresses liminality with regard to the traditional matrix of "race, class, and gender," as Howells implies, but also with regard to age, a category of difference that needs to be included in the critical scholarly discussion of what constitutes the text's definition of "otherness." The intergenerational relationship depicted in the novel is a central element for the constitution and redefinition of the protagonists' identities. When Howells writes, "[i]t is through the stories of these two protagonists who are struggling to formulate their identities on the boundaries of social definition that concepts of liminality are explored" (149), the liminality of age must also be included in the discussion.

In *Cereus Blooms at Night*, spaces and places play major roles in the development of personal life-course narratives. The village of Paradise on the fictional Caribbean island of Lantanacamara initially prompts associations with the Garden of Eden—not least of all because of the village's name. Associating Caribbean landscapes with paradise has a long history in the development of Caribbean literature, Lorna Burns asserts (52), arguing that this trope was already recognizable in the testimonies of Christopher Columbus, Amerigo Vespucci, and others. Such a conflation of the New World with the Garden of Eden, she argues, served to disguise imperialist exploitation and masked colonial power relations (52). Mootoo, however, subverts idealized representations of the Caribbean landscape as paradise (the village's name is both ironic and subversive), and distances herself from any idealization by portraying a paradise lost when describing the garden of the main character, Mala Ramchandin.

While this garden, in which the eponymous cereus blooms, has received special attention as a symbolic landscape (see, for instance, Burns; Casteel; Hoving, "Gardening"), the nursing home, which serves as a setting in the story's extensive frame, has been largely overlooked as a symbolic, liminal space.[7] This is all the more astounding because the Paradise Alms House is central to the protagonists' development, enabling the marginalized characters to come to terms with their sometimes traumatic pasts. It is revealing that the narrator describes the home's location as a heterotopic space outside the city limits, a space elsewhere and in the middle of nowhere at the same time, with a lane that ends long before it reaches the home: "The Paradise Alms House is not en route to anywhere. To get there, one must leave the main road, cut through a cane field and carry on up a lane that ends on top of a small hill. The home with its excellent view of the cane fields is in the shallow valley below. There is nothing beyond" (122). The home, as Nurse Tyler describes it here, is literally located "over the hill," at the periphery, far away from the center of the village's social life. In this way, the nursing home represents a place beyond the present,[8] which Bhabha has described in *The Location of Culture*: "'Beyond' signifies spatial distance, marks progress, promises the future; but our intimations of exceeding the barrier or boundary—the very act of going beyond—are unknowable, unrepresentable, without a return to the 'present' which, in the process of repetition, becomes disjunct and displaced" (4). As Howells observes, this excerpt reads like a "sketch for Mootoo's novel" (148). The characters go "beyond" all boundaries to return to their origins, but also return to the present, a place from which they can continue, travelling "beyond" into a future (148). Interestingly, the starting place for this journey, clearly a progress narrative, is a Catholic nursing home. Contrary to conventional representations of nursing homes, the home in *Cereus Blooms at Night* is a place of improvement and growth, which is also illustrated by Mala Ramchandin's development: a few days after being delivered to the home, tied to a stretcher, and unable to move, she soon recovers: "After a few days in the wheelchair,

7 Linda Chris Fox, in her article "The Paradise Alms House: Siting Literary Thirdspace in Shani Mootoo's *Cereus Blooms at Night*, actually does refer to the nursing home.

8 Here, I adapt Coral Ann Howells' interpretation, in which she uses Bhabha's study of the postcolonial diaspora to explain how the text itself, as a "Canadian" novel set on a Caribbean island, is positioned "in-between" the Caribbean and Canada "by its narratives of desire for escape and its transformations of identity" (Howells, *Contemporary* 148).

Miss Ramchandin was strong enough to walk" (Mootoo 46). Both Mala and Nurse Tyler develop new life course identities after getting to know each other in the Paradise Alms House. The novel "traces a particularly harrowing late-life journey from silence and insanity to human interaction and sharing," as Perrakis asserts (19).

In Mootoo's novel, the narrative of a care-giver is again used to introduce readers to the troubled life story of Miss Mala Ramchandin, an old woman. Tyler, the homosexual Afro-Caribbean nurse at the Paradise Alms House, "the only Lantanacamaran man ever to have trained in the profession of nursing" (6), is exclusively assigned to the care of Mala, an Indo-Caribbean "crazy lady" (7). She is said to have murdered her father who, having been left by his wife and her lesbian lover decades earlier, takes revenge for this humiliation by brutally raping and abusing his then young daughters, Mala and Asha, for several years before mysteriously disappearing. While Asha eventually manages to escape to Great Britain, "the Shivering Northern Wetlands," as Mootoo names it, and later on to Canada, the trauma-related guilt that Mala suffers prevents her from leaving her father's house. She remains with him for several years before killing him during a violent fight.

The novel begins decades after Chandin Ramchandin vanishes, when Mala, after years of dwelling in the wild garden around her family house beyond the margins of society, is taken to Paradise Alms House. There, she is "to receive proper care and attention until the end of her days" (8), as is the ruling during her murder trial at court. She is exonerated for want of evidence because her own house, and with it her father's dead body, has burned down: "No victim, no evidence, no witnesses—no crime" (8). As Paradise is a small village, however, Mala remains a suspect, "the nurses' gestures were loud enough. They recoiled several paces" (19), when the helpless woman is brought to the home. Because both characters, Mala and Tyler, are "scandalous figures," as Coral Ann Howells states (149)—Tyler, because of his homosexuality and Mala, because of her status as a social outcast—none of the nurses wants to interact with them. Neither skin color nor race, however, are the primary identity markers in this context, as Howells observes (149). She affirms that "issues around sexuality and gender are much more socially relevant. The old colonial mechanism of violent othering has not vanished, but has only been transformed into the social ostracism of certain individuals who are seen to transgress the heterosexual norms of their community" (Howells 149). "Miss Ramchandin's care was therefore left in my hands," Tyler explains (Mootoo 13). The nursing and nurturing care Mala subsequently receives in the home not only changes her own life, but also Tyler's. The relationship they develop is as crucial to the transmission of the story as it is to the survival of the two characters, as Sally Chivers contends (*From* 75).

The effect of nurturing on their connection also affects the community on a larger scale, which is revealed by Tyler's observation that, upon Mala's admission to the home, the thick, black cloud of smoke that had been hovering over the village begins to disappear: "[i]t is said, incidentally, that [...] the life-robbing cloud began to break up and shift south over the ocean, letting light shine in Paradise once again" (8). The complete destruction of the eerie house, a symbol of sin and moral decay, not only frees the townspeople from the uncanny "other" hovering at the community's edge, but also rids them of their own guilt: although Chandin Ramchandin's violence and his incestuous relationship with his daughters was an open secret in the community, nobody ever openly confronted him. Instead, Mala is ostracized by the community, and victimized yet again. Even Asha's letters, in which she begs Mala to join her in Canada, are never delivered to her "because the righteous postman, deeming the Ramchandin house to be a place of sin and moral corruption, refused to go up there" (Mootoo 243). After killing her father and hiding his body in the basement, Mala never again enters the house. She remains in the garden, living with the animals and plants that completely hide and shelter her. She is considered a mean, magical creature, an evil witch parents warn their children about, and the townspeople almost forget about the crazy, wild woman dwelling on the hillside.

When Mala is finally taken to the nursing home, this is done "out of compassion for her health and welfare" (8) by Judge Bissey, who, also having grown up in the small town, still guiltily remembers bullying Mala and her little sister when they were all young children. It is also Judge Bissey who finally gives Mala her sister Asha's letters, which had been kept in a box at the post office all these years. Moving into the care home means re-entering social life for Mala. Contrary to her family home, the Paradise Alms House is a nurturing environment, which enables both Mala and Tyler to re-narrate and reevaluate their life course narratives not only with regard to their "queerness," but also within the larger framework of the novel as a postcolonial text "that confronts the binary structures inherent in colonialism and in sexual politics through a narrative that first explores the traumatic effects of such polarization on individual lives across several generations, and then in an effort of displacement sets out an alternative narrative of transgressive desire, which opens up spaces for new identity constructions" (Howells 148).

Mootoo narrates the heterotopic space of the care home as a nurturing place in such a way as to facilitate a process of re-identification with the protagonists. This re-appropriation of their life stories is only possible because of the specific characteristics Mootoo ascribes to the nursing home. She crafts it as a place that, as L. Chris Fox states, "provides a locational frame within which cultural meanings are reworked so that characters may perform self-coherent versions of themselves and be appreciated as themselves by others" (73). Fox also positions the home as central to the story, and reads "the alms house and its residents' garden as a place of productive literary thirdspace" (70). Her argument resonates with Homi Bhabha's definition, who sees the process of identification as a process of hybridity, which "gives rise to something different, something new and unrecognisable, a new area of negotiation of meaning and representation" (Rutherford 211). The liminal space is described by Bhabha as a "productive space of the construction of culture as difference" (209), and this is, I also argue, the home's primary function in the novel. In this sense, the home itself operates as a "third space," because it facilitates the formation of a productive hybridity for the subjects inhabiting it.

The presence of the cereus plant, a key image of the novel, indicates that the nursing home and its surroundings present a nurturing environment in which growth is possible. The care home not only ensures Mala's survival, but also that of the cereus plant, which had once grown next to her house. Otoh Mohanty, a central character in the novel, saved a clipping of the succulent before setting fire to the house and garden. He does so to destroy any evidence of Mala's crime, trying to protect her from being convicted for murder. Together with his father, Ambrose, he brings the clipping to the Paradise Alms House, where the gardener plants it and where it develops its symbolic bloom.

Ambrose Mohanty, Mala's childhood friend, plays a pivotal role in Mala's development. When he comes back to the village after several years of studying, he begins an affair with Mala. Her father Chandin, incidentally observing Ambrose as he leaves the Ramchandins' house, is extremely jealous. He severely beats Mala, and brutally rapes her several times during the night. He demolishes the entire kitchen, and attempts to kill Mala with a cleaver. Ambrose, returning to the house the next day, finds Mala severely wounded. Suddenly, Chandin attacks him with the cleaver. Mala trips Chandin so that he falls, and sinks her teeth into his wrist. Ambrose "saw the opportunity to go for help" (227), and dashes out of the room in an act of cowardice, unintentionally slamming the door against Chandin's head, stunning him. Feeling "as though he had been betrayed by Mala, and at the same time wrestling with the notion that she could not possibly, not conceivably have been agreeable to intimacies with her father" (227–28), Ambrose distances himself from Mala. He ponders running for help, but is stopped by his fear of being associated with "the shameful goings-on in the house" (228), thereby siding with members of the island's community in blaming Mala for the incestuous relationship. Before he leaves, he hears a dreadful crashing and notices Mala calling his name. Ambrose runs back upstairs to see, "instead of the woman he had made love to the day before, an unrecognizable wild creature with a blood-stained face, frothing at the mouth and hacking uncontrollably at the furniture in the drawing room" (228). Mala, in a state of absolute confusion, oscillating between her childhood memories and the present, returns to Chandin, who is still lying on the floor, and hits his head with the door until she is exhausted. Although Mala begs him to stay, Ambrose again fears for his own life, and bolts from the house. Mala then drags her father's body down the stairs, and locks it in the basement. Utterly confused, she returns to the house to look for her mother, re-living the moments of her departure, which had traumatized Mala as a child. Mala does not dare re-enter the house for fear that her father might return: "She never lit a lantern in that house again. Nor did she, since that day, pass a night inside its walls" (230). During the following years, Mala dwells in the garden next to the Cereus plant, immersing herself in nature, and discontinuing her use of spoken language:

> Eventually, Mala all but rid herself of words. The wings of a gull flapping through the air titillated her soul and awakened her toes and knobby knees, the palms of her withered hands, deep inside her womb, her vagina, lungs, stomach and heart. Every muscle of her body swelled, tingled, cringed or went numb in response to her surroundings—every fibre was sensitized in a way that words were unable to match or enhance. Mala responded to those receptors, flowing with them effortlessly, like water making its way along a path. (127)

In contrast with examples given in other Canadian novels, such as Margaret Atwood's *Surfacing*, this immersion in nature is not a healing experience. Mala's withdrawal into the wild garden isolates her completely, separating her even further from human society. Howells argues that "Mala becomes a living ghost as she abandons language and leads a truly liminal existence, teetering on the borderline between human and natural worlds" (155). In the garden, Mala remains frozen in her childhood trauma, unable to escape without outside help.

She exists in the wilderness around the house, detached from the city: "With its yard-long, bean-like purple pods, the mudra had taken over the side of the yard, completely blocking out the road beyond and glimpses of town" (154–55). As Howells notes, "her residence on the verandah is a sign of her in-between existence: she is still human, a woman who may speak the language of the animals, but who wears clothes and sits on a chair in her garden" (157), which grants her invisibility and, at the same time, isolates her. Isabel Hoving reads the garden as an "ambiguous paradise" that is neither an Edenic site, nor an obscure jungle: "At first sight, the yard recalls the image of the lost Garden of Eden, which European explorers wanted to recognize in the lush Caribbean islands they visited for the first time. At second sight, however, there is something seriously wrong with this lost jungle paradise. There is something very eerie about the garden" ("Moving" 154). The uncanny atmosphere is reinforced by its peculiar, nauseating smell, "[a] ghost of scent" (Mootoo 154) that hovers over the yard. When Otoh, Ambrose Mohanty's son, approaches it, he is aware of the "double recognition" (Burns 56), and notes that "except for the odors he would have sworn he was in paradise" (Mootoo 155). Mootoo here deliberately subverts all clear-cut boundaries, including those defining paradise and hell, and, as Burns also observes, deconstructs any binaries by conflating house and garden (56):

> Fruit trees and hot pepper trees had sprung wherever birds and insects dropped their seeds. A patch of bright orange, sweet-smelling roses and a profusion of night-blooming cereus plants were the only ornamentals in the yard. The roots of the cereus, like desperate grasping fingers, had bored through the damp wall of the house. It was no longer the wall that supported the succulent but rather the other way around. (Mootoo 115)

The odors that pervade the garden stem from the dead body of Chandin Ramchandin in the basement. Worms and maggots have started consuming his body as well as the wooden frame of the house:

> Termites had gnawed a board barring the window and sunlight beamed through throwing a brilliant gash on the opposite wall and illuminating the insects. [...] The insects that had fallen crunched beneath her bare feet. They were fodder for a vibrating carpet of moths, centipedes, millipedes, cockroaches and unnamed insects that found refuge in Mala's surroundings. Death feeding life. (130)

Nature has started to take over, controlling the garden and the house, and blurring the border between inside and outside.

This image is contrasted with the garden of the Paradise Alms House, which is clean and professionally maintained by the institution's gardener, Mr. Hector. Here, a clear separation exists between inside and outside, the yard and the house. Mr. Hector is in control of everything that grows there: "He was carrying a full gerbera plant, flowers, leaves and roots protruding from a large ball of soil in one hand, a spade in the other" (72). Assuming that it might humor Mala, Mr. Hector suggests that she should do some gardening in the newly arranged flower beds. Tyler remembers that a clipping of a cereus plant had just been left for Mala Ramchandin by two visitors, but as the head nurse had turned them away, he had forgotten about it. When he suggests planting the succulent clipping, Mr. Hector only accepts it reluctantly because he deems it too ugly. While he digs a hole to plant the cereus, a conversation develops between the two men. Mr. Hector tells Tyler how he reminds him of his older brother, who was sent away years ago, "He was kind of funny, he was like you" (73). Mr. Hector misses him terribly: "Is like I recognize you but is a sad feeling" (72), he tells Tyler. This short sequence deepens the relationship between the gardener and Tyler, and strengthens Tyler's self-esteem: "[I]t suddenly lifted a veil between us. Unexpectedly, I felt relief it was voiced and out in the open. I had never before known such a feeling of ordinariness" (73). This is the first feeling of normalcy and an initial hint of Tyler's liberation from the traditional sexual identity categories described, which from then on takes root in him, like the cereus plant takes root in the garden.

The two visitors who left the cereus clipping are, as readers learn later, Ambrose Mohanty and his son Otoh. Ambrose, after running from Mala's house, married another woman, Elsie, "for solace" (109), because she reminded him of Mala. They have one daughter, Ambrosia, who eventually transforms into a son and becomes Otoh, an acronym for "on the other hand." This was given to him as a nickname because of his "ability to imagine many sides of a dilemma [...] and the vexing inability to make up his mind" (Mootoo 110). Otoh literally embodies the conflation of binaries, which is also expressed by the fact that his gender transformation was so "flawless" (110) that "even the nurse and doctor who attended the birth, on seeing him later, marveled at their carelessness in having declared him a girl" (110). Again, Mootoo blurs all boundaries, and Isabel Hoving reads Otoh and his father as another embodiment of the transgression of borders:

> Father and son form a curious pair, and they embody the novel's most remarkable instances of border crossing and mirroring. Ambrose is a former suitor of Mala, but he proved unable to save her from trauma and he has slept away most of his life ever since. Otoh is his remarkable son: he is a transgender boy who succeeded in letting even his parents forget that he was born a girl. But Otoh is crossing not only just the border between genders but also that between generations: he takes over his father's place by bringing Mala food, sometimes even dressed like his father, in an effort to make amends for his father's betrayal. The cereus is therefore a gift from two people who cross borders between genders and generations, past and present, sleep and waking life. ("Moving" 162)

Otoh crosses yet another boundary when, dressed up in his father's clothes, he sets out to the enchanted garden to bring Mala food. He feels obliged to continue on in his father's tradition when Ambrose has to stop visiting the house after an accident that confines him to a wheelchair: "Otoh, intrigued by his father's devotion to a woman whom he had not seen in more than thirty years, accepted his inherited task" (Mootoo 111). After bringing food to Mala for several months and being fascinated by her, Otoh eventually dares to speak to the strange woman his father has adored all his life. He is her "first human visitor in at least a decade" (150). Mala, using words for the first time since moving into the garden, mistakes him for Ambrose. In this passage, focalization shifts between the two characters, and the narration uses a "language of magic realism, offering a kind of suspension between two modes of apprehending the world, where neither realism nor magic is cancelled out," as Howells (158) analyzes the scene in which Otoh and Mala start dancing in the garden.

The fairy tale turns into a "Gothic nightmare" (158) as Mala leads Otoh down into the basement through mounds of dust, clouds of stench, and around a huge pile of furniture several feet thick that hides the doorway of yet another locked door, behind which she shows him her father's decayed body ("an indecipherable mass," Mootoo 163). The horrible sight and smell overwhelm him. He faints, and only wakes up again as Mala carries him upstairs. During a scene that mirrors his father's flight decades ago, he escapes from the house, leaping through the wall of shrubs, bushes, and plants, and runs as quickly as he can towards the village road, where he finally collapses. People quickly gather around him, misunderstanding Otoh's stammering comment of "A body, it have a body in she house" (Mootoo 166). They wrongly conclude that a murderer has entered Mala Ramchandin's yard. The rumor spreads and changes quickly, finally reaching Ambrose, who is terrified that his son might have been the victim. Ambrose stands up from the wheelchair for the first time in years, and pushes it into the street in order to look for Otoh. When he finds him, Otoh tells him what had happened. Both father and son now share the concern that Mala will soon be accused of having murdered Chandin. Otoh's fear of having betrayed Mala is resolved by Ambrose, who remarks, "Clearly you did not cause trouble. It seems that trouble was lurking like a diseased phantom, waiting to be revealed, and you had the misfortune to come upon it" (Mootoo 170). Upon hearing that the police have taken Mala into custody, Ambrose, again unable to save her, sinks back into motionless passivity, while Otoh sets out to burn Mala's house in order to destroy any proof of her crime. He sets fire to the house, burning it entirely, so that the house and trees and "every bit of live and dead matter that had thrived on the Hill Side property remained floating through the town in an irritating dust, suspended in a thick, black cloud above the town and blocking out the light of the sun" (188), restoring the previously secluded space, albeit transformed, to the public view and serving as a reminder, for almost a week, to the community of the house's dark history. The only living remnant from Mala's property is a clipping from the cereus plant, which Otoh takes with him.

After Otoh's flight from the scene, Mala becomes the main focalizer of the narration. Filled with despair due to Otoh's (and, due to the case of confused identity, Ambrose's) abandonment, she realizes that she might be in danger, and decides that "her first duty was to save and care for Pohpoh" (172). Her childhood self has become a split personality, a separate individual in need of her protection. This separation enables her to stay alive by allowing her to construct alternative narratives of rescue and escape (Howells 157). Howells notes, "In her distress, Mala's identity fractures completely into a condition of schizophrenia where she is divided between the adult Mala and the child Pohpoh, caught in a time loop between present and past as she leads the police downstairs to her father's body" (159). The story is now related through Mala's focalization, who perceives Pohpoh to be a child that she needs to protect from Chandin, who in her eyes is still alive and a threatening presence. She considers herself in control of the situation, safeguarding imaginary Pohpoh. While the policemen interpret her whispering off to the side as a sign that she has gone mad, Mala has only one aim: to help Pohpoh escape. In her fantasy, she sees Pohpoh fly away: "Down below, her island was soon lost among others, all as shapeless as specks of dust adrift on a vast turquoise sea" (Mootoo 186). Mala is taken into custody while her house burns down, and while any proof of crime is destroyed. She is not convicted of murder, but is sent to the almshouse. Here, the narrative switches back to the beginning of the book when she arrives at Paradise Alms House tied to a stretcher. The book opens with Tyler addressing the reader in what seems to be an explanation for the story and its aim, that of finding Mala's sister, Asha. Mootoo creates a narrative meta-level, and establishes Tyler as a narrative voice with an agenda—to draw the reader into the story and help look for Asha:

> By setting this story down, I, Tyler—that is how I am known, simply as Tyler, or if you wanted to be formal, Nurse Tyler—am placing trust in the power of the printed word to reach many people. [...] Might I add that my own intention, as the relater of this story, is not to bring notice to myself or my plight. [...] Forgive the lapses, for there are some, and read them with the understanding that to have erased them would have been to do the same to myself. (4)

With these statements, Tyler ascribes meaning to his role as a nurse; he is the one who knows Mala Ramchandin, and he is the one who communicates her story to the world outside the home, "fashioning a single garment out of myriad parts" (105). By pleading for "trust in the printed word" he shows that without his narration, Mala's story and her life—and with it, his own—would disappear. Because Mala is almost dying and does not speak when she is first admitted to the home, readers must already assume that not only a process of recovery, but also a process of developing trust and understanding, must have taken place in the home that enable Tyler to tell her story (Chivers, *From* 75). At the same time, Tyler's account draws attention to the fact that Mala's voice is interpreted by someone taking care of her, pointing to an act of representation that "in itself risks reinforcing frameworks of oppression" (Burns 61). Burns continues,

> Mindful of the complex politics of representation, *Cereus* both draws attention to the risk of reinscribing oppression and the necessity of speaking for or about vulnerable members of society. While the risk remains that Tyler projects something of his own agenda on to Mala's story in the act of retelling it, by highlighting the opacity of Mala's past, her inability to identify with her own memories of her childhood self (Pohpoh), Mootoo nevertheless underscores the necessity of Tyler's mediating perspective. (61)

Without Tyler, Mala would not be able to make herself understood to others, nor would she be able to come to terms with her own traumatized past, and she understands that she needs him in order to survive. From a feminist perspective, it may seem problematic that Mala loses her voice, and the re-construction and interpretations of her life-course narrative are dependent upon a man. Mala seems to be constructed as a "madwoman in the attic"—a "monster" and an "angel" at the same time (Gilbert and Gubar 17). Yet, the novel also subverts this binary, and highlights both the need for Tyler to tell Mala's story and their relationship as a "model of alliance or co-belonging with a conscience, one that protects vulnerable members" (Burns 61). Tyler both accepts and is himself already in need of this role of translator when he first touches Mala, and notices her transformation: "This one touch turned her from the incarnation of fearful tales into a living human being, an elderly person such as those I had dedicated my life to serving. I needed to know the woman who lay hidden by the white sheet" (Mootoo 11). First, he must get used to her acts of communication, since she does not speak, interpreting her small movements, making sense of her wailings, her perfect imitations of animal sounds, and the seemingly absurd utterances ("Pohpoh") as well as single words that she slowly begins to use.

His dedication to care for her to the best of his abilities, and his devotion to listen and respond to the old woman's needs clearly differentiates him from caregivers described in the stories in Edna Alford's *A Sleep Full of Dreams*, such as Arla, who rarely displays the patience and dedication her patients require. Although Tyler is not sure whether his attempts will ever be fruitful, he tries to be as sensitive as possible: "There was still no recognition that she heard me. I became acutely conscious of my movements and the subtleties of my tone, which may have been all that communicated with her" (Mootoo 16). Every slight improvement is meticulously recorded in Tyler's little notebook, and he learns to understand her gestures and sounds, and begins to grow "[a]ccustomed to reading, as if by Braille, her twitches and gasps" (100), and "to recognize in her mutterings elements of the legendary rumors" (99). "I felt like an explorer charting her life in murky, unmapped waters. I was not sure what I was discovering beyond her voice but I felt it would not be long before I would have the privilege, and honour, of entering her world" (72), Tyler describes the process that, in the end, leads to the success he has wished for, resisting any praise that he had "performed miracles" with Miss Ramchandin, "knowing the change in Miss Ramchandin was only a result of humane treatment" (97). In the nursing home, Mala progresses from a "crazy woman tied to a stretcher" to a woman sitting in a wheelchair, mumbling syllables and emitting animal sounds, and then to a woman walking freely and talking to her former lover, Ambrose, who has become her frequent visitor at the Paradise Alms House, by the end of the book.

This is clearly an example of a progress narrative rather than a decline narrative: Mala reverses the traditional development of a person entering a nursing home. She adopts speech again, and is brought back to life in the nursing home after "everyone in the village seemed to have finally forgotten about Mala" (113). On the book's last page, Tyler reports that Mala "trembled with joy" (249) sitting on a bench during a reunion with Mr. Mohanty, and "uttered her first public words: 'Poh, Pohpoh-poh, Poh, Poh, Poh'" (249).

Tyler's investigations and the "restoring and re-storying of Miss Ramchandin" (Howells 150) also restore his own self-confidence, and strengthen the bond between the two individuals, which is proven when Miss Ramchandin successfully protests against the home administration's plans to take Tyler away from her by devastating her room. When she understands that Tyler may have to give up his exclusive caregiving for her, she starts to build mountains of furniture in her room. To stop Mala's seemingly crazy behavior, Tyler gets to maintain his care of her, which leads, with reference to the blooming plant, to the "affiliation blossoming" (48) between Miss Ramchandin and Tyler. Tyler's act of coming out as a homosexual is facilitated by Mala, who steals a female nurse's uniform for him. She wordlessly encourages him to secretly put it on in her room, only to ignore his new outfit when he shows himself to her: "She knows what I am, was all I could think. She knows my nature. [...] The reason Miss Ramchandin paid no attention to me was that, to her mind, the outfit was not something to congratulate or scorn—it simply was. She was not one to manacle nature, and I sensed that she was permitting mine its freedom" (76–77). Tyler, for the first time, feels "natural," "normal:" "I had never felt so extremely ordinary, and I quite loved it" (78), he states. Mala's unconditional acceptance permits him to recognize his agency in terms of questioning social norms and values. From the privacy of Mala's room, he will soon step out into the public space of the Alms House and its garden. He comments early in the novel,

> [o]ver the years I pondered the gender and sex roles that seemed available to people, and the rules that went with them. [...] I was preoccupied with trying to understand what was natural and what was perverse, and who said so and why. Chandin Ramchandin played a part in confusing me about these roles, for it was a long time before I could differentiate between his perversion and what others called mine. (47–48)

Tyler's explorations here include his own revelations, but also relate Mala's history. Howells notes, "Tyler's investigation provides an important dynamic in the restoring and re-storying of Miss Ramchandin, reconstructing her history of sexual abuse from the victim's perspective against the falsity of social opinion, while at the same time Tyler's self-confidence is restored through Miss Ramchandin's unconditional acceptance of him" (Howells 150). By reconstructing Mala's life, Tyler not only transmits her story, but also manages to carve out a niche for himself in the narration. The act of storytelling, in fact, enables him to position himself "as the center of his own life story" (Howells 151) despite the fact that the narrative situation changes frequently. Although Tyler remains the main storyteller during large parts of the novel, the narrative voice shifts from that of an omniscient narrator to Miss Ramchandin's indirect inner monologue, especially when her confused state of mind is described immediately before her admission to the nursing home. It is highly unlikely that Tyler can know all the details he relates throughout the book, but I agree with Rebecca Ashworth, who, instead of viewing him as an unreliable narrator, reads him as a "reader of narratives" (Ashworth 37), arguing that "unreliable readings and even misreadings are far less important than Tyler's attempt to read" (37). In order to read people or characters, she contends, Tyler, as well as readers of the novel, must learn to empathize with them. Tyler's ability to do so stems, as he explains it, from his relationship with his own grandmother: "The relationship between Nana, my Cigarette Smoking Nana, and me, her Peculiar Grandson, was special, for we both had secrets from my mother, her daughter. Miss Ramchandin and I, too, had a camaraderie: we had found our own ways and fortified ourselves against the rest of the world" (48). Tyler's grandmother is the one who first tells him, during his childhood, about the Ramchandin family, thus introducing him—and the readers—to Chandin Ramchandin's history, which is crucial to the plot. Howells claims in this context, "[s]torytelling has mutually restorative functions here as it weaves different kinds of sexual transgressiveness into the wider context of Tyler's grandmother's tale told twenty years earlier about one of the casualties of colonial history" (150).

In the nursing home, the characters feel Tyler's empathy; their constant "in-between-ness" can only change into a productive site of identity development through Tyler as a caring person. Yet, Tyler's account "falsifies the novel—not the facts but the structure," as Howells notes, "for this is a very fractured narrative, with its multiple voices, its temporal dislocations, and its hesitations between realism and fantasy, 'with neither managing to subordinate or contain the other. This sustained opposition forestalls the possibility of interpretive closure through any act of naturalizing the text to and establishes system of representation'" (Slemon 12, qtd. in Howells 159). The rejection of a linear plot is a deliberate strategy, she maintains, which "creates the sensation of being caught in the middle of proliferating narrative versions where resolutions are promised but endlessly deferred. The protagonists' condition of always being 'in-between' is mirrored in the reader's own experience of the text" (159). The act of placing in-betweenness in the foreground relates to both postcolonial, as well as gender and age identities, because Tyler not only relates the story of an old woman's social marginalization on the island, but also that of homosexuals (160). Tyler provides a voice for this state of in-betweenness when he describes what he felt when wearing women's clothing for the first time: "Not a man and not ever able to be a woman, suspended nameless in the limbo state between existence and nonexistence" (Mootoo 77). Tyler's liberation from this limbo state is facilitated by Mala (who also enters the home in a limbo state, the "fourth age"), on the one hand because she offers him a way to recognize his normalcy as a homosexual, and on the other because she is the reason why Tyler gets to meet Otoh, her visitor. Due to his own ambiguous sexual identity, Otoh contributes to Tyler's liberation. Their romance at the end of the novel disavows all binaries regarding sexual identity categories: "I was about to cross his line" (247), Tyler reports when deciding to approach Otoh. Wearing pink lipstick, a flower-patterned scarf and "enough scent to make a Puritan cross his legs and swoon" (247), Tyler picks a bouquet of flowers, and presents it to Otoh who "deliberately cupped [Tyler's] hands and held them to his chest" (248). Holding hands, they wait for the cereus to bloom to consummate their love for the first time: "From the cereus hung pink buds on the ends of long stems. […] 'The cereus will bloom in just another few nights. Can you wait?' I whispered to him. 'Yes, yes. Just barely, but I will wait'" (248).

The ending of the story is filled with hope, as Howells argues, "precariously balanced against loss as it is poised on the cusp between present and future, with everybody at the Alms House waiting for something to happen" (160). While Tyler and Otoh are holding hands for the first time, Ambrose, whose wife Elsie left him before he visited Mala in the home, tells Mala, "No time to waste, not a moment to be wasted" (Mootoo 248). Hearing this, she starts to speak "her first public words" (249) which, although it is not quite clear what her stammering means, can be interpreted as her acceptance of their late reunion. Through Tyler's account, readers learn that Mala is still waiting for Asha to return. The last sentence of the book in which Tyler (as in large parts of the novel) addresses Asha, reads, "[s]he expects you any day soon. You are, to her, the promise of a cereus-scented breeze on a Paradise night" (249). In this scene, Mootoo subverts conventional assumptions of old age as a state of decline. Mala, despite the fact that her age is unknown, is a nursing home resident who progresses.

The nursing home represents a third space that allows the cacophony of voices to be disentangled, leading to what seems to be euphony in the end. It is contrasted with Lantanacamara, which is represented as a place where such healing is not possible. The people inhabiting the town suffer from different sorts of identity crises because they are caught in their "in-between" spaces, trapped between different identity categories in situations that do not allow for creative renegotiation. As Tyler, addressing Asha, observes, "I wonder at how many of us, feeling unsafe and unprotected, either end up running far away from everything we know and love, or staying and simply going mad" (90). Those who find their way to the alms house, which, as a symbolic space, breaks up all binary oppositions over the course of the story, manage to overcome their crises. Others, such as Mala's father who is himself a victim of the island's colonial oppression, die, or like Mala's mother and sister, emigrate. Within the caring and nurturing space of the Paradise Alms House, the characters of Tyler, Otoh, Mala, and Ambrose can develop, and with them the cereus plant, which also depends on the benevolence and care of Tyler, Otoh, Ambrose, and ultimately Harry, the gardener, to survive. As Fox puts it:

> Through performing, witnessing, and accepting themselves and others the effects of the past on each are recognized and cared for in the present while webs of interconnection are formed that will serve in the future. Intergration,[9] both within and between this group of individuals, is the basis for a radical interconnection that makes hybrid community not only possible, but productive: the cereus has rooted and will bloom.

Cereus Blooms at Night is an example of nursing home narratives that counter the assumption that such institutions are merely sites of decline. The interpersonal and intergenerational encounters that are portrayed in the novel show the importance of nurturing relationships and mutual listening and understanding in order for the characters to develop, as well as for readers to be able to reimagine care homes differently. As Chivers puts it, the depiction "encompasses a reimagination of the possibilities of what most people think of as a last

---

9 Fox here deliberately misspells the word "to parallel Bhabha's 'international' which places the emphasis on relation, on between-ness, on 'inter.'"

resort in frail old age" (*From* 77). Mootoo's novel is one of the few books that place the caregiver in a prominent position. Even though it is not a documentary or an auto/biographical text, a genre which, as Kathleen Woodward argues, might be better suited than fiction to press for changes in social policy because it "draw[s] us closer to what is real" ("Public" 46), the novel calls attention to the "public secret" of the caregivers, lifting them and the old people out of "the one-dimensional frame of victimhood. Isolated and separate, caregivers and elders are vulnerable. Together, caregivers and elders are strong," Woodward maintains ("Public" 46). *Cereus Blooms at Night* portrays Mala, despite her frailty, as a strong and pivotal character, and reverses the conventional assumption of aging as a state of decline. Both Mala and Tyler find a home in the liminal space of the Paradise Alms House.

2.3 Challenging the Nursing Home Specter: Joan Barfoot's *Exit Lines*

Joan Barfoot's novel *Exit Lines* (2008) also focuses on the difficulty of renegotiating one's identity within the context of long-term residential care. The novel introduces readers to Sylvia Lodge, one of four protagonists, who has to negotiate the difficult transition from the privacy of her own home to the semi-public space of the Idyll Inn retirement lodge. In her struggle against an overly well-meaning nurse on the one hand and an overbearing administrator on the other, she resists becoming a "patient" and prefers to be seen as a paying customer. "Here, people are *residents*, at least to their faces," Sylvia contends, not without a hint of bitterness (29). She sees the Idyll Inn as a hybrid space—a hotel, light-flooded and customer-oriented from one perspective, and a "genteel, open-doored prison" from another (16). "'I am Sylvia Lodge,' she announces at what, in a hotel, would be the front desk; in a prison, the guard post. 'I have arrived'" (10). The novel starts with Sylvia Lodge moving to the Idyll Inn to avoid becoming a burden for her daughter Nancy. She has moved to the lodge on her own initiative and—in a passive-aggressive mode—did not even inform her daughter about her decision. Most importantly, however, she is aware of the fact that this is not yet the ultimate destination she will move to: "Depressing, really, and this isn't even a nursing home, the next step downwards en route to incapacity's basement" (20), she says to herself.

The novel tells the story of three women, Sylvia, Greta, and Ruth, and one man, George, who meet—or meet again (George and Greta had actually had an affair when they were younger)—as they become residents of the

Idyll Inn. Soon, the four characters become friends, and undermine the rigid rules imposed by the management by "forming an alliance, downing early-evening glasses of chardonnay to the consternation of the administrator" (Wheelwright n.p.), as one of the reviewers put it, while they are more or less enjoying their "community of fate." The story reaches a climax when Ruth, the "baby of the place" (Barfoot 55) only 74 years of age, announces her intention in a theatrical gesture to leave "the stage of life" by committing suicide exactly on her 75th birthday. To prepare for her exit, she carefully crafts her speech (hence the title) with which she intends to ask her three friends for euthanasia as she cannot carry out her plans without them. "Dry cleaner bags, duct tape, little scissors – primitive tools, but as Ruth says, 'Simple is best'" (263). After being rather shocked at Ruth's request, her three friends decide to help her. Having a common goal, their friendship deepens and there is a certain sense of purpose now that makes them overcome their mental disabilities and physical difficulties. When the set moment for Ruth's assisted suicide has come, they gather in her room, trying to convince her once more to re-evaluate her decision. But Ruth is determined to go through with her plan. Just before they actually set out to wrap plastic around Ruth's head, Greta suddenly collapses with a severe heart problem. Sylvia instantly runs for her medicine, while Ruth gets up from her bed to let Greta lie down in it. Together, they competently manage to save Greta, thus also demonstrating, as Patricia Life also observes (113), their ongoing ability to react to new situations and to alter their consequent opinions and actions. Ruth, recognizing the new significance friendship has given to her life, determines to put aside her earlier suicide wish. Instead of assisted death, the situation in a comical turn of events develops into one of assisted life. The plot is resolved in almost a cliché ending when Ruth realizes that the support of her new friends makes life meaningful (Life 113).

Joan Barfoot first thematized the care home back in 1985 with her novel *Duet for Three*, which portrays Aggie, an old woman who is afraid of being moved into a nursing home by her daughter. In her most recent novel, *Exit Lines*, Barfoot modifies the depiction of the care home to some degree, making it more luxurious and hotel-like. In this respect, *Exit Lines* can be placed in the tradition of stories such as *The Best Exotic Marigold Hotel* (2011) or *Quartet* (2012), which also portray residents in their "third age" who are able to afford an affluent lifestyle, and decide to leave their long-time dwellings, making provisions for the time when they will eventually need assistance.

The differentiation between a traditional nursing home and a hotel is emphasized at the beginning of the novel when Sylvia, through whom the passage is focalized, describes her new home. She is fully aware that, despite its hotel-like ambiance, the residence is in fact a caregiving institution and, therefore, a move away from independence:

> Unlike nursing homes, with their particular standards for the amount of actual medical care required in the course of a day, not to mention a considerably less elegant ambience, this is a *retirement lodge*, the Idyll Inn—hard to imagine who dreamed that name up. "Sounds like one of those twee cottage names," Sylvia told her friend Mabel when she was deciding to move here. "Dun Roamin. Bide-a-Wee. You know? The Idyll Inn, my rear end. The Belly-Up is more like it." (20)

Joan Barfoot sets her novel in a luxurious place that boasts a sun deck, large private suites, a shuttle service into town, and birthday cakes for people "with healthy incomes but varying hopes, despairs, abilities and infirmities" (231). Despite the lavish ambience, the Idyll Inn remains a caregiving institution that interpellates individuals into the role of resident-patient.

Like many other care home novels, *Exit Lines* illustrates how the experience of transitioning from home to institutional care changes a person's sense of self. Anthropologists such as Renée Rose Shield have observed that care home residents often experience an incomplete *rite of passage* when moving into a long-term care institution, as they have to leave old roles behind, but do not have any new roles they can assume (Shield 103). In *Exit Lines*, this process can be clearly traced with all four protagonist residents as focalization oscillates between the four characters (and Annabel Walker, the manager, in some instances) who all develop different coping strategies. As Sylvia Lodge functions as the prime focalizer in large parts of the book, I will concentrate on her perspective. The novel opens with her account of the transition:

> She must learn not to think home of the place she has left, even if she lived there for half a century and has been here for maybe ten minutes. So much will need swift redefining; for instance, what's referred to here as the living room, with its sturdy bluey-grey spillproof carpeting and pale yellow blank walls […] it will be her sitting room. That being, she expects, her main activity in it. (13)

What used to be "living"—connoted with activity—is now reduced to mere "sitting," which can in itself be very emotionally and mentally active, but is here, through its opposition to "living," connoted with dying, or at least idleness. The residence's ambiguous name "Idyll Inn" that can also be heard as "Idle Inn" foregrounds this stereotype of inactivity in old age and emphasizes a decline narrative. Equally, Sylvia's interpretation of the spill proof floor-cover underlines the narrative of physical decline. Although the room does not have a linoleum floor as common in a hospital or nursing home room, the easy-to-clean carpeting has been put there for reasons of institutional efficiency and hygiene.

Sylvia has moved into the retirement lodge on her own initiative, a sign of agency in late life, and tries to justify this move by imagining a positive future for herself, forcing herself to see the home in an optimistic light: "Her suite is the seventh door on the left down this wide hallway. Her sanctuary; her vacant sanctuary at the moment, pending the arrival of her possessions. The remains of her life. Don't think of them that way" (12). Always having been very disciplined, Sylvia forbids herself to let herself go and tries to shut out even the smallest doubt that moving into a home eventually means that she will have to deal with thoughts about the finiteness of her being. Clinging to her independence, she is determined to enjoy life in her new home, imagining herself on her private sundeck that she will furnish with "her own private lawn furniture [...]. She sees herself out there in loose trousers and shirt, a book and binoculars, the world of the sitting room left well behind" (13). Sylvia imagines a space of her own, outside of the home and at the same time part of it—a transitory space that allows her to benefit from both places, uniting aspects of institutional care-giving and independence. She feels the need to reinforce her freedom and stresses the fact that she will be able to move around freely between institutional and private space as she intends to replace the "clinically white vertical blinds" with "a second door to the outdoors and her own private deck" (13). Sylvia will decide herself to what extent she is symbolically and literally inside or outside the institution, and the door, more substantial than mere blinds, will reinforce this borderline. Although she feels that her freedom to move about is jeopardized, she still tries to convince herself that keeping up a good spirit is what she needs to do. Determined to think positively, she tries to reformulate her concerns and fears into affirmative ideas, giving them "[t]he most positive possible spin" (16).

In her fight to remain independent despite institutionalization she wins an argument with the institution's manager Annabel Walker who tried to talk her into moving to the second floor "where the most lucid and able are supposed to gather in merry segregation" (14). As in *Half Life*, the residents' or patients' abilities determine which floor they live on. In the Idyll Inn, the upper floors are allocated to those who only need little help while the main floor rooms are kept for residents who, as Annabel expresses it, "can't move so independently" (14). Sylvia sees them as "other" and defines herself as not being part of them, which she underlines by insisting on moving into a suite on this particular floor: "Having a deck suits me best. Have you considered that your plan is entirely backwards? Of course that's up to you. And your other residents. But as for me, this is my choice" (14), Sylvia tells Annabel Walker. She will not simply be allocated a space, reduced to her body that is placed in the institution. She has a self-understanding as a paying customer and thus insists on her freedom to choose. The aspects of freedom and choice are linked to keeping personal control, which the narrative highlights when Sylvia cannot help noticing the small differences that seem to foreshadow her future as a more dependent person: "The toilet and shower feature bars to hold on to and lift off from as need be. It's the little things, isn't it? While other little things can turn at the flip of an ankle into quite large things" (12). As this passage shows, Sylvia's move to the Idyll Inn redefines her first and foremost in terms of physical abilities. It is primarily her aging body that will be taken care of, and she learns that the decision on which floor she may reside are usually left to nurses and medical practitioners who cite physical aspects as a basis for such decisions. Sylvia's adjustment process in the facility and the consequent redefinition of her identity are difficult, and although she is aware of the process and manages to subvert many of the institution's strategies, the transition is experienced as threatening to her identity as an independent and self-determined person.

The Idyll Inn as a place also structures Silvia's relationships and exerts its power on new inhabitants, as the opening paragraph of the novel reveals:

> At three o'clock in the morning, that defenceless hour when anything feels possible and nothing human or inhuman out of the question, the Idyll Inn's only sounds are the low hum and thrum a complicated building makes to keep itself going. Like any living body, even a sleeping or unconscious one, a building has to sustain its versions of blood and breath, so there's a perpetual buzz to it, white noise to the night. With only those faint sounds of companionship, three o'clock in the morning is an uneasy hour for the wakeful. (1)

The simile ("like any living body") and personification emphasizes the important role the building plays in the narrative. With its human characteristics it literally embodies institutional power and links spatiality to the social as it determines its residents' relations.

Another perspective of the Idyll Inn that relates the building to the body is also presented in the next chapter: "This Idyll Inn, if viewed from the unlikely vantage point of the air, more or less resembles a sperm: a rounded head with a long two-storey tail" (4) with all the "friendly, communal, well-intentioned features located in the part of the building which would, from the air, form the plump head of the sperm" (5). Whether the shape of the building should underline the fact that it houses active life or even represents a new start in life, or whether the metaphor alludes to an eternal circle of life and death, it seems absurd and certainly bears some irony which is reinforced by the description of what the sperm's head contains: it houses the staff office with "harried people, women, on a steep learning curve" (6) and the "ill-named library, a dark paneled room with no books" (6)—descriptions that highlight the fact that the emotional aspects of care-giving are not very well taken care of in the Idyll Inn. There is no point in complaining to anybody because "[c]omplaints risk retribution," (76) as Greta observes with an air of disillusionment and fear at some point—a phrase characteristic of the relationships between residents and staff at the Idyll Inn. Relationships among residents themselves are to be formed in the unwelcoming common areas such as the dining room with "a certain draftiness around some of the windows" (7), the crafts room and the coffee lounge where all sorts of gatherings can remain within the control of the staff. Sara Jamieson observes in this context,

> The novel's emphasis on the intentions and expectations underlying institutional design draws attention to how the built environment functions, particularly in its more public areas, as the expression of specific ideas about how the elderly should best manage the leisure time that the facility has made available to them. The pastoral focus on leisure in *Exit Lines* frames the novel's engagement with gerontological debates concerning the optimal level in old age of activity and engagement with the world. (373)

With reference to Katz (*Cultural* 121) Jamieson points out that "'the association of activity with well-being in old age' is one of the dominant ideologies of contemporary gerontology" (373), observing that the importance of activity and interaction was more compatible with the ideal of positive aging than what came to be known in the 1960s as "disengagement theory" (373), an approach that regards the desire to withdraw from any activities and the attenuation of former relationships as natural aspects of aging (374). *Exit Lines*, she argues, "participates in a rehabilitation of concepts associated with disengagement, suggesting that the choice to cease participation in certain activities, and to focus on certain relationships while letting others lapse, has at least as much to recommend it as maintaining high levels of activity and social contact in old age" (374). Sylvia as well as the other characters literally embody disengagement theory. She is suspicious of activities that are forged by planned encounters: "Relationships are bound to develop, but obviously it will be necessary to hold out against forced jollity. Presumptuousness. The sort of thing that leads to sing-alongs, and clumsy exercises from a seated position to the tunes of old ballads" (11). These disciplinary acts, as Sylvia understands them, reflect Michel Foucault's notion of the institutional gaze (*Discipline* 174), but Sylvia and her friends radically undermine all kinds of disciplining ("Honest to God, we're just old, we're not morons" (EL 51)) and refuse to participate in "all the promised fun" (31). For this reason, Annabel Walker, the embodiment of institutional discipline, is suspicious of the group meetings in Sylvia's room—and she is right, as they are actually held to prepare for Ruth's assisted suicide.

It is precisely here that *Exit Lines* subverts the Foucauldian panoptical gaze as well as discourses of normalization. While the consciousness of being surveyed has also been induced in the residents of the Idyll Inn, they still reject and even reverse, as Patricia Life has pointed out, institutional discipline and any attempted administrative gaze. "They boldly move about the residence in the middle of the night in the dark, and they know more about the administrator's private secrets than the administrator herself does," Life argues (118), alluding to the fact that Annabel Walker's father used to be Sylvia Lodge's secret lover, and Sylvia is well informed about Annabel's turbulent family history. When they finally set out together to euthanize Ruth, the rejection of the institutional gaze is at its peak. They manage to carve out a niche of independence and self-determinacy, and although the mutual euthanasia pact of the residents presents a questionable twist in the plotline, the text here suggests that the residents seize the ultimate agency, agency over their very existence (Life 124), challenging the institution's surveillance practices as well as the assumption that they have become "institutional bodies" (Wiersma and Dupuis).

Exit Lines can be read as a powerful and self-confident assertion of strength, endurance, and energy in old age. The characters "defy the outmoded social expectations of passive senescence by taking charge of their lives. [...] By leading 'young' lives in middle and old age, these fictional heroines [and heroes] undermine the conventional binary opposition between young and old," as Barbara Frey Waxman has stated with reference to what she calls *Reifungsromane* in the context of feminist literary gerontology (*Hearth* 183). Sylvia and her friends in

Exit Lines reject the negative cultural stereotypes of what it means to be old in a caregiving facility. Joan Barfoot uses the space of the care home as a setting metaphorically to critique traditional assumptions that are discursively anchored in such spaces. The value of such a text is to be found, therefore, not only in its literary quality, but also, and more importantly, in the ways in which it contributes to deconstructing metaphors and discursive formations that represent the care home as a place where the focus is directed first and foremost on the aging *body*. Instead, such texts widen the focus to the whole person, and consequently invite diverse readings that provoke questions of identity and the life course as well as about inter- and intragenerational relationships, questions that naturally include bodily aspects, but are not limited to them.

Like feminist scholars who address the gendered construction of space and the spatial construction of gender (McDowell and Sharp; Massey), I argue that the intersection of age and space, for which the care home novel can be used as a paradigm, needs to be addressed by literary gerontologists in order to facilitate a change in attitudes toward old age. Both the creation and the analyses of such sites in care home narratives can contribute toward that end. As literary gerontologist Sally Chivers states in a similar context, "These depictions of institutional care, more than commenting on the possibilities of such facilities to provide improved care, demonstrate the complicated process of forming attitudes toward the frail old and help to counter the impetus to think of age as either positive or negative. They provide examples of how narrative fiction can offer a perspective on the individuality of elderly residents that differs from clinical interaction" (*From* xlvi).

2.4 Celebrating Life: *Rhonda's Party*

The 8-minute Canadian short film *Rhonda's Party* was written by Christine Comeau, directed by Ashley McKenzie, and produced by Nelson MacDonald as part of the Atlantic Filmmakers Cooperative's FILM 5 program for emerging filmmakers. It premiered at the Montreal World Film Festival in September 2010. It has won several prizes[10] and was included in Air Canada's flight

10 The film received awards at the Montreal World Film Festival, the Atlantic Film Festival, the Worldwide Short Film Festival, St. John's International Women's Film Festival, the En Route Film Festival (*Best Cinematography*), the Young Cuts Film Festival (*Best Cana-*

entertainment program as a winner of the airline's film festival "EnRoute,"[11] reaching a relatively wide audience for such a film.

Rhonda's Party recounts a tragic and, at the same time, touching incident in Rhonda's life as a nursing home patient. She has spent months planning a party to celebrate her friend Margaret's 100th birthday. Rhonda is still busy with the final preparations when she learns that Margaret, the guest of honor, has passed away. Before Rhonda, played by Marguerite McNeil, can cancel the party, the samba band arrives and starts to play. Tightly clutching a red feather from Margaret's scarf in her fist, she finally chooses to join the "birthday" party, making it a farewell celebration in honor of her best friend.

In *Rhonda's Party*, the intersection of space and identity is emphasized on several levels. The sterile corridors in which some of the action takes place are highlighted in the opening and closing scenes; a doctor with a stethoscope and a nurse in her white coat reinforce the hospital-like atmosphere, and close-up shots of a room full of mobility and health care devices such as canes, crutches, walking frames, wheelchairs, and bedpans underline the aspects of limited mobility and disability. The film's opening sequence is unsettling. With a silent shot of a long and dimly lit aisle and its closed doors, a very dark and clinical atmosphere is created. No paintings or any other decorative objects, nor any signs of life, are displayed. The sterile setting suggests that the comfort of the residents is less important than the efficiency of the institution, as is signaled by the laundry bins on wheels that stand in front of some doors. The dismal, gray scene, completely lacking sound or color, and the cold neon ceiling lights that reinforce its sad ambience, create an uncanny feeling, and evoke common associations such as sickness, dependence, dementia, and death. After a few long seconds, the title of the film appears in large, superimposed, white letters: *Rhonda's Party*. The almost ironic juxtaposition of the *tristesse* presented during the first seconds with the "party" in the title invokes the curiosity of the viewer. How will "Rhonda"—yet unknown to the audience—celebrate, or be celebrated, in such a sad place? What sort of party is going to take place here?

The next scene shows a low-angle shot of a dilapidated radiator and window, wind softly stirring the thick, white, hospital-like curtain. This is the only noise apart from that of what we learn a little later is of scissors cutting paper, which continues while a close-up of a calendar month—although the specific

---

dian Short), and the CBC Short Film Faceoff 2011 (*Telefilm People's Choice*) (see http://www.grassfirefilms.ca/#645/custom_plain)

11 http://enroute.aircanada.com/en/film-festival

month is not recognizable—is shown, with all the days up to the eighth of the month crossed out. Obviously, the day on which the scene takes place is the marked 8th. It is circled with what looks like a black-and white representation of a red felt pen. Still, and although the film was not shot in black and white, no colors except for shades of gray or sepia have been introduced.

The first scene featuring color is an extreme close-up of a woman's wrinkled face, and in particular, her eyes concentrating on the green, red, and blue paper stars she is cutting out with yellow scissors. Red and blue balloons sway silently above her desk while the woman completes what seems to be a handmade birthday card, "Happy 100th Birthday, Margaret" is written on the front. The camera focuses on the woman's hands, marked with age spots and eczema, as she clumsily writes "For Margaret" onto the card. The yellow and blue birthday card has an eye-catching red ribbon, foreshadowing that from now on every item in the film that is related to the birthday is yellow, red, blue, or green, and stands out from the sandy gray background of the entire nursing home and its equally grayish patients.

In the next scene, the camera follows a young nurse as she walks towards the reception desk, which is centrally located in the home, overlooking both the aisle and the adjacent sitting room. The first word spoken in the short film is "sorry"—the nurse apologizes to a doctor and receptionist for having kept them waiting. They need her to sign an official "Registration of Death" form. The receptionist, a middle-aged woman dressed in beige like everyone else, is seated in a small space behind her desk, and does not seem particularly friendly or patient with the young nurse. That the nurse is dealing with her first death and is still very new in her profession can be concluded from the fact that the receptionist has to help the her find the signature line on the form. The stark white of her coat also stands out against the beige surroundings, indicating that she has not yet been "institutionalized." While she signs the form, the camera zooms in on the letters just long enough to reveal—not without irony—that the nursing home is called "Trodden Hills" and is in Nova Scotia, and that the name of the dead person (in an ironic nod to the film's director of the same name) is "Mackenzie, Margaret Ashley." The camera moves to the adjacent sitting room, which is decorated with several yellow, blue, and red balloons and a large banner saying "Happy 100th Birthday Margaret." Two women, one with a walking frame, the other also supporting herself on it, approach the young nurse whom they call Amy, suggesting that someone should take down the birthday sign. "And what about Rhonda?" they ask. At this point, no one has yet told her what has happened.

Rhonda, the woman who has been cutting paper stars and inflating balloons in her room for hours, is now visited by Amy, who tries to deliver the sad news very gently, "Rhonda, I know how special you wanted to make the party," Amy begins. "Oh, well," Rhonda answers, still cutting stars. "I ordered the best cake from Ricardo's. A full slab cake. I didn't care how much it cost. You see, here, they would use a cake mix. A cake mix! For Margaret!" Rhonda does not conceal her dissatisfaction with the place, referring to the "cake mix" as a *pars pro toto* for the indifferent and careless treatment she disdains.

After several tries, Amy eventually manages to tell Rhonda that her friend Margaret has passed away. Rhonda, in shock and denial, answers, "No, no, you don't understand, sweetie. We've been planning this party for six months now. Where is she? I want to talk to her." This scene explains the film's title. "Her" party, the capstone of the project that had produced meaning in the gray everyday life of the nursing home for six months, is now jeopardized by Margaret's death. For Rhonda, the celebration has been a project—an "escape world" (Goffman, *Asylums* 309) in which she could lose herself, "temporarily blotting out all sense of the environment which, and in which, [s]he must abide" (309). Rhonda pushes Amy out of her way, and walks briskly into Margaret's room.

Margaret's few personal belongings have already been packed up, only a few hours after her death. The room with its hospital bed, stripped of all individuality, will soon be ready for the next patient. Rhonda is shocked at the emptiness, which reinforces the heterotopic institutional aspects of the setting. "Where are all her pictures? Who gave you permission to do this?" she asks and takes a red feather from something that looks like a feather boa—the only colored item in the scene—from the open suitcase, symbolically holding on to her friend. "She must be very upset," Rhonda states, still in denial. While she tries to come to terms with Margaret's death, the other patients are still "patiently" and passively waiting in the sitting room, still wearing their party hats although they are by now all aware of what has happened. It seems as though they remain inert, seated like spectators, curious to see how the situation will develop; nobody has told them to go back to their rooms. The group is depicted as a beige conglomerate of old people that all look alike, which again reinforces the aspect of homogeneity, another facet that invokes the "nursing home specter."

In this scene, the filmmakers represent the nursing home "as a place where individuality disappears alongside the more obvious loss of independence," as Chivers claims in a different context (*From* 58). "That homogeneity typifies the way in which old people relegated (as it is so frequently expressed) to institutions are considered primarily if not solely as old (and therefore dependent)," she continues (58). It is often stated that it is "nice for old people to be among themselves," a statement that presupposes the assumption that being old is a more significant identity marker than any other factor. But after having lived long lives, the people's differences might actually be more striking than their commonalities arising from various forms of dependence or frailty. As Paul Higgs and Chris Gilleard note:

> At first sight, the increase in the numbers of older people might suggest greater opportunities for intragenerational solidarity [...]. Precisely the opposite seems to have happened. Age is more a site of contradiction than of community. [...] It is increasingly meaningless to consider age as conferring some common social identity or to treat older people as a distinct social group acting out of shared concerns and common interests. (*Cultures* 8)

Similarly, Sally Chivers has noted, the institutions' "biggest flaw" is "a tendency to homogenize the very old" (*From* 60). This homogenization is in direct opposition to the cultural narrative of individualism that, even if more dominant in the U.S. than in Canada, is a central theme in novels that deal with aging and identity. Roberta Maierhofer maintains that "the quest of the individual for a self-determined life in opposition to the norms of society has often been defined as the central cultural narrative, in which the desire of the individual to seek and define an identity within or without the community is the driving plot" ("Crossing" 250–251). *Rhonda's Party* is an example of such a quest. What makes this quest special is that it is set in a nursing home, the heterotopic setting of which changes the preconditions. Moving into institutional care redefines notions of individualism and self-determination and impacts the development of a life-course narrative. The processes that lead to this "mortification," Goffman notes, are "fairly standard in total institutions" (14) and include everyday chores such as bodily care performed by staff, which can be particularly threatening, "rendering older people as bodies that need to be cleaned, dressed, maintained, and treated" (Ryvicker 13). In Foucauldian terms, these bodies are subject to the clinical or social "gaze" (*Discipline* 174), and positioned as "other" in relation to the staff (Ryvicker 13).

In *Rhonda's Party*, the mortification of the home's residents is expressed through more or less subtle means, first and foremost on the level of aesthetics. In one example (fig. 2), a close shot focusses on a woman whose shirt seems to reiterate the chair's cover pattern, suggesting that she blends in perfectly, not only with the group, but also with the furniture.

Fig. 2: Stills from the Short Film Rhonda's Party

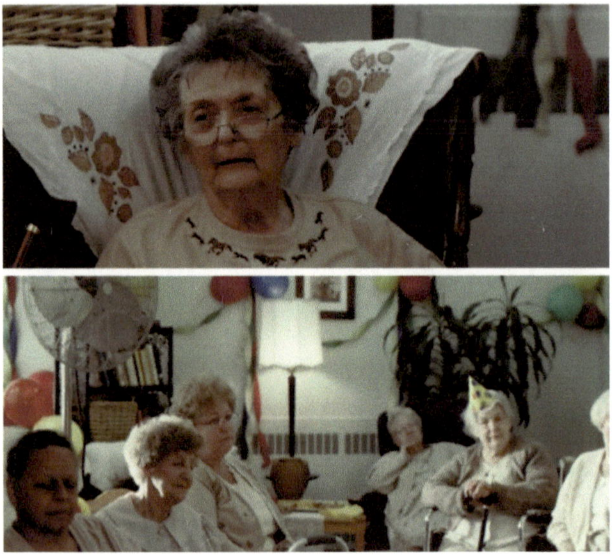

The only patient who seems to resist this homogenization to at least some extent is Rhonda. Although she, too, wears a beige vest, the rest of her clothes are black, and by organizing the party, she has injected the colors red, blue, green, and yellow into the residence—if only for one day. The party she has been planning is an overt sign of resistance against the institutional gaze. The staff, with the exception of the understanding nurse Amy, Rhonda's only supporter, is not in favor of activities that deviate from the routine of the institution. The bad-tempered, beige receptionist, for instance, likes to keep her distance from the inmates, signaling this by putting a stop sign on the cabinet drawer at the boundary of her enclosed space from which she can, almost as in a panopticon, survey the aisles and the sitting room.

The receptionist embodies the nursing home's authority, and she is irritated when the cake is delivered to her desk, intrudes into her space, closes in on her, and violates the boundary she has put in place against the patients. When Amy, rudely ordered to take it off, tries to move it somewhere else, she holds it such that the candles read 001 instead of 100. On a metaphorical level, this reverted cake could be interpreted as celebrating a new beginning—on the one hand, of Margaret's "new life," and on the other hand, of life on a more abstract and general level: life goes on—and even though Margaret is no longer with her, Rhonda will not be defeated. By taking agency, she has successfully resisted mortification, and seems to know that Margaret would not want her to cancel the celebration—hence the title of the film, *Rhonda's Party*.

Exactly at this moment, the samba band enters, making a huge amount of noise with their whistles and drums. The celebration has started. While Amy is at first shocked, a close-up shows how her facial expression suddenly changes, and she starts to smile, as if she has understood the importance of celebrating Margaret in her absence. Rhonda, still sitting on a bed, also hears the samba drums from a distance. The camera zooms in, showing an extreme close-up of her tightly closed fists. Encouraged by the rhythm, Rhonda slowly opens them, releasing the red feathers, indicating that she is symbolically letting go of her friend. She fetches a red balloon from her room, and determinedly walks down the long, nearly black-and-white corridor, the ceiling lamps of which highlight the balloon as if it were a blinking red light. In the final scene, a long shot, Rhonda turns the corner, pulling the balloon behind her, presumably to enter the sitting room where the band is playing, and joins the party. Now, as opposed to the opening shot, the doors are all open, movement and color is visible, and the former silence has given way to raucous samba sounds that fill the aisle and the entire home with life.

With the use of the concrete space of the nursing home as a setting, Comeau, McKenzie, and MacDonald have contributed to the newly emerging genre of the nursing home narratives. The film encourages viewers to evaluate their own attitudes towards aging and old age in institutional care. Rather than emphasizing Rhonda's or Amy's perspectives through the use of camera techniques such as a simulation of the characters' sight-lines, the camera imitates the position of a participant-observer, inviting the viewer to enter the home. Unlike the inmates, the viewers are not committed to stay. *Rhonda's Party* taps into the fear of an aging population of finally ending up in institutional care, and initially offers no respite from this dread. The movie's potential to challenge the nursing home specter lies in another quality: it broaches the topic of individuality and collectivity, underlining an individual woman's efforts to subvert institutional power structures through an act of defiance. With her initiative to organize a colorfully decorated birthday party, complete with a fancy banner, party hats, a cake, and a samba band in the

"Trodden Hills" nursing home, Rhonda counteracts the mortification of her identity in the nursing home, resisting the clinical gaze and emphasizing her individuality in contrast to the homogenized group of people that characterize the "Institution." Through Margaret's death, Rhonda's plan develops an even more strongly subversive aspect. She challenges the nursing home specter, and insists on celebrating life in the face of death, despite the intimidating institutional surroundings that interpellate her as a patient with only little influence on everyday matters. She defies objectification and homogenization and, with the help of Amy as her ally, manages to appropriate the nursing home's space for her celebration. Rhonda takes agency, carving out some individual niches for herself, and reading the film within the context of second wave feminism that points to the interrelatedness of the personal and the political, she acts as a positive example for all women.

The position of the young caregiver is also important in this context. In Foucauldian terms, she subverts the normalizing discourse that renders the bodies docile (*Discipline* 135), and encourages the patient's resistance. Through her understanding and empathy, Amy supports Rhonda's plans, and acknowledges her individuality, takes her seriously, and sees her not only as a patient, but as a person. Amy has gone out of her way to help Rhonda organize the party very much against the will of the other staff members, as the critical remarks of the receptionist reveal. Although Rhonda might have been strong and independent enough to pursue her plans without Amy's help, the nurse's support is crucial, and leads to the development of a closer relationship between the two women. Furthermore, it reinforces the change Rhonda is able to bring about in the home because Amy, a staff member, takes sides with Rhonda, a patient, crossing the boundaries of her professionally inhabited space—a separation characteristic of total institutions (Goffman, *Asylums* 19). By presenting Amy's perspective, the film emphasizes the need for individualized care from the caregiver's point of view.

The relationship that develops between the two characters, Amy and Rhonda, is important and comforting for both, and transforms not only Rhonda's, but also Amy's identity. While Rhonda might see Amy primarily in her role as a nurse, Amy manages to understand the importance of Rhonda's resistance, and sees herself in relation to the old woman. This relational understanding of identity is also referred to by Roberta Maierhofer, who argues that in a rapidly aging society, a shift in cultural values will be necessary to foster understanding of the interdependence of generations. She emphasizes "the necessity of mutual and supportive relationships as a key to the development of a personal identity" ("Crossing" 251), and points to the need to redefine individuals "not only as independent and self-supporting, but also as necessarily relying on the help and assistance of others" (249). Applied to questions of eldercare, such an approach that takes a life-course perspective and subverts the binary opposition of young and old by a concept of "self-in-relation" (251) has the potential to challenge the nursing home specter. The film *Rhonda's Party* offers a strong and life-affirming expression of individuality, despite the bleakness of institutional care.

3 Captives of Care—Prisoners to the Palsy?

Resisting Confinement from Within

> Most prisoners foresee a time when they will get out. Here we know there is no way out, only down, little by little, till death do us join with whatever comes next, if only dust to dust. Hope is one thing of which we are deprived.
>
> — May Sarton, *As We Are Now*

May Sarton's novel *As We Are Now* (1973) is one of many literary examples that illustrate the fear, hopelessness, and despair commonly associated with nursing homes. Such portrayals usually represent the home as a prison from which death is the only escape. This chapter will focus on the nursing home as a fictional space that expresses the peripheralization of old age, its physical limitations, and the restricted mobility often associated with it—what Shakespeare's Edmund of Langley aptly calls being a "prisoner to the palsy" (*Richard II* 2.3.124–25). Extending Susan Braedley's concept of the "ruling metaphor," I argue that the prison metaphor serves as a powerful discursive framework that guides all social interactions. The texts demonstrate isotopies of confinement, repeated themes, images, and motifs that reinforce the experience of restriction, even incarceration. Helen Small discusses this as part of what she terms *care noir*, a "broad and inventive mode of perverse imaginary in which the institution looms all powerful and 'care' provides the thinnest of covers for licensed abuse" (Small 179). Within this framework, the nursing home is depicted not as a place of comfort and support, but as an oppressive institution that isolates and infantilizes its residents, stripping them of agency and dignity (179).

While portraying the institution as a bleak space of confinement, many texts also offer powerful counter-narratives of resistance to imprisonment. As this chapter will show, these counter-narratives bear witness to the protagonists' individual agency, independence, and growth, and help to deconstruct stereotypical notions of old age as merely a time of dependence, decrepitude, and disease. The protagonists presented in this chapter struggle against abuse, homogenization, and infantilization from *within* the confining walls of the care home, thereby challenging the nursing home specter and the ruling metaphor of imprisonment. Such narratives have the potential, as Sally Chivers puts it, to "revise cultural scripts that attempt to hold elderly characters firmly in place" ("On" 204), and contribute to ongoing debates of what long-term care should ideally be.

As Chivers points out, "[t]he popular press focuses on nursing homes as contemporary 'gulags,' sites of increasing use of chemical restraints, places of abuse and violence, and locations of tragedies that reveal high levels of neglect" ("Blind" 134–35). Such representations function as powerful and pervasive metaphors for the experience of old age in "heterotopias of deviation" (Foucault, "Of" 24). But texts that portray old people as "appropriately contained" (Chivers, "Road" 213) in long-term care institutions can also have a negative impact on the social and cultural construction of aging. Both literature and film play their distinctive, but interrelated, roles in deconstructing stereotypes, myths, and established assumptions with regard to aging and old age as a state of containment. The analysis of fictional narratives and their subversive power is crucial to our understanding of what it means to grow old in institutional care—and, of course, to its possible re-imagination.

This chapter offers a close reading of four texts, May Sarton's famous novel *As We Are Now,* Leslie Larson's novel *Breaking Out of Bedlam,* John Mighton's play *Half Life*, and Margaret Atwood's short story "Torching the Dusties," four works that show how the homes' residents/inmates, each in their own way, rebel against their confinement from within. Written at a time when few texts employed the care home as a setting,[1] *As We Are Now* is one of the earliest texts exemplary of the genre, which as it begins in the 1960s and early 1970s, depicts the home as a dreadful place. Four decades later, *Breaking Out of Bedlam* (2010), *Half Life* (2005), and "Torching the Dusties" (2014) still represent the home as a place of docile dependency. These representations are still rooted in the collective memory of the institution's history, as discussed in the introductory

1 Among them are John Updike's *The Poorhouse Fair* (1959), Margaret Laurence's *The Stone Angel* (1964), Alice Munro's short story "Spelling" (1978), and Edna Alford's short story collection *A Sleep Full of Dreams.* While Alford's collection appeared only in 1981, individual stories already came out in 1976.

chapters, and continue to conjure up the "nursing home specter" to which Betty Friedan dedicates a whole chapter in *The Fountain of Age*: "In ten years of my research, no data has emerged to counteract my impression of nursing homes as death sentences, the final interment from which there is no exit but death" (510), Friedan maintains, perpetuating the discourse of the home as horror in her influential work. "Even at their very best, nursing homes," she continues in an interview in 2002, "remove people from the society of the living. […] It's just assumed they are no longer people. Too often they are treated as helpless children, sedated or put in restraints" (Luddington 151).

Topics such as abuse, infantilization, and sedation feature prominently in Sarton's *As We Are Now*, Mighton's *Half Life*, and Atwood's "Torching the Dusties." Even if Larson's *Breaking Out of Bedlam* does not feature physical violence, residents are still infantilized and homogenized. In all four texts, the protagonists struggle, fight, and find means and ways to undercut (even if not always entirely successfully) the authoritarian regimes that interpellate them into their roles as patients. The protagonists of Sarton's text escape institutional confinement only on an imaginary level through sexual fantasy (Standish Flint) and death (Caro Spencer), and even though one of the protagonists in *Half Life* manages to repeatedly break the door code in order to leave the home and go drinking, his escape plans are always frustrated within a few hours. Larson's text seems to rewrite the journal that Sarton's protagonist wrote forty years earlier; while Caro Spencer dies within the confining walls of the home, Cora Sledge manages to "break out of Bedlam," and the novel ends just as she is about to move back into her old house. In Atwood's "Torching the Dusties," the last story analyzed in this chapter, the heterotopian nursing home becomes a death trap for all but two characters, when a group of young people wearing baby masks burns down the home.

3.1 Embodying Imprisonment

Before analyzing these texts, I would first like to elaborate on the figure of confinement as a metaphor and on the nursing home's synecdochical significance, a recurring guiding theme across the representations discussed. Representations of aging often closely intertwine notions of body, identity, and home, and the following section explores these connections in detail. Indeed, the aging body itself can be interpreted through Bakhtin's concept of the chronotope, as it embodies the passage of time. The visible changes in the aging body reflect the accumulation of lived experiences, memories, and personal histories. The body can therefore be read as a spatiotemporal narrative, physically manifesting an individual's life journey and serving as a tangible representation of time itself. In line with Bakhtin's concept of the chronotope, physical limitations in old age can be interpreted as a spatialization of time, concretely illustrating how the aging body itself becomes a site of imprisonment.

Kontos observes that older persons frequently describe illness or disability as imprisoning an "imprisoning of their inner youthfulness" ("Multi" 34), suggesting the aging body acts as a constricting, confining space. Similarly, Featherstone and Wernick argue that "for those who are in deep old age, who are weak, frail or disabled, the body is not only a masking device which conceals and distorts the self which others interact with, in addition the lack of mobility and functioning capacity may make the body seem to be a prison" (11). This resonates in Edward Hays's impressive depiction of aging as incarceration, where the body's decline metaphorically strips away identity, autonomy, and dignity—an experience that embodies the intersection of space (the body as prison) and time (the loss of memories, capacities, and selfhood). I cite it here extensively because it illustrates the abject character old age can assume in an extreme manner:

> One day you awake to find yourself behind barbed wire fences as a prisoner of an escape-proof concentration camp—old age. You have been seeing all the warning signs of your dreaded deportation in the mirror and knew soon you would be next. [...] The essence of entering prison is loss. The possessions of those entering are confiscated. As they are stripped of clothing, lost too is their dignity. Elders experience this confiscation of dignity as well by examinations in doctors' offices and in various medical procedures. These losses increase as they age, as slowly hair color goes, and for some, hair itself. Bodily strength and agility are taken away, then teeth, eyesight and hearing. Painful losses of later years can include the fabulous freedom achieved at 16 of having a driver's license. At any time in aging comes a profoundly dreadful confiscation—loss of memory. When memories of loved ones, dear friends, adventures in life, one's work or profession are taken, the elderly are stripped naked to the bone. (Hays n.p.)

In addition to Hays's shocking comparison of old age with a concentration camp (a comparison that May Sarton also uses in *As We Are Now*), this passage reveals several negative assumptions about what it means to grow old. Hays interprets old age to be an external threat that strikes a person at a certain point in time, and often seemingly unexpectedly during the night. He generalizes the experience of loss, decline, and illness—or what he simply calls terror—as universal. Yet, at the same time, he argues that there is a kind of miraculous agency in trying to "turn old age's prison into a time of forgiveness and gratitude," as the title of his article suggests. Regardless of Hays's moralistic attitude, his essay is an example of the metaphor of old age as an imprisonment, which prevails in many cultural representations, including most of the long-term care narratives discussed in this book, and especially those presented in this chapter.

Don Fidencio, for instance, the 91-year old protagonist of *Amigoland* who escapes a care home to travel to Mexico and die there in peace, expresses his frustration about the futility of his escape: "He had escaped one prison only to discover that there was no way of escaping his own failing body" (Casares 285). Don Fidencio sees his decrepit body as an oppressor to whom he is hostage, and his comments can be likened to those of the Duke of York in Shakespeare's *Richard II*, who describes himself as "prisoner to the palsy" (Woodward, "Instant" 55). Likewise, Joan Barfoot's *Exit Lines* presents George, who is angry at his own body for failing him after he suffers a stroke: "Pathetic. It's not just lost words and leftward vision that frustrate, it's a body that won't let him whip around to check what's behind him. . . . A man shouldn't be so defenceless" (35).

This oppositional relationship to one's aging body is based on a Cartesian dual perception of the self and the body, which is often experienced as alienating, as Kathleen Woodward contends in her theory of the "mirror stage of old age". She develops this theory with reference to Jacques Lacan's concept of the mirror stage of infancy:

> It is not surprising that the image of the mirror should dominate literary representations of the aged body. The horror of the mirror image of the decrepit body is the inverse of the pleasures of the mirror image of the youthful Narcissus. As we age we increasingly separate ourselves—what we take to be our real selves—from our bodies. We believe our real selves, that is our youthful selves, are hidden inside our bodies, not commensurate with them. Our bodies are old, we are not. Old age is a state in which the body is in opposition to the self and we are alienated from our bodies. ("Instant" 55)

Woodward's observation has been confirmed by several literary accounts of the experience of old age. The alienation that occurs when the body is no longer experienced as self, but as other, enables the use of the metaphor of the body that both houses, and hides, the self. In *The Portrayal of Old Age*, Heather Gardiner writes that "the image of the house of the ageing body as a form of confinement is common in the literature of old age" (26–27). Gardiner also sees the nursing home as a metaphor for the fears and feelings that growing old and dependent evokes:

> Old age is frequently expressed in literature in the language of confinement and imprisonment. Either imprisonment is portrayed literally, such as confinement in a nursing home or other limited space, or the process of building a "stone house" of self-imprisonment is suggested, one whereby the elderly protagonist carefully orders and controls what he or she chooses to present to the outside world. (24)

One of the examples that illustrates Gardiner's point is Alice Munro's short story "Spelling" in which Rose, a young woman, visits the Wawanash County Home for the Aged and is shown an old woman who is confined behind the bars of her crib. This old woman's language is reduced to "spelling" occasional words; she is otherwise unable to speak. Gardiner argues that the "description of her imprisoned in her crib and the focus on her speech suggests the caging of another language in old age" (27).

Another example Gardiner's analysis led me to discover is that of David Waltner-Toews's short story "A Sunny Day in Canada" (1980), which portrays an old married couple, Prometheus Koslowski, the narrator, and his wife Rachel, who lives with dementia. They are confined in a nursing home to a "two-bed inescapably pastel-pink room. Nursery, nursing home, the choice of names is no accident" (Waltner-Toews 240). Prom, while observing a fellow resident who fantasizes about having an affair with one of the nurse's aides, focuses on his body: "His body had a stroke on the left side, his big fat quivering body. He does not admit inhabiting that body. He lives in another body, young and muscular. A body that will go with Betty, the chubby blonde aide, to the lake this weekend" (243). Like Munro's "Spelling," Waltner-Toews's story also describes the failing language of the oldest old: "We progress, in this place, from long sentences to short phrases to a few key words and finally to silence and eternal peace. The staff help us in this unlearning of language, this progression which is the reverse of childhood. By now, most of us here speak in simple sentences" (241). Prom's observation, which also contains a critique of the taciturn nature of the staff, is based on a narrative of decline and reduction. As Gardiner observes, "[n]ot only does confinement of the old occur in smaller and smaller spaces, but the body shrivels in its space and, as the old man points out, so does language" (30). She underlines the difficulty of adequately representing the experience of old age with this statement.

Prom describes his old body in spatial terms, not only by using the cultural narrative of the circle of life, but also by describing how his body is placed, and "tucked in a cave" that resembles a womb:

> Let me tell you about my body. My body is a skeleton wrapped in parchment. The orderly discovers this archaeological artifact every morning, tucked into a cave of white sheets and woollen blankets: bald as a plucked chicken, the legs bent up towards the chest, twisted around each other. Doctor Toews says the body is reverting to fetal posture, which just shows how far removed from the womb he is. (Waltner-Toews 241)

Waltner-Toews describes the experience of the end of life as a preparation for a final birth—which is death—that closes the circle of life. Prom knows that Rachel will soon be released from the confining space of the home and her own body, and he visualizes the end of their life as a journey to heaven (which is also mirrored in the collection's title, *One Foot in Heaven*):

> But her lightness, that is what I love. One morning, she will lift up through the window like a kite, up, up, growing smaller and smaller into the blue prairie sky. I shall be holding the string. When she arrives up there, she will give a little tug, and I too will be pulled loose. I shall float up after her, unstuck from earth. (Waltner-Toews 241)

The story ends with Rachel's death, and rests on Prom's hope that he will soon be able to follow her. The nursing home in this story is presented as a waiting room for death, a *pars pro toto* for the "foreign country of old age," as Sarton puts it (23), or the "banished existence in the land of the fourth space" as Haim Hazan theorizes it ("Beyond" 91).

The physical limitations that are experienced by an aging person are also described by Gardiner in her analysis of *Redwork* (1990), a children's book in which Michael Bedard describes the restricted world of old Mr. Magnus: "The house Mr. Magnus lives in no longer has its own shape, but has taken on the shape of the old man, now in his nineties, 'settl[ing] around him like a second skin'. The movements of Mr. Magnus are limited to this house, where a 'few sad rooms' become an 'old man's world' and 'horizons' are reduced to 'walls' (178)"

(Gardiner 27). May Sarton has Caro Spencer describe her situation in a similar way in *As We Are Now* (1973). Caro feels entrapped both in her own aging body and the dreadful, prison-like nursing home: "I am walled in" (111) she describes her situation, "[t]he walls close in on every side. I do not remember things very clearly" (115).

The body as spatial entity is also foregrounded in Margaret Laurence's novel *The Stone Angel*, where Hagar Shipley is afraid of the care home: "Is it a mausoleum, and I, the Egyptian, mummified with pillows and my own flesh through some oversight embalmed alive?" (96). She leaves her own home, and escapes to a village on the beach, but instead of the summer house she remembers, she only finds a dilapidated ruin in which she seeks shelter, sick and exhausted. Heather Gardiner connects Hagar's aging body with its surroundings:

> By placing the ninety-year-old Hagar in a deteriorating building next to the ocean, Laurence presents the image of an old woman with a failing body sitting on the edge of the formlessness of eternity, far removed from the security of the bodily house which has offered her shape and form for most of her life. [...] Hagar's sense of identity is closely tied to the house she lives in. At Shadow Point, Hagar is separated from her house and the "shreds and remnants of years" (36) it contains, and new voyages into realms away from physical objects remain the only possibility. (86–87)

When Hagar, after her long and exhausting escape from Silverthreads, the care home in which she was placed, is hospitalized at the end of the novel, and moved from the geriatric ward to a semi-private room (281), she remarks that "the world is even smaller now. It's shrinking so quickly." The next room will be "the smallest of all," with "just enough space" for herself (282), Hagar says, anticipating her own death.

In her analysis of "Ageing in the 21st Century," Catherine Du Toit analyzes the metaphor of shrinking space by means of the aging body:

> Contraction or shrinking is another recognizable figure of ageing which is adapted to contemporary conditions. Brought about by the physical inability to move, the reluctance to abandon a familiar setting, the decay of the senses or the progressive loss of contact with the world outside, the ageing subject finds himself in a shrinking space. [...] The ageing body itself is also subject to physical contraction. Degenerative diseases such as osteoporosis cause shrinkage in height. In Alzheimer's disease, parts of the brain atrophy

> as neurons and synapses die. This "process of reduction", as Philip Roth calls it in *Everyman* (92) transcends the physical, and the experience of ageing, whether accompanied by physical suffering or not, is often expressed as diminishing and belittling. (285–287)

All these examples, including parts of Du Toit's explanation, define aging as illness, loss, and decline and are part of a cultural narrative of aging. Faced with such limitations, the protagonists in the novels discussed here respond by creating an escape world for themselves in their imagination, challenging the confining structures of old age and the care home, which serves to illustrate these limitations in other ways. "Writing can be construed as an attempt to root oneself in the present, in other words, to confirm one's continued presence in the world by creating an existence that will allow a certain appropriation of time [and space] through the iterative remembering the reception of a text brings about," Du Toit argues (294).

3.2 Writing Against Confinement: May Sarton's *As We Are Now* and Leslie Larson's *Breaking Out of Bedlam*

> Do not go gentle into that good night,
> Old age should burn and rave at close of day;
> Rage, rage against the dying of the light.
>
> — Dylan Thomas, "Do Not Go Gentle Into That Good Night"

As We Are Now (1973) and *Breaking Out of* Bedlam (2010) each present an old woman's struggle against institutional confinement through the act of journaling. Writing in their diaries, Caro Spencer, the protagonist of *As We Are Now*, and Cora Sledge, the protagonist of *Breaking Out of Bedlam*, chronicle their lives, hopes, and fears in secret diaries that are only made public after their deaths. For both women, writing becomes an act of defiance, a means of reclaiming their voices and resisting the inhumane treatment they endure in long-term care. Their pens serve as sharp weapons, wielded in protest and revenge against the institutions that seek to silence them. More importantly, the women's journals help them overcome traumatic experiences, and enable them to reclaim personal freedom and agency—each in their own way. *As We Are Now* and *Breaking Out Of Bedlam* present two women's creative acts of writing that lead to a "composing [...] of the self" (Woodward, "May" 111). Both novels can be read as *Reifungsromane* (Waxman, *From* 2). The similarity between the protagonists' names as well as other parallels in the stories may be coincidental, but as the following analysis will show, *Breaking Out of Bedlam* parallels *As We Are Now* on several levels, and can be read as a modernized, re-written version of Sarton's more than fifty-year-old novel. Albeit with very different style and tone, the novels offer proof of the two old women's resilience, and their search for self in institutional long-term care.

As We Are Now records the last days of 76-year old Caro Spencer, who is taken to "Twin Elms," a "Dickensian nursing home" (Woodward, "May" 118) in rural New England by her older brother and his young wife after having suffered an incapacitating heart attack. Caro, a former high-school math teacher, is a single, educated woman determined to fight against the ageist treatment she experiences in the small, unkempt, privately owned place. When she feels she finally cannot bear the humiliating treatment any longer, she sets fire to the home, killing all its residents, including herself. Her diary is found hidden in a fridge, as is indicated in the afterword, which, although it first looks like a meta-text, is actually part of the fictional world of the novel: "AFTERWORD: This manuscript was found after the fire that destroyed the Twin Elms Nursing Home. In a letter found inside the cover, Miss Caroline Spencer requested the Reverend Thornhill to have it published if possible. This has been done with the permission of her brother, John Spencer" (134). Caro writes down her testimony to warn others, and raise awareness regarding the marginalization of the old, frail, and sick: "Perhaps if this story of despair could be published it would help those who deal with people like me, the sick in health or mind, or the just plain old and abandoned" (112). She calls it "The Book of the Dead" (10), her "*memento mori*," (10) not only to hint at her own finiteness, but also to raise the readers' attention to the fact that her fate may also be ours as we age (Maierhofer, *Salty* 328). As Maierhofer also writes, Caro places herself in a larger social and intergenerational context for which the novel's title is also significant: "As you are now, so once was I; Prepare for death and follow me" (Sarton 5) the epigraph reads from which the title is adapted. She finishes the journal while thinking of her intended audience: "Only one thing, THE important thing I must manage to do is place all the copybooks in the frigidaire. To you who may one day read this, I give them as a testament. Please try to understand" (133).

While Caro Spencer addresses her wish to shed light on the horrible conditions of institutional care to anyone who will find her journal after her death, Cora Sledge in *Breaking Out of Bedlam* addresses primarily her children (and readers) to whom she intends to reveal the secrets of her traumatic past, begging them for their understanding, and inviting them to reevaluate her story:

> I'm going to take all three books, seal them in an envelope, and write OPEN UPON MY DEATH on them. I'll put them in my linen closet where I keep all my best pillowcases and towels, things that's too nice to use. When I die and you come to clean out my house, you'll find them. You can do whatever you want. I've pictured you reading them and finding out the truth. If you see any mistakes—spelling or wrong words—you can fix them. You have my okay. (Larson 310)

Cora, an 82-year old feisty widow, initially documents in her journals her suffering in The Palisades, an assisted living institution in Phoenix, Arizona. Deciding that because she has "nothing to lose" (4), it was now time for her to tell the truth about her life, she begins to write down her story: "I hope those that put me in this place read it when I'm dead—which I have a feeling won't be long. Maybe then they'll see" (Larson 4). At first, her writing is also an act of revenge. She is furious at her three middle-aged children, who decide that she can no longer properly take care of herself in her own home where she had lived with her late husband, Abel. Actually, since his death, Cora has become addicted to pills and junk food, cannot walk but a few steps at a time, is forgetful, depressed, and has become heavily overweight. Her children's concerns about their mother's well-being seem justified. Cora has been excluded from any decision-making process regarding her future, and feels that her citizenship rights are being violated in an ageist manner: "My mistake was thinking an adult could make her own decisions. Thinking I was still an American citizen with rights that couldn't be taken away. [...] They talked to lawyers and looked at places to put me. They got everything in order. I was the last one to know" (Larson 7).

In a tradition of literary self-reflection, Cora, like Caro—also begins writing a diary. Her writing becomes a routine that keeps Cora alive amidst the institution's "droolers," who are "wheeled along or plod like zombies" (Larson 9). In her tell-all journal, she interweaves two narrative strands, past and present, that reflect and explain each other. While the strand narrating the present provides her with a means of catharsis in, subversion of, and resistance to her current situation in the care home, the strand that chronicles her memory enables her to make a "life review" (Butler). This allows her to come to terms with past conflicts, and to reevaluate and re-narrate them in order to integrate them into a positive life course narrative. While Caro Spencer in *As We Are Now* finally burns down the home and commits suicide, *Breaking Out of Bedlam* ends with Cora leaving the home, and moving back into her old house after the two narrative strands, past and present, have been connected to create a future for Cora.

Hellish Total Institutions

In this context, the ambiguity of the novel's title needs to be mentioned: "Bedlam" is the nickname of Bethlehem Royal Hospital in London, the oldest psychiatric institution in the world (founded in 1247). The hospital's website refers to its history:

> From Shakespeare's time onwards the word "Bedlam" has been widely used to conjure up images of "turmoil, confusion and cacophony." Unfounded myths about the hospital's early history include claims that exorcism was used to treat some patients, and that up until the late nineteenth century as many as 96,000 people visited "Bethlem" each year, and paid to see patients being "exhibited" on Sundays. (South London and Maudsley NHS Foundation Trust n.p.)

While these myths may be "unfounded," the conditions were certainly far from humane. In colloquial, modern English, "Bedlam" has come to stand for chaos and madness. The novel's title refers to both meanings of the term—the very structured, rigid institution Cora is sent to, and the chaos of her life prior to her institutionalization.

Cora lives in an assisted living wing of "this hell they call The Palisades" (Larson 49), but fears that she will eventually have to live "in B Wing, locked up in bedlam with those lunatics and half-deads" (158). Even though she is not "state," i.e., relying on Medicare support like some of the poorer people who share wards, where "more than half the bare fluorescent lights were out, and the ones that *were* working sizzled and flickered like a scene from hell" (91), the room she inhabits is small and impersonal. Her view includes only chains of laundry carts and daily truck deliveries, and she feels choked by the fumes: "My room even has a number, 136, like a motor lodge or a doctor's office" (49). The home is run by "Bigbutt and her henchmen" (233), as Cora calls the head nurse and her helpers, and is described as a "place that's no more than a warehouse, a storage bin where people are tossed until the next shipment comes in" (49). Several times she refers to the "disinfectant smell" that "didn't cover up that piss stink" (80) and the "nasty plastic dishes [...] covered in chewed up food and cold gravy" (79), "half hospital, half prison" (296)—"except you got to break the law to end up in there and here your only crime is you lived too long" (37). Institutional life lacks dignity:

> [F]luorescent lights in the hall reflect on the floor that's white, too, everything white, but a dirty white—like snow that's piled up beside the road. You see one horror after another walking by the open doors of people's rooms. Nobody pays any mind to decency. I've seen bare-ass old men with their balls dangling down to their knees, and tattered dog-ear tits like socks with rocks in the end. It's enough to turn your stomach. (50)

During the first months after her institutionalization, Cora seeks comfort in her sleeping pills: "The first few months I was here, I didn't want to come out of my room or see anybody or even get out of bed. I could not get my mind around what happened to me. I took whatever pills I could get my hands on and half the time I didn't know my own name. Then I got pneumonia. Good, I thought. I finally found a way to die" (37). At least, Cora would have had a role in her own death.

Caro Spencer in *As We Are Now* describes her institutionalization in a similar way, but without the irony and sense of humor that reveal a certain distance to what is going on around Cora. Caro Spencer is at best bitter and cynical. "I am in a concentration camp for the old, a place where people dump their parents or relatives exactly as though as it were an ash can" (9), May Sarton has her protagonist complain, also using the over-exaggerated and inappropriate image of the concentration camp[2] to express her extreme frustration about the poor standards of the home and her treatment, but also, and more importantly, with her suffering in the foreign and forgotten place.

2 In *Understanding May Sarton*, Mark K. Fulk explains that Sarton frequently uses the Holocaust as a subtext in her writing (49; 98; 101). This comparison seems particularly out of place because Sarton refers to concentration camps in other contexts throughout the novel, making it clear that she is well aware of the abject horror of such places. While such comparisons are not uncommon (Shapiro 237; M. O'Neil) and extend back to 1930, they are clearly questionable.

Writing as Self-Defense

Sarton calls *As We Are Now* "her 'J'accuse'"[3] (Springer 48) in which she articulates her indictment of society's inhumane treatment of dependent elders. Caro Spencer's diary is equated with an open letter that rebels against the inhumane conditions under which old people are forced to live in nursing homes. Her journal is a "life-testimony" that she wants to use to reach out to the world, bringing the perpetrators to trial, as Shoshana Felman theorizes the act of witnessing with regard to the act of writing and reading. "A 'life-testimony' is not simply a testimony to a private life, but a point of conflation between text and life, a textual testimony which can *penetrate us like an actual life* [...] something crucial takes place which is of the order of a *trial*" (Felman 1). Caro Spencer appoints herself as a witness, and speaks for others to others (Felman 3).

Caro Spencer's home Twin Elms is run by an authoritarian nurse, Harriet Hatfield, and her daughter Rose, depicted as two overweight and uneducated women. Harriet leaves no doubt as to who has the upper hand: "She has been trained to treat the inmates as inferiors to be ordered about, controlled in every possible way. I escape the control simply by being myself. However meek I am, I am still myself. This, I presume, is what has to be destroyed" (Sarton 95), Caro writes in her diary. Kathleen Woodward reads the relationship between the nurses and Caro as follows: "Spencer is abandoned to die. Worse, at Twin Elms, [...] she is initiated into evil. She confronts the corruption seemingly inherent in the relationship between master (the administrator) and slave (the patient)" ("May" 120). The text here resonates with Goffman's description of a person's entry into a total institution. Goffman (using only male pronouns throughout the text) writes that a person

> comes into the establishment with a conception of himself made possible by certain stable social arrangements in his home world. Upon entrance, he is immediately stripped of the support provided by these arrangements. In the accurate language of some of our oldest total institutions, he begins a series of abasements, degradations, humiliations, and profanations of self. His self is systematically, if often unintentionally, mortified. He begins some radical shifts in his moral career, a career composed of the progressive changes that

3 The term "*J'accuse*" is attributed to French writer Émile Zola who wrote an open letter in 1898 in the newspaper *L'Aurore* in the context of the Dreyfus affair (Essig 173).

> occur in the beliefs that he has concerning himself and significant others. (*Asylums* 14)

Caro Spencer rebels against the institutional pressures that threaten, as Goffman expresses it, her moral career. In fact, many passages in the novel can be read as descriptions from the inside of a total institution, as if to illustrate Goffman's case studies further: "There is a connection between any place where human beings are helpless, through illness or old age, and a prison. It is not only the heroic helplessness of the inmates, but also what complete control does to the nurses, guards, or whatever" (Sarton 49), and "[i]f keepers are corrupted by having absolute power, what about those they keep? We learn to ingratiate ourselves [...]. So if I am punished, I deserve it" (74–75). She has already internalized her guilt—she is guilty of being old.

From the first week of her institutionalization on, Caro tries to defend her sense of self against the humiliating mortification she experiences in the home. Once, after speaking up against the nurses' inhumane treatment of a fellow resident, she is locked in a dark room, which is a devastating experience for her: "They shatter me. I am not worthy, a leper—an old woman without control over herself" (Sarton 42). She is well aware of the processes that endanger her identity ("Don't let them steal your mind," 29) and tries to resist being mortified (Goffman, *Asylums* 14) by writing down her thoughts and experiences as best she can in her little book:

> I am forcing myself to get everything clear in my mind by writing it down so I know where I am. There is no reality now except what I can sustain inside me. My memory is failing. I have to hang on to every scrap of information I have to keep my sanity, and it is for that purpose that I am keeping a journal. Then if I forget things later, I can always go back and read them here. (Sarton 10)

Caro knows she cannot fully trust herself: "The borderline between reality and fantasy is so thin in this confined, dreadfully lonely place" (26). It also becomes clear to the reader that Caro is not always a reliable narrator, and that she oscillates between reality and imagination, rationality, and senility (Maierhofer, *Salty* 331). Whether her narration is an accurate description of the nurses' sadistic dictatorship or if this is how Caro conceives and interprets what could merely be sloppiness and carelessness on the nurses' part is not important. What is more important is that the novel reveals the significance of her maintaining integrity in that she maintains her identity in life and death and counteracts the fragmentation of self (Maierhofer, *Salty* 331).[4]

Caro's journal serves as her map (a repeated image) that allows her to navigate the borderland between rationality and imagination: "So, in this way, this path inward and back into the past is like a map, the map of my world. If I can draw it accurately, I shall know where I am" (Sarton 10). I agree with Woodward, who reads this passage of knowing "where I am" as a "rejection of paternalism and the adoption of a conscious political position" (Woodward, "May" 122). By locating herself on this map, Caro Spencer strives to make the horrible conditions of her existence at Twin Elms, but also the way old people are treated in general, accessible to the public. Caro equates her experience of oppression to that of the African Americans' resistance: "I have my own ideas of what those beyond the pale do—the blacks, for instance. They finally come to see that violence is the only answer to oppression. They make bombs" Caro states (Sarton 107). Her diary "leads to an act of *guerilla warfare* inside the closed world of Twin Elms and, Spencer hopes, may have an influence outside it," Woodward notes ("May" 122). Not death itself is horrible, as Maierhofer puts it, but a life without dignity preceding death, and this is why Sarton argues for a dignified way of aging in spite of physical and mental restrictions (*Salty* 328).

Cora Sledge's writing in *Breaking Out of Bedlam* is also an act of "guerilla warfare," with her new pen used as a weapon in the fight, sharp as a knife: "You might notice I'm using a new pen. [...] It writes small and pointy, so I can fit more on the page. [...] I feel like I'm using a needle, or a knife, when I'm writing with it—like I'm ready to get down to business. [...] The black ink is good, too. Makes everything I write look important" (Larson 111). Hoping that their pen may be mightier than a sword, both Cora and Caro fight for self-determination. Finding words to write and re-write their life-course narratives is extremely important for them. Cora, especially, indulges in the process, and describes the act of writing with an expensive new fountain pen she finds in her drawer as an almost sensual pleasure. "It's beautiful: a deep wine color with a gold nib. The ink is *brown*! When you write, it looks like a treasure map" (Larson 111). In fact, her writing, like Caro Spencer's, maps out her life in front of her and shows her the way to a hidden treasure: her own life story, her identity. This metaphor recurs in the chapter "A Way Out" when Marcos, the gay Latino

4 „Deutlich wird im Roman, dass es vielmehr darum geht, die Integrität der Identität im Alter und im Tod zu bewahren und der Fragmentarisierung des Selbst entgegenzuwirken" (331).

technician who comes daily to bring Cora her inhaler (before secretly smoking cigarettes with her, a paradoxical visit), gives her a "big book of maps from the Day Room" (159). Cora, black and blue after a fall, has to stay in bed and puts it across her knees, using it as a writing table to state, "I'm making the best of it and catching up on my story" (159).

Cora also uses the pen to practice writing her own name, which is printed in the novel in what looks like her handwriting to emphasize the importance of this sensual act. "Coral Spring," she writes her maiden name, and below it "Cora Sledge," and finally "Mrs. Cora Kovic" (112). The names not only trace the development of her past marital status but also map out a future pathway; Kovic is the last name of Vitus, an Eastern European fellow resident with whom she has fallen head over heels in love. She secretly dreams of getting married to Vitus, who literally embodies life, and who encourages Cora to change hers. A very active and good-looking charmer, Vitus also seems to fancy Cora, and pays her frequent visits in her room. But Vitus Kovic is also presented as a trickster with a certain uncanny and mysterious aura around him. His handsome appearance makes him stand out from the other men in the home. There is no obvious reason why he would be in an assisted living facility since he is very fit, active, and healthy. He appears and disappears in unexpected places, and Cora can hardly ever locate him when she wants to see him in his room. When she does try to visit him, she gets lost in the home's hallways:

> There were little square plaques with the room numbers beside each door, odd on one side, even on the other. They could have been milestones for as long as it took me to get from one to the other, but I just kept plodding along, taking it one step at a time. I could feel that group behind be watching. Seemed like I was disappearing down a tunnel that kept getting darker and darker, and the smell got worse, too—the pee so shrill and strong it made my scalp tingle. (Larson 93)

The imagery used to describe her path is uncanny, and the description reads as if Cora were going further and further towards a forbidden place. The exhausting walks Cora undertakes in the home parallel the wanderings of her mind into her past; while she initially gets continuously lost, she manages to walk a little further every day, and the farther she gets, the closer she comes to being able to verbalize her repressed memories so they can find their way into her journal. On her first exhausting walk, she eventually manages to find Vitus's room, but he is not there. She keeps helplessly wandering about until she is exhausted and collapses into a wheelchair. "That mean nurse, Tanya" (97) eventually finds Cora in the hallway and pushes her back where she belongs. With her last remaining energy, she gets out her key to open the door (she had locked it because a couple of things had recently been stolen from her room), and finds Vitus sitting there, watching TV, eating her trail mix, and grinning. "You left it open," he says (98).

Social Death: Feeling Out of Place

Similar to Cora Sledge, Caro Spencer is also lost and "out of place" in the small, rural facility of Twin Elms. In contrast to Cora Sledge, she is the only woman resident among several men. Also, she is the "odd one out" because of obvious class differences: "It is terrible to have to admit that even here, one does not change one's class. I am a snob. I went to college, taught school for forty years, come of gentle people. [...] I have no peer, no one I can talk to" (Sarton 17). The nurses notice the difference as well, and ridicule her sophistication: "Of course she's a lady and we are a bit rough and ready for someone like her" (18) they contest, making it clear to her from the beginning that she should not expect special treatment (18). Caro cannot find any allies in the other residents, and feels isolated: "I look at them from very far away as if they were in the distance, across a wide river. We have nothing in common. Why pretend that we do?" (82). Her loneliness is particularly hard to endure, and the constant threat and paralyzing pressure put on her by the head nurse makes her life almost unbearable. This leads to what Haim Hazan has called "social death"—a death that precedes biological death: "A person begins to lose social roles and cultural identity prior to the termination of biological existence. The interval between social death and physical death may span a period of many years, and it is one of the fundamental elements of our culture in relation to the aged," Hazan states (*Old Age* 69). Caro writes in her diary to prevent herself from suffering a "social death," but her efforts to resist and keep a "social life" become more difficult every day.

After a few days, she has already internalized the institutional gaze in the panoptical world of surveillance: "After a short time, even a very few days here, one begins to feel like an animal in a cage. Even if the door were open, one would not dare move" (Sarton 22). The novel mirrors what Michel Foucault writes in *Discipline and Punish* when he describes the effect of the panopticon "to induce in the inmate a state of conscious and permanent visibility that assures the automatic functioning of power [...] in short, that the inmates should be caught up in a power situation of which they are themselves the bearers" (*Discipline* 201). Caro is constantly aware of the surveillance, which makes it difficult for her to communicate with her only ally, Mr. Standish Flint, a retired farmer who is almost deaf and suffering from cancer and bedsores, but who is appreciative of Caro's clear mind and resistance. Despite his lack of hearing, Standish Flint is as angry as Caro, and rebels against the nurses Harriet and Rose by hiding his tranquilizers, refusing food, and offending them by shouting obscenities at them. Rose is particularly offended by Flint's "expatiat[ing] on their enormous bums and breasts" and his "repertoire of dirty jokes" (Sarton 26). Waxman (*From* 151) interprets the narration of Flint's survival tactic ("his chief escape is sexual fantasy," Sarton 26) as a deconstruction of the stereotype that sexuality and senescence are mutually exclusive, an interpretation that Woodward, in her interpretation of Sarton's text, reads as part of "a critique of our cultural devaluation of elders" ("May" 115, also quoted in Waxman, *Hearth* 151).

While sexuality is an integral component of their very being for both Caro and Standish Flint, it is an absolute taboo in the institution. Flint's dirty jokes make Rose cry, Caro, on the contrary, finds them "quite funny" (Sarton 26), but regrets that she cannot tell him about her life in return: "I suppose he imagines I am an old maid—I could tell him some things but they are not to be shouted. [...] The conversational opportunities here are certainly at a minimum" (Sarton 26). Sexuality has always been an important aspect of Caro's life; for instance, in the journal she narrates how she followed her secret (married) lover, Alex, to France. But because Standish Flint needs to be shouted at, developing any closer friendship is difficult; the walls seem to have ears. She can hardly talk to him openly as "there is a house law that doors must not be closed. The two women are always in and out of every room, and one never knows when they are listening" (18). The panoptization of the inmates transforms them from human beings into subjects, and creates their "otherness," as Caro asserts: "We are talked about always as 'them,' as if we were abandoned animals thrown out of a car" (16).

When Standish Flint dies lonely "in the ambulance among total strangers" (70), Caro is depressed and feels guilty for having betrayed him; after all, it was she who initiated a medical inspection of the facility through a comment to Reverend Thornhill. The inspectors take Mr. Flint, who wants nothing but die in peace, to hospital against his will. "His battle to die with dignity in his own way was lost" (70), she writes, and her description of the dehumanizing procedures to which dying Mr. Flint is subjected is evocative of psychiatrist Elisabeth Kübler-Ross's famous book *On Death and Dying*, in which she emphasizes the importance of "interpersonal human relationships" (9) at the end of life through which the fears, anxieties, and hopes of a dying person can be expressed.

Twin Elms defies all such principles, and undermines all human relationships. After her only ally's death, Caro feels extremely lonely. The nurses, she believes, punish her for triggering the home's medical inspection, and prevent Reverend Thornhill's daughter Lisa from visiting her, arguing that a visit would not do Ms. Spencer any good. Caro had been looking forward to the young girl's visit, which she sees as a lifeline to the world outside. "The door that had opened a crack is being slammed shut," Caro writes (77). She craves the Thornhill family's visits because they are the only meaningful communication she receives. "The fact is that I am dying for lack of love. Exactly as though the oxygen in my lungs were being slowly diminished" (116).

Reclaiming Agency

For Cora Sledge, Vitus is the bearer of meaning. The more she sees of him, the more she feels alive: "When I'm around him, my whole body feels like it's covered with little mouths sucking in fresh air" (139). She here uses a similar metaphor—that of breathing—which connects love to life. Cora craves Vitus: "I can hardly contain myself. Vitus is like a new place I got to go" (173), she writes. She wants to discover his body, and indulges in sexual fantasies. As in Caro Spencer's journal, sexuality also plays an important role in Cora's. Not only does she narrate her past sexual life, but also focuses on her strong desires in old age. She notes down her fantasies very explicitly, and once even manages to push Vitus onto her bed, but is disappointed. He escapes, excusing himself politely, and leaves Cora wondering whether his impotence has to do with her obesity or his age. In her journal, Cora expresses her sexual wishes, and merges her present urges with past memories, emphasizing that her old age and physical weakness have nothing to with her sexual desire.

Together with her sexual activity, which serves as a catalyst, her wish to live a full life again is reinforced by Vitus. With the help of her diary she develops a three-step plan: "Before I get too far in this book, here's a list of things I want to do: 1. Wean myself off these pills. [...] 2. Get to walking [...]. 3. Get me some new clothes" (117–18). Cora's cutting down on pills initially allows her to go cold turkey:

> I wake up in the middle of the night with the sweat pouring off me and the feeling that I been chased up and down dark alleys by an army of zombies.

> Sometimes the terror in my chest is so strong I have to curl up like a cutworm and pull the blankets over my head. I been that far from pushing the panic button. [...] There are times when [...] my head is a storm of black water swirling like a whirlpool. (116).

In contrast to the feelings of terror that assail Caro Spencer, Cora knows that the nightmares she endures actually are indicative of progress. She gets better and better, starts a short walking routine, and loses weight. Soon, her children begin to congratulate her on her rejuvenation, as does the home's doctor: "Mrs. Sledge, according to these records, you've lost sixty-one pounds in six months. Your blood pressure has dropped twenty points. Your heart rate is down over 10 percent and you haven't refilled your prescriptions for tranquilizers, antidepressants, or sleeping aids" (Larson 190). Her diary helps her to recuperate even further, and soon she is ready to work through her buried and partially repressed memories:

> I wish I could see everybody's faces when they lay eyes on all these pages, every one of them covered with words I wrote myself, with no help from anybody. I marvel at it myself. Sometimes I flip through just to see all that ink. I can't help but think how miserable I was when I started that first book, the one with the lavender on the cover. I would just as soon have died as go on living. What a whole different world it is now. Still, with all that's happening here right now and so many things to think about, I got in the back of my mind that other story, the one that happened so long ago. It's with me night and day, in my dreams, in my every waking moment. I'm getting that story straight for the first time in my life. I'm *letting* myself see what happened, watching myself like I was in a movie. Sounds crazy, but for the first time I see a person who was struggling, groping in the dark. (Larson 196)

Cora Sledge prepares to confront herself with her past, and the process of writing is a conscious one: "It feels so strange to write this down. To pick the words and set them down next to each other [...] when all those years I've only seen it in pictures" (227). Up to that point, she had had no words for her trauma. Cora goes through a phase of abjection and panic, but finally manages to say her dead baby's name again: "*Alice.* I haven't let myself say that name for so long, much less write it. Shape it, writing the mountain of that first letter, lifts the corner on a whole world of sorrow" (225). Cora recounts the story of how she found her first baby, Alice, dead in the crib, and how she has blamed herself for Alice's death, believing it happened because she had not wanted the baby when she first learned of her pregnancy. Alice's death, her subsequent guilt, and nauseating self-hatred lead to Cora's panic attacks and almost lethal depression. However, she also recounts how Abel always stood by her, and never mentioned that Alice, for whom he also grieved, was not his child. Neither he nor Cora ever told their younger children about their half-sister—a secret she anticipates that they will learn while reading the journal.

The thought of Abel comforts Cora, although narrating her trauma pulls her back into the past: "Writing about Alice plunks me right down in the middle of those tormented times" (232). Cora is comforted by Abel's ghost who begins to appear, rushing to her help whenever she needs him, just as when he was still alive: "You might think this part was a dream, too, but you'd be wrong. [...] I could tell without him saying a word, that he'd come to take care of me [...] I felt such comfort having him there" (234). Cora is able to remember more and more details of her repressed past. As Larson obviously pays attention to her characters' names, it could be argued that just like Vitus makes Cora come alive again, Cora's memories of Abel make her "able," in a way he always had.

Cora resumes writing, and recognizes it as an act of creativity: "I love the look of these books, every damn page covered with my writing that I labored over sitting alone here in this room, casting my mind back to all them places, recalling things I didn't know I remembered. The books are thicker when I fill them than they are when they're brand-new. The pages suck up my life and get fat with my thoughts" (235). As her story gains weight, and she loses weight, her books take up more and more space, and so does Cora herself:

> Ever since that night I walked up to Vitus's room, I found out how far I can go by just putting one foot in front of the other one. Let me tell you that seeing the people around here, people with their legs swollen up, or missing altogether, or dangling like limp noodles from their bodies—not to mention the ones stuck in wheelchairs parked in a puddle of piss—has convinced me that, hard as it is, I got to keep moving. They'll never let me out of here if I can't get around, so every day I go a little farther, even if it's just a few steps. I stop and rest whenever I need to, but I'm finding out that I can do more and more. I walk out there in the courtyard, down the hall, even out to the lobby. (117)

The only danger she now fears is that the brown ink stemming from the new pen might get her into trouble. As a lot of things have recently gone missing from residents' rooms, including Cora's, and the administration accuses her of having stolen the beautiful pen. As a matter of fact, the thefts have been going on for quite a while, and when Cora's crystal, a very important talisman, goes missing, it slowly becomes clearer to the reader that Vitus may have had something to do with the thefts. Cora has to get rid of her journal and the pen, and just when she is about to throw both items into the dumpster, Abel suddenly appears, and advises her to tape the pen to the underside of her nightstand, and to put the book under the rug by her bed to conceal it, saving her memories, her past, her present, and her future.

Caro Spencer in *As We Are Now* also briefly learns how love can change her life, and the bleakness of the institution is relativized. A lifeline is cast to her when a new nurse, Anna Close, whose name suggests intimacy and care, substitutes for Harriet, who goes on holidays for a fortnight. For the first time during her stay at Twin Elms, Caro feels understood and truly taken care of: "It is being cared for as though I were worthy of care. It is being not humiliated but treasured" (92), she writes in her journal. Anna, the "angelic person" (82) is "pure human goodness" (100), and Caro literally flourishes along with her surroundings: "The rose has opened during the day. I have lain here for an hour really paying attention to it. And now I think I'll go and sit outdoors" (84). She allows herself to expand her radius of action and leave the house to sit in the sun outside. Her change of mood is triggered solely by Anna's understanding of Caro's situation. "These are wonderful days. […] I do not really want to die at all these days. I am avid for life" (92). Her narrative is a clear expression of the intertwining of identity and place; as her mood changes, she also describes her surroundings in a drastically different way. Caro is overwhelmed by the way Anna treats her, stating, "[s]he seems to understand me in a way I have needed for years. The room feels airy and clean when she has been there with her magic touch" (92). "We can read this politically," Woodward argues, "a temporary alliance with a trusted, honorable half-member of the administration is possible. Sisterhood can be sustaining" ("May" 123). Caro's bond with Anna intensifies during the brief period, and she falls in love with her.

Soon, the walls again seem to close in on Caro, because Anna's departure approaches. "I am about to die," Caro writes, "Harriet comes back on Saturday […] When Anna told me this morning, […] I was falling through space in a state of uncontrollable panic" (Sarton 97). She cannot stop crying because she is aware of the fact that the institution's structure will inevitably reassert itself (Woodward, "May" 123). Caro can no longer sit outside—the sun has disappeared, and it is too cold (Sarton 103). Caro's mood is expressed metaphorically through the weather, the surroundings, and the light. She feels the threat of slipping back into the uncanny empty space, devoid of communication: "I endure in a vacuum" (102) she writes after Harriet returns, reinstalling her hellish regime (100). Thinking of Anna, she states, "she is 'outside,' safe. I am inside, in danger of despair and madness" (103). In order to stay "close" to Anna, she writes her a letter that she copies into her diary. Harriet, wanting to control her residents, reads Caro's journal, and exposes her relationship with Anna. She humiliates her, accusing her of being a lesbian, and calls her a "dirty old woman": "'This is no place for queers,' she said. 'We'll have you in the State Hospital" (106). By threatening to send them to the State Hospital, the administrator keeps her residents under control. Homosexuality, in the head nurse's eyes, needs to be punished; it is seen as a "stigma" (Goffman, *Stigma* 13), as is frailty or dementia. If the amount of care required by a patient increases, or if they misbehave, they can no longer stay at Twin Elms. In a traditional American narrative expressing fear of state institutions, the State Hospital is represented as even worse than Twin Elms: Caro knows that going to the State Hospital, where Standish Flint was also sent, means entering a kind of limbo state, the "banished existence in the land of the fourth space" (Hazan, "Beyond" 91). There, she fears she would be drugged, "put to sleep, [...] kept in a state of lethargy" (Sarton 107). Caro is aware of the mortifying practices of the institution, of her impending social death. Annette Leibing's work resonates with this passage. She draws on Giorgio Agamben's concept of bare life—a body stripped of personhood (Agamben 4)—to describe a "space without rights located between life and death, [...] a frightening no man's land" (Leibing 249). Someone who inhabits this space, she explains, becomes a "living dead" person, leading what Agamben calls "a life devoid of value" (Leibing 249). Caro expresses this state in her diary: "I have been murdered. Murdered in the most cruel of ways possible. [...] I do not address myself any more as Caro. Caro is dead [...] that person has ceased to exist. Someone else, mentally ill, tortured, hopeless, has taken over my body and my mind. I am in the power of evil" (107–09), she writes in her journal. Twin Elms, Caro begins to understand, may never become a place where she will be allowed to die in dignity. She also suffers because what she ultimately learns from this experience is that "it is virtually impossible to make oneself whole and die intact, uncastrated, in this institution" (Waxman, *From* 151).

Epiphanies of Self-Determination

With this awareness, her frustration reaches a peak, and turns into pure anger. "The institution's systematic repression of the positive, uniting forces of love necessarily generates an equal and opposite force that eventually erupts in violence," Woodward asserts ("May" 123). While the first part of Caro's diary is dedicated to her wish to reach wholeness, to grow mature, and ripen towards death, the second half is given over to an expression of anger and frustration. It culminates in a moment of epiphany after Anna's departure: "But with it came a flash of insight. [...] It was that things can be changed here, but only by violent action. If I lose my temper I will be put in the dark again. But if I burn the place down some day I can open this locked world. [...] I was staggered by the flash of what I conceived" (Sarton 89).

This moment of epiphany, during which Caro Spencer decides to burn Twin Elms down with cans of lighter fluid, is mirrored and distorted in Larson's novel as Cora Sledge's "eyes lit on the gasoline" (114) in the garden. While Sarton's Caro talks about death, Larson's Cora comes alive. She sits outside in the sun, watching the gardener take the lawn mower apart, with the gasoline can beside him:

> You've seen them—they're metal, about the size and shape of a toaster, bright red. I don't know how long I'd been looking at it when my breath caught in my throat. My chest heaved, my chin wobbled, and before I knew what was going on, I was sobbing. Tears streamed down my face like a river. You know why? Just that goddamn color. *Red*. The red of that can was the purest, brightest red I'd ever seen. I'd forgotten that color, and right then it all came rushing back to me. [...] (Larson 114)

A wave of the memories about the color red sweeps over Cora, among them memories of her mother's lipstick and a candy apple from Halloween, but most importantly the "frost of blood that covered my little angel the very first time I laid eyes on her. [...] All that. And me, too. The stone I'm named after. Coral" (115). Her daughter's birth is equated with her return to life:

> I hadn't seen a color like that in years. That's when I realized, plain as day, that them drugs was leaving me. I was waking up from a long sleep. I sat on that metal chair still as a statue, my eyes fixed on that red can, while I thought about all the things I'd missed living in a world with colors as bleached out as a faded snapshot. [...] The sun shifted and a breeze came up. It played in the hair on my arms and the back of my neck. It tickled the creases of my arms and the corners of my eyes like God himself breathing on me. The branches of the trees quivered, the leaves twirled, the clouds slipped across the sky. Everything around me moved and breathed. I was in the middle of it, sitting in the metal chair." (Larson 116)

As opposed to the home in *As We Are Now*, Cora is not mortified by the institution. On the contrary, her "social death" had occurred at home, while the institution provides the framework that enables her rejoin life. Although the home is—perhaps as a matter of convention that is determined by the genre of the nursing home novel—portrayed as a panopticon in terms of its floor plan, described as a "half prison, half hospital" (296), and the surveillance ("They slept with their doors open. Maybe it was a rule," 307) is depicted as a number of debatable institutional safety regulations enforced in the nursing wing, Cora Sledge is aware of the fact that she was lost, and is only now finding herself while in the home. *Breaking Out of Bedlam*, the novel's title, can, thus, be read as not only a description of Cora's liberation from the home, but as her escape from her own mental turmoil. Cora finds keeping her journey extremely painful, but she sees her time in the home and the journal she keeps as a way to complete her life, and to complete herself:

> I was a stranger to myself, somebody I hardly recognized. I try to figure out when I lost track of myself. Must have been my late twenties, early thirties. Now that my brain is clearing up, I'm getting to know myself a little now. Thoughts passing through my mind, they're new to me. Feeling things, seeing things. Like a newborn baby. It scares the living shit out of me. You might wonder, Why now? and believe me, so do I. Something happened to me is all I can say. Vitus is part of it, and coming to this place. Getting to this age of my life. Thinking I got to the end and finding there's still a ways to go. It's only these flashes I have, flashes of remembering myself like I used to be, that make me feel that some part of me is still out there somewhere, alive. (Larson 117)

Cora's relationship with Vitus serves as a catalyst for her self-determination. Although she knows hardly anything about him, and despite her children's warnings, she agrees to marry him. He proposes to her while giving her an emerald ring—a ring she feels she cannot wear because something is wrong with it, but the prospect of getting married, and moving back into her own house together with Vitus changes her life entirely. She does not think that she will stay in The Palisades until the end of her life anymore, and asks her daughter to tell the lodgers living in her house that they will have to move out because she is coming back: "I ain't senile and I ain't crippled! For all you know I could live twenty more years" (Larson 212).

Cora's children are alarmed and mistrust Vitus. As the novel soon reveals, they have a reason to do so. Larson here plays with a motif frequently employed in nursing home novels—parents fighting against staying in the home, and children fighting against new relationships that could endanger their inheritance. In this case, Cora's children are presented as having no choice. Vitus is a crook who has been to jail, he has been married to three wives and, as is soon revealed, is the thief that the home's administration has been looking for. The necklace, emerald ring, and fountain pen, which were Vitus' gifts for Cora, have all been stolen. Cora is devastated when her children finally manage to convince her that she has been tricked by Vitus. The worst disappointment occurs, however, when she learns that Vitus had been officially blaming all the thefts on Cora in order to conceal his homosexual relationship with Renato, a twenty-year old Filipino nursing student, whom he had also been supporting with sales of the stolen goods.

Cora is shattered and withdraws into her room for five days, numbs herself with sleeping pills, and prays that she will never wake up again. But on the sixth day, she knows she will not give up: "Not yet. I am not ready to go away yet" (291). She runs a bath and lies down in the hot water—literally and metaphorically cleansing herself, and rethinks her relationship with Vitus. "When I was clean and dry, with fresh clothes and combed hair, I felt light, like those astronauts floating around in space" (291). She finds Vitus and confronts him. When he tells her that he is leaving, she sees him "walking out of [her] life forever" (295). "I had just the tiniest bit of breath in my lungs. 'At least I loved you true,' I said as he walked past. 'Everybody makes mistakes.' Without turning around, he raised his hand and twiddled his fingers good-bye" (294).

The next two chapters of the novel, named "The Key" and "The Hole," finally weave the two narrative strands together and reveal the last details of Cora's secret. Instead of being devastated and heart-broken, she realizes that she has managed to find her own strength, a strength that is not dependent on anybody else. Cora does not see her love for Vitus as having been a mistake. Rather, she now knows that she is capable of true feelings again. "I loved him pure, and no matter what he did or didn't do, that feeling made me well. It brought me back to life" (304). She is happy to have met and loved Vitus: "It was so simple, I laughed. Vitus, I thought. He gave me the key. He might not have known what he was doing, but he set things in motion, bought me my ticket out of here" (297).

After Vitus leaves for good, Cora sleeps well for the first time in years, and talks to Abel, who keeps appearing as a ghost. "'It ain't over, Toad,' he said. 'You got things to do.' [...] I never meant for you to be shut up in a prison. It ain't right. Don't let them kids jerk you around, Toad. Take matters into your own hands. Do what you need to do'" (296). Cora's decision to move back into her old house provides the last piece of the puzzle, which fills a gap in her memory. "The Hole" narrates how Abel and Cora buried a baby, Alice. "Nothing in my life could have prepared me for the sinister sight of that gaping pit. Seeing a wood box lowered into the ground with your own child inside is something you can't fathom unless it happens to you," she writes in her journal (299). "Two days later, here I was. A different person in a different world" (299). Cora verbalizes the shame, guilt, and love that she felt for Alice. After the funeral, Alice becomes a secret that neither Abel nor Cora ever speak about, and Cora states, "This is what I'm starting to realize as I write all this about Alice, like my eyes have slowly been opening" (300).

> Talking about Alice has been like burying her all over again, but this time I feel like I'm putting her to rest, like she can finally sleep. She can stop this feverish living inside me and go be with her own kind, go to that other place and leave me be. Now that I have told my story, it's like I was looking down on myself from up above, like there's no ceiling to my room and from the sky I saw me in the middle of this cinder-block square, sitting here in this chair with my book in front of me. It has been my lifeline, the rope pulling me back to myself. Cora Sledge, I forgive you. I pity the girl you were and the shame you've suffered. I'm not feeling sorry for you like I've done year after year. I'm opening my heart to the sorrow I feel. Though the tears are sluicing down my face and I'm rocking back and forth here in my chair, I feel a calm because I forgive you. A space is opening in my heart. I didn't know how much pain there was until now, when it melted away and peace came in to take its place. (300)

In this passage, Cora calls out to herself, names herself, and forgives herself, which can be read as a process of re-claiming of her own identity. She has learned to accept herself, which has been a painful struggle that has now come to conclusion, leading her to a peaceful wholeness from which she can start anew. This passage shows that even in old age (Cora is 82) reclaiming one's identity, and re-narrating the course of one's life is possible. As she says to her daughter Glenda, "[f]or all you know I could live twenty more years" (Larson 212).

As Glenda is reluctant to let her mother move back into her own house, Cora needs to find her own way to take care of things. In a final act of revenge against "Poison Ivy," the table mate she hates so much, Cora wears the emerald ring Vitus had given her. She knows by now that it has been stolen from Ivy, but displays it, glittering, on her finger in the dining room. Ivy furiously reports Cora to the administrator. Cora is called into the head nurse's office, but denies having had anything to do with the theft. Soon after, Glenda phones Cora to tell her that she has to come and pick her up. "The little click when she hung up sounded like a key unlocking a door" (304), Cora writes, enjoying her newly won freedom. Almost nostalgically, she walks towards the Day Room she had hated so much. "I'm proud of myself for coming out the other side," she states. During her tour, Cora suddenly feels that she needs to go to Vitus's room:

> It wasn't until I got inside and the door slid closed again that I wondered what in the world I was doing. There I went again—down, down, down, to the bowels of the earth, even though it was one floor up. When the door slid open, I'd traveled back to the time when lunatics were chained to the walls of deep, dark dungeons. The empty corridor stretched out in front of me. A dark echo clanged in my ears. The smell of piss and sweat was thick. Down toward the end of the hall someone yelled, the icy sound of a nightmare. I stepped out in the hall and started walking. (306–07)

In a setting that resembles hell, she finds Vitus's empty room, and is magically drawn towards his bed and dresser. This journey into the "dungeons" is comparable to a psychological journey into the underworld of Cora's own psyche. Only by fighting the demons there (she has to get past Vitus's roommate, Daniel, who looks like a vampire with his apnea sleeping mask: "His skin was the color of skim milk. He flashed his fangs at me," 308), can she overcome her sense of fragmentation, fear, and self-loathing. The space of the care home is metaphorically used to emphasize Cora's journey. Opening all the drawers, she finds her crystal, the rock her father gave her before she married Abel, in the bottom one. It had always represented a treasure to her, and was a thing she could hold on to, which gave her strength. She was devastated when it was stolen from her room, and is now filled with of happiness as she regains it. Finally finding the crystal makes Cora whole, so that she can prepare to leave the home.

The book ends with "My Prayer," the final chapter, in which Cora waits for Glenda to pick her up. "Can you picture me sitting at my own kitchen table, drinking coffee out of my own cup? [...] Climbing into my own bed at night and in the morning stepping out on the porch and looking out across the yard?" she writes as one of the last entries (310). "There are some blank pages left in this book, clean and white without a thing written on them. I got no more use for it. I am going home" (310). The journal has fulfilled its function: Cora is making peace with her life. "Now I have a prayer," she ends the journal, "Heal my heart. Please, I ask. Calm its pain, soothe its scars. Keep it open, Lord, despite everything—reaching for life, ready to love" (311).

Similar to Cora Sledge's narration, *As We Are Now* can and has been read by age critics such as Waxman (*Hearth*), Woodward ("May Sarton"), and Maierhofer (*Salty*) as a provocative narrative of an old woman's search for identity. It is through the creative act of writing, they argue unanimously, that Caro's strength and resistance manifest themselves. Even when she portrays herself as a helpless old woman, she impressively counteracts society's treatment of old people. The same holds true for Cora in *Breaking Out of Bedlam*. For both women, the creative act of writing leads them to acts of self-composition, and "serves to critique our cultural devaluation of the elderly" (Woodward, "May" 146). Whereas at the beginning, Caro Spencer still sees the home as "the house where I have to come to terms with everything, sort it all out, accept it all, I think that it might be salvation, a rock in which to stand at least" (Sarton 24), the salvation takes on a different shape than she had expected. Like Cora Sledge, she sees her time in the home and the journal she keeps as a way to complete her life, to complete herself: "There are things I have to do inside myself before I can die. And I have the belief that [...] we ripen toward death, and only when the fruit is ripe may it drop" (19).

Ripening and Liberation

Barbara Frey Waxman uses this image of maturity in her definition of the genre of the "novels of ripening," "I call this genre, in a feminist literary critic's act of naming, the *Reifungsroman,* or novel of ripening—, opposing its central tenet to the usual notion of deterioration in old age. The name is inspired by septuagenarian writer May Sarton's optimistic concept of 'ripening towards death in a fruitful way'" (Waxman, *From* 2). Both *Breaking Out of Bedlam* and *As We Are Now* are novels of ripening that emphasize aspects of growth in their main characters. Through the creative act of writing the journal, Maierhofer argues with reference to *As We Are Now*, Caro confronts herself with her own identity and her finiteness (*Salty* 329). Like Cora Sledge, Caro Spencer writes, "I am interested in me. I am a long way still from the fulfillment, the total self-understanding that I long for now. I remain a mystery to myself. I want to get right down to the core, make a final perfect equation before I am through, balance it all up into a tidy *whole*" (Sarton 24). She sees fulfilment as a goal. She expresses this through the use of spatial terms ("a long way," "to the core"), terms that suggest that after investing an effort, she might arrive at the goal, which is both a spatial and temporal expression. As soon as she realizes that the institution does not facilitate, but blocks her attainment of this goal, a moment of epiphany reveals new insights to her: "I have believed since I came here that I was here to prepare for death, but I did not yet know how to do it. [...] I see, now that death is not a vague prospect but something I hold in my hand, that the very opposite is required from what I thought at first" (Sarton 126). It is Caro's own responsibility—she can locate her life and death, again spatially, herself. In other words, to reaffirm her integrity and to liberate herself, as Waxman contends (*From* 156), she must take control of her own life—through suicide and collective euthanasia, which she understands her act of burning down the home to mean. From this perspective, the two novels are fundamentally different, although both advocate personal agency. While Cora opts for life, Caro chooses death—the most radical form of agency. By controlling her own death, she becomes "ripe or fully mature at the end of her life" (*From* 156). Disengaging herself from any relationships, Caro describes her liberation from her worldly existence:

> It is strange that now that I have made my decision I can prepare for death in a wholly new way. I feel free, beyond attachment, beyond the human world at last. I rejoice as if I were newborn, seeing with wide-open eyes, as only the old can (for the newborn infant cannot see) the marvels of the world. [...] Everything mundane falls away. (Sarton 125–26)

She also liberates herself in terms of spatial confinements ("beyond the human world"), placing herself deliberately outside the symbolic order. The association she draws between her newly achieved freedom and that of a newborn invites a Lacanian reading of her identity development. Kathleen Woodward has masterfully expanded the Lacanian concept of the mirror stage of infancy to old age. In "The Mirror Stage of Old Age" she argues, "[i]n the mirror stage of infancy, the infant enters the imaginary. In the mirror stage of old age, the subject enters the social realm reserved for 'senior citizens' in the western world. But the point is that the subject *denies* this identification rather than embraces it. The mirror stage of old age is the inverse of the mirror stage of infancy" (*Aging* 67). The infant perceives the image of his or her body as a harmoniously whole and ideal unit, simultaneously experiencing the body as uncoordinated.

The mirror stage of the infant is a stage prior to socialization, and the mirror stage of old age is its exact opposite; it is a stage during which the *image* is experienced as fragmented, threatening, and alienating:

> Alienation characterizes the mirror stage of old age (alienation is embedded in language, of course) but in a different sense as well, and the terms are reversed: the harmonious whole resides within the subject, and the *imago* prefigures disintegration and "nursling dependence." If the infant holds his mirror image in an amorous gaze, the elderly person resists it. The narcissistic impulse remains—it imposes itself upon all our desires—but it is directed against the mirror image. (Woodward, "Instant" 60)

In Sarton's text, Caro Spencer experiences herself as whole, but perceives the image of her face in fragments:

> Can this worn-out, haunted old body be me? My eyes used to be so blue, but now they have faded. And my mouth, rather stern at best, looks thin-lipped. Deep lines pull it downward. My neck anyway is pretty good for an old bird—none of these scrawny tendons showing. My pearl choker hides the wrinkles. But time at a mirror is worse than wasted time, Caro. It makes you feel depressed. Better turn the mirror to the wall. (Sarton 29)

As the child passes through the mirror stage, he or she becomes a social being, but the old person dissociates him- or herself from society during this stage, which may "precipitate the loss of the imaginary," as Woodward writes. "Where would we then be located? Outside the mirror?" she asks (*Aging* 69). Here, Woodward makes it explicit where old women are, in Kristeva's terms, located; they are pushed beyond the symbolic order—outside the social body, rendered "abject" (Kristeva 4). Sarton argues against this abjection of old people, who are hidden from sight in nursing homes. As she planned in the beginning of the book, Caro now arrives at the core of her existence, albeit in a different way than she had expected. As Caro feels her soul will not be able to grow in the dreadful institution ("I treasure my soul as something given into my keeping, something that I must keep intact—more, in a state of growth and awareness whatever the odds," 19), she realizes that she can only find fulfilment by preparing for her own rebirth through death: "Impending death is the catalyst that makes Caro appreciate life and brings her to fruition," Waxman observes (156). Her act of setting fire to Twin Elms can be seen as an act of social criticism, Waxman continues to write:

> [It is] a moral gesture of resistance to its evil and her humiliating treatment there, a gesture asserting her humanness, courage, integrity, and self-completion. In cleansing the place, she also acts as a social critic, sounding the clarion against society's cruel treatment of the dependent elderly: Caro "transforms her death into an indictment of society's attitudes toward the aged and the infirm" (Bakerman 21). (Waxman, *From* 156)

She symbolically and literally incinerates the home, and therefore has the power to act; her agency is not undermined by the symbolic order or by institutional rules and regulations, and the panoptical structure she observes still cannot prevent her from rebelling against ageism, "a nod to Foucault's insistence that the possibility of resistance and revolt are embedded within disciplinary discourses of power," as Gravagne puts it (46).

In 1973, Sarton's novel touched a nerve with regard to institutional eldercare. It was written at a time when nursing home inspections had just become mandatory. After the change in Social Security Laws (1950), which required the establishment of a standard-setting or licensing agency that would set minimum standards for nursing homes (Garvin and Burger 54) and also reinforce them, inspections became more frequent. The first official accreditation program for nursing homes was created in 1966 by the Joint Commission on Health Care Organizations (JCAHO), an organization that has long been known for accrediting hospitals (Stahl). These standards included fire prevention mechanisms, such as sprinklers, which were previously not common in homes. Garvin and Burger in their book *Where They Go to Die: The Tragedy of America's Aged* dedicate a whole chapter to nursing home fires: "The deadliest place in America today is not the highway or the slums of Harlem—it is the nursing home," (97) they contend. It can claim all the superlatives (98): "During the sixties, a reportable nursing home fire has occurred at an average of more than one a day. [...] Nursing home fires have increased—with a sudden upsurge in 1961 starting the trend" (98).

Because many newspapers reported nursing home fires that occurred in the late 1960s and early 1970s, it is very likely that Sarton's book drew inspiration from these events. While the majority of fires were reported to have been started accidentally, for instance by cigarettes, after a patient smoked in bed and fell asleep, as Garvin and Burger point out (99), Caro Spencer's deadly rebellion goes a step further: it is an act of rebellion performed to catch attention from society.

Sarton's story strongly urges for a reform of eldercare. Caro Spencer's identity, as Maierhofer claims (*Salty* 337), is not endangered by the threat of death, but by the inhumane treatment she experiences in old age. Although she is at her caretakers' mercy, she manages to write a manifesto of her identity, hoping it will reach a large audience of all ages. The book, Maierhofer contends, is an angry demand for an adequate place in society for old women as well. Equating strength and power with sickness and death might initially seem contradictory, but the text itself proves that such equality is possible (337).

The different versions of the book's cover that appeared when it came out in 1973 and 1992, respectively, also highlight the re-interpretation of the novel in terms of the protagonist's individual identity. While the first edition's black-and-white cover made by Penguin in 1973 shows a gray, wintery landscape against which a tall, old tree and parts of the façade of a small brick house in the countryside stand out, which emphasize the aspects of space and place, the later version (Norton 1992) graphically supports an approach that focuses on the protagonist's life-course narrative. Maierhofer points out the difference between the two covers in *Salty Old Women* (338): the newer version contains various items that are colorfully arranged in what looks like a scrapbook. A picture of a young woman looking straight at the camera has been placed in the center; a clock face; several dried leaves and roses; some postage stamps; a delicate necklace with little hearts; several matches (both burned and unused); and some singed pages from what looks like a journal, hinting at the novel's plotline ("a lapis lazuli pin, a faded rose petal, once pink, slipped into the pages of this copybook" (121) are displayed. The change in the design of the covers not only supports a different reading experience, but also points out aspects of social development with regard to the way women's aging is interpreted (Maierhofer, *Salty* 338). Maierhofer particularly emphasizes the importance of a women's search for self during old age. Sarton's protagonist, she maintains, is a "salty old woman" (a term also used by Waxman), who refuses to adapt to social norms. By consciously emphasizing these aspects of the novel, Maierhofer argues, we as readers can overcome one-sided interpretations of such stories, and open up to new methods of interpretation in order to do justice to the female protagonists with regard to their dignity and integrity, with all the inconsistencies this entails (*Salty* 338–39).

Sarton skillfully employs the nursing home as a setting of a fight for justice. Twin Elms serves as a spatial metaphor that localizes the horrors of a life depraved of social and cultural recognition, through the "othering" of old age. It literally represents the social and cultural "metaphorical black hole" of the fourth age, the "shadowlands of disability, diminishment, and death" as Peter Laslett describes the "fourth age" in *A Fresh Map of Life* (Gilleard and Higgs, "Aging" 126). Haim Hazan's concept of the "fourth space" resonates with Caro Spencer's existential crisis. Caro finds herself in danger of being drawn into the "fourth space" when she writes, "[a]mong all the other deprivations here we are deprived of *expression*. The old men slowly atrophy because no one asks them what they feel and why. Could they speak if someone did?" (Sarton 82). Caro Spencer, however, fights against being colonized, as Hazan expresses it, by writing her diary.

While *As We Are Now* takes a political stance, *Breaking Out of Bedlam* primarily focuses on an individual's traumatic past. Larson's text also advocates for a woman's individualism, self-determination and agency in old age. In this sense, both novels can be read as powerful narratives that overcome the confinement and challenge the borders of the "unknown country of old age," as Sarton famously spatialized this experience.

3.3 Sentenced to *Half Life*

The setting in John Mighton's play *Half Life*,[5] which won the prestigious Canadian Governor General Award in 2006, is an old fashioned, prison-like facility, and its residents are treated as inmates rather than as patients, clients, or residents. In fact, the play, like Sarton's novel, can be read as a portrayal of a "total institution." It tells the story of Clara and Patrick, two octogenarians who live in a nameless Canadian home for veterans and their families and form a romantic relationship. While Clara is developing dementia, Patrick's identity as a veteran is linked to national memory (Goldman 118). Whether they had actually been lovers earlier in their lives or whether they only imagine having had a wartime love affair becomes increasingly unimportant throughout the play. What counts is that they now enjoy each other's presence. Although their relationship seems to give meaning to their lives and makes them very happy, their love is seen as intolerable by both the institution's management and their respective children.

Patrick's 40-something year old daughter, Anna, an artist, finds it only a little less difficult than Clara's son, Donald, a psychology professor and expert

5 I am referring to the original script, not a performance.

in artificial intelligence, to cope with her feelings about her father having an affair with Clara. Especially Donald is immensely concerned about his mother's and Patrick's "misbehavior" and prefers to ignore the fact that his mother is actually very happy. Donald's relentlessly scientific worldview (he works on a project on artificial memory in machines) makes him unable to understand how his mother's apparent loss of memory which enables her to live happily in the moment makes her more human, not less (Scotten 9). He is determined to prevent the old couple from getting married.

In the meantime, Patrick's daughter Anna seems to have understood what the romance means to the old lovers. "He is taking his medication regularly for the first time in his life. He hasn't tried to escape or go drinking since he came here. He's even started to talk to me. He's told me stories about his childhood and the war that have made me see him differently," Anna argues in favor of her father's marriage plans (Mighton 63). But she only tries half-heartedly to convince Donald, who has power of attorney over his mother, to support the couple's engagement ("You may not understand it, but it means something to them. It's his last chance to share a life with someone" (62)). Donald, however, does not even think about changing his mind. When Patrick learns about Donald's decision, he rebels by breaking out of the home and drinking, but is soon apprehended. Donald, who comes to visit his mother, finds him tied to a chair with restraining straps and with a large bruise in his face. He refuses to untie him, also to underline his decision not to let him marry his mother: "I wouldn't be living up to my responsibilities as a son. She is not fully herself," he maintains (65). As a result, Patrick further provokes Donald's anger by telling him how he had made love to Clara. Anna, having learned about her father's recent escape and drinking, now also turns against him and agrees that he be moved permanently to the closed ward ("They have decided he's a danger to himself" (67)), keeping him from seeing Clara. The play here critiques the disindividualization of care home residents by foregrounding the power struggle between the institution (to which Donald and Anna also belong), on one hand, and its old residents on the other. As in many care home narratives, the struggle is resolved by means of spatial separation.

In *Discipline and Punish*, Foucault talks about the effect of the panopticon to "induce in the inmate a state of conscious and permanent visibility that assures the automatic functioning of power" (210). As residents of the nameless Canadian nursing home, Clara and Patrick have become "docile bodies" (Foucault, *Discipline* 135) that are subject to a panopticon-like "institutional gaze" (174), and are supposed to behave according to the rules and codes imposed by an institution that patronizes and infantilizes them. The play showcases numerous examples of ageist practices such as elderspeak, elder abuse, and the continual invasion of the residents' privacy in their own rooms.

The institution exerts its power on the level of space: "Patrick," Nurse Tammy warns him, "if anyone finds out you've been going out to buy cigarettes, they'll lock you upstairs!" (Mighton 43). Being moved to the upper-floor closed ward is used as a constant threat, and even in the residents' rooms, no guarantee of privacy is given. This lack of privacy is one of the prime and most frequently criticized characteristics of care-giving facilities. As opposed to "home," the quintessential private space, institutions are semi-public spaces inhabited by medical staff and care-takers with the right to enter their clients' rooms. In the play, however, Clara is stripped off her privacy and agency not by the medical staff and not only due to her early-stage dementia, but by Reverend Hill, a character who literally embodies institutional power. Although he is not a care-taker, he seems to have access to the home and any of its rooms at any time, exposing Clara to an asymmetrical and omniscient institutional gaze.

As the following situation shows, Clara's autonomy, privacy, and personal freedom are constantly undermined, not by doctors or nurses, but by visitors who intrude on her private space without allowing her to decide whether she wants to allow them access. "Knock-knock. I hope everyone is decent," Reverend Hill says as he enters Clara's room, just as she finishes bathing and puts on her dressing gown (50). "I'm just putting Clara to bed," nurse Tammy explains, demonstratively looking at her watch to indicate that he is not welcome. Tammy is generally not very friendly towards Reverend Hill. She does not approve of his morals, is critical of his sermons ("No wonder you're losing your congregation" (52)), and defends the old couple's affair against him as best she can. Although she is generally very understanding, she still represents the institution and has to keep with its rules. Straightening Clara's sheets and sighing, "My goodness, Clara, your bed is a mess. Have you been having an affair?" (51), Tammy, in an absurd interchange, scolds Clara in front of the Reverend. "I don't believe in sex before marriage," Clara retorts. "Then you'll have to get married," Tammy says. "Aren't I too old to get married?" Clara asks, upon which Reverend Hill states, "I am not sure Clara is ready for marriage quite yet. She would have to ask permission from her son. He has power of attorney" (52). Tammy, enervated by Reverend Hill's comments, cuts this conversation short by stating "It's past Clara's bedtime" (52). Clara, who does not have much to say during this conversation, is infantilized in this scene. When Patrick suddenly shows up in Clara's room, Tammy again says that they could, and should, be left alone. "They're adults," she argues (53). Reverend Hill, however, points to the strict house rules but agrees to let them have a little time together, provided he and Tammy stay in the room. Tammy then takes a tape and cassette deck out of her bag and encourages the couple to dance, which they enjoy. She seems to be the only person who understands Clara's and Patrick's love, but is quite unexpectedly replaced by a new nurse, Diana. A conversation between Donald and Anna indicates that Tammy's sudden disappearance has to do with the fact that she has broken more rules than just those of keeping Clara and Patrick apart: Donald suspects her of stealing money from his mother. Whether or not this accusation is accurate cannot be verified, but Tammy seems to spend Clara's money on clothes that she buys for the old woman without being asked to do so, and without producing any bills and change for her (50).

In the play's final scene, the new nurse, Diana, comes to put Clara to bed. Clara is slightly confused because she has never seen Diana before. Diana explains that she usually works upstairs and tells Clara, who says that she wants to go there, that it is actually a very sad place that people would prefer to leave. Alluding to Patrick, whom Diana does not yet know, she says, "There's one old gentleman who stands by the door all day asking if he can go out. [...] He's a drinker. No one will let him out [...]" (75). Patrick, however, does know how to leave, because he was a mathematician and worked as a code breaker for the Special Services during World War II—useful skills that enable him to return to his love. In fact, soon after Diana leaves, he enters Clara's room. Diana, returning, is surprised to see him:

> DIANA: Hello, Patrick. What are you doing here? You're on the wrong floor.
> Pause
> How did you get down here?
> PATRICK: I broke the code.
> DIANA: You're very naughty. Now we'll have to change it. (79)

Diana asks another nurse to take Patrick upstairs again. Her evaluation of the situation is based on the space he inhabits, and she misinterprets Patrick's escape from the upper floor as mental confusion rather than capacity: "I'm sorry, Clara, I don't know how he got down here. He seemed very disoriented" (79). Clara tells nurse Diana that she did not have to show Patrick out ("I didn't mind. We're married" (80)). Because she does not yet know Clara very well and tries to keep the conversation going while putting her to bed, Diana plays along, asking whether he was a good husband, which Clara confirms (80). An instant later, however, when the nurse leaves, Clara again shifts to her past: "I knew a Patrick once during the war..." (81). The play ends with Clara repeating incoherent childhood memories to herself. The lights fade with Clara gratefully reminiscing what a nice day she had had with the children's choir visiting.

The play's ending leaves open whether Patrick will again be able to break out to see Clara, but what has become clear is that by resisting institutional rules, he has finally been separated from his beloved Clara. The "system," represented by Donald and the home, cannot tolerate the fact that Patrick will not allow himself to passively slide into quiescent old age: he refuses to be just another old person abandoned by the rest of society. He has decided to fight for what he wants, and in the end this is what separates him from Clara (Scotten 10–11). The two older characters' happiness is not important to the "system" represented by Donald, Reverend Hill, and the institution as a whole. His fight against institutional power is represented as futile.

The care-facility, with its rigid rules, as presented in this play, can be seen as a prototype of Goffman's "total institution" (xiii). Entering such institutions results in "role dispossession," Goffman argues, as the "self is systematically, often unintentionally, mortified" (14). Life within the limits of the institutional space is, as the title of the play indicates, only a "half life;" the nursing home is a world separated from the outside, where different rules and regulations apply, and contribute to interpellating individuals into their roles as patients, stripping them of personal freedom and choice. This is illustrated by the following humorous episode involving Agnes, another resistant patient:

> AGNES: Where is Mrs. O'Neill? Why isn't she here?
> TAMMY: She died last night.
> CLARA: Oh, that's terrible.
> AGNES: How did she die?
> TAMMY: She died very peacefully and quietly in her sleep.
> AGNES: At least she doesn't have to do crafts anymore.
> (Mighton 44)

In this brief scene, Agnes expresses her discomfort with the institutional schedule to which she must comply. Desiring more personal control, she asks the nurse whether she can go to her room rather than doing crafts. Her frustration with the confinement in the home becomes evident as she recounts how as a child, she enjoyed her freedom: "I was one of the children who would disappear and find a hill somewhere just outside of town. I'd spend the day writing stories in my head" (45). Here, she uses spatiality to critique the confinement and dependence she now experiences in old age.

The care home's separation from the outside world and its realities are expressed not only on a spatial, but also on a temporal level. The first scene already addresses the difference with regard to frames of reference and aspects of space, time, and experience between the inside and outside of the home:

> ANNA picks up a paper and starts reading.
> ANNA: Oh my God!
> DONALD: What is it?
> ANNA: Three hundred people died yesterday. In Nepal.
> DONALD: You should check the date on the paper. It's two years old.
> ANNA: Oh.
> (Mighton 4)

The irony expressed in this scene, which in the play serves as comic relief, indicates that real events do not have much, if any, impact within the microcosm of the home. This may especially be the case for some residents, such as those who have dementia. In relation to aspects of memory, the term "half life" acquires another meaning, that of the disintegration and decay of memory. Donald, in particular, as an expert in artificial intelligence, finds his mother's increasing memory loss extremely hard to accept. Daniel Brooks, who directed the play at Toronto's Tarragon Theatre, says in the production notes:

> John Mighton's *Half Life* is a play about memory—or more precisely—forgetting. The central idea is that we are defined as much by what we forget as we are by what we remember. And given that identity is contingent on what we remember, how does the loss of memory affect identity? Under investigation is the following: What is it that constitutes self, and what might be this thing we call the soul? (Jones 1)

The themes of memory and forgetfulness are central to the play. Social practices defining the nursing home in *Half Life* contribute to the way the characters renegotiate their identities through an ongoing dialogue involving the past, present, and future. The system does not allow for Patrick's and Clara's life course narratives, which are constituted not by what they are actually able to remember, but what they are able to imagine. Especially for a scientist like Donald, who believes in the existence of an absolute truth and has little tolerance for ambiguity, a reconstruction of his mother's life course narrative is unacceptably threatening. The couple's wish to create a new joint narrative in which they belong together and share happiness is not compatible with Donald's, Anna's, and institution's agenda, and is consequently rejected.

3.4 The Chrono-Heterotopia of Old Age in Margaret Atwood's "Torching the Dusties"

> We face a threat more grave and certain than those posed by chemical weapons, nuclear proliferation, or ethnic strife: the "age wave."
>
> — Peter G. Peterson, former chairman and CEO of Lehman Brothers

In this chapter, I examine the care home as a paradoxical space of exclusion, designed less to provide genuine care as a safe space for the protagonists (Snaith 122) than to contain the perceived "burdensome" aspects of old age. Using Michel Foucault's concept of heterotopia, I explore the marginalization of old age and ageism manifested through spatial segregation in Margaret Atwood's apocalyptic short story, "Torching the Dusties," the concluding tale in her 2014 collection *Stone Mattress*. The story explicitly engages with a chronotopic structure through its apocalyptic and dystopian setting, aligning precisely with Elizabeth Barry's interpretation ("Glut"). She states,

> The discrete locations of older-age care as they are described in these stories are not only an indictment of the marginalisation of older people, however, but also the occasion for a particular aesthetics that makes creative play with the tensions between inside and outside, private and public, care and control. I read these spaces here in line with the logic of Mikhail Bakhtin's *chronotope*, which as noted earlier is a feature of narrative that brings time and space into explicit relations; where, in Bakhtin's words, time "thickens, takes on flesh, becomes artistically visible" (84). The spaces of the stories in question institute and impose their own temporal laws and rhythms. (Barry 146)

Arguing that Bakhtin's concept of the chronotope emphasizes how temporal and spatial dimensions intersect within narrative form, generating meaning, Barry analyzes how in Atwood's narrative, the compressed, crisis-driven temporal frame—marked by imminent catastrophe, economic distress, and generational hostility—directly mirrors the limited temporal horizons experienced in old age. "Old age seems to serve in this context as a metaphor for a contemporary society on the brink of financial implosion or environmental extinction," she states ("Glut" 145). The old and frail protagonists are trapped spatially (within the retirement home) and temporally (awaiting inevitable violence), evoking a sense of imminent, collective ending. Thus, the story's dystopian setting becomes a chronotope embodying contemporary fears—such as environmental collapse and economic instability—that intersect specifically with anxieties surrounding aging populations. Barry's reading highlights how the short story form itself encapsulates this convergence, reflecting how old age is symbolically situated within broader social anxieties about diminished futures and societal collapse. In short, Atwood leverages the chronotopic fusion of temporal crisis and confined, heterotopic space to dramatize intergenerational tension and the cultural narrative of aging as part of an approaching apocalypse.

The narrative follows Wilma and Tobias, two companions trapped inside Ambrosia Manor, an upscale, gated retirement community that is besieged by a violent mob—an anti-old age movement called "Our Turn." Members of the movement operate internationally in large numbers ("They say millions are rising up," "Torching" 245). They gather at nursing homes, wearing baby masks, with the intention to literally "torch the dusties" (256). They set care homes on fire all across North America, seeking, they announce, to clear away "the parasitic dead wood at the top" and "the dustballs under the bed" (256). Public discourse here has shifted towards a normalization of the old as "other." The role of the media in perpetuating this attitude is witnessed by the story's focalizer, Wilma, as she listens to a panel discussion on a radio show: "There is rage out there, and yes, it's sad that some of the most vulnerable in society are being scapegoated, but this turn of affairs is not without precedent in history, and in many societies – says the anthropologist – the elderly used to bow out gracefully to make room for young mouths by walking into the snow or being carried up mountainsides and left there" (257). The talk show pits young against old as the anthropologist and an economist debate the actions of Our Turn. Remarkably, it is the student of humanities who argues that geronticide might be a solution because the older people are "eating up the health-care dollars" and the economist who interrupts him/her to observe "that is all very well, but innocent lives are being lost' – to which the anthropologist counters: 'that depends on what you call innocent…'. At this point, 'the host announces that they will now take calls from their listeners'" (257). As in Atwood's other work, her use of sarcasm as a means of social critique is evident. Her tale problematizes the way in which old age is "othered," stigmatized as useless, inefficient and burdensome in a society that is based on production and consumption—and the solution portrayed in the story is radical. Old people are being constructed in Atwood's tale as a new target group against whom injustice is gradually becoming discursively legitimated.

Even though Atwood's dystopic story is fictional, age studies scholars such as Margaret Morganroth Gullette have emphasized that the othering of social groups, including the old, can indeed lead to extreme forms of violence. Gullette dedicates her latest book, which bears the telling title *Ending Ageism, or How Not to Shoot Old People* (2017), to the problematic issue of the scapegoating of old people. The work fights against "increasingly grave instances from the array of ageisms. [...] [for example] glaring neglect in private or public life, grossly hostile speech, abusive images, cruel practices, threats, incitements to self-harm, or violence" (xxii). As Gullette explains, "People tend to distance themselves from individuals or groups that frighten them. Fear can be taught, heightened, or redirected: after World War II, against communists; after 9/11, Muslims; today, immigrants. Social-identity and terror-management theories, informed by age theory, explain how fear can be manipulated against old people. A handy new group to target" (Gullette, *Ending* xxi).

Atwood's text deals with exactly this process and carries it to the extremes: the old become a new target group of a life-threatening form of ageism culminating in geronticide. They are seen as an economic and social challenge—what is commonly described as a "burden" on society. Atwood's tale problematizes the way in which old age is "othered" and stigmatized as unproductive, emphasizing the way old people are seen as "parasites expensive to maintain" (Cruikshank, *Learning* 25) in a society that is based on production and consumption. It highlights the relationship between the space and identity of the aging body as it is increasingly isolated from social interaction. As this analysis will show, "Torching the Dusties" resonates with Haim Hazan's concept of "social death" (*Old Age* 69).

"Torching the Dusties" illustrates the corporeal and spatial dispossession of nursing home inhabitants. Ambrosia Manor has become a Foucauldian heterotopia—a place which excludes the old "within the social fabric they inhabit," as Stanka Radović writes in a different context.[6] The tale invites a reading of

6 Radović analyzes the heterotopia of old age in Beryl Gilroy's *Frangipani House* in her book *Locating the Destitute. Space and Identity in Caribbean Fiction* (2014).

the exclusionary space and its effect on identity. As Radović asserts, "[a]s a site of spatial alterity, heterotopia connects to Lefebvre's theorization of the spatial effect of the body, namely its ability to produce difference. [...] When it emerges as disruptive, as in the case of old age, the body is certainly one such excluded social element, radically other and thus capable of mobilizing and reappropriating otherness as a form of spatial practice" (Radović 132). With reference to Lefebvre, Radović claims that "the excluded body is thus reflected in the spatial function of the heterotopia, itself an excluded space" (132)—it is open but at the same time isolated, with controlled access and exit (132). Lefebvre states, "[d]ifferences endure or arise on the margins of the homogenized realm, either in the form of resistances or in the form of externalities (lateral, heterotopical, heterological). What is different is, to begin with, what is *excluded*" (*Production* 373). The burden narrative of old age is part of the discourse of exclusion, which manifests itself in the heterotopic space of Ambrosia Manor. The story highlights the relationship between the space and the identity of the aging body as the aging person is increasingly isolated from social interaction owing to the body's discursively constructed otherness. This aspect of the story invites a Foucauldian reading. In his essay "Of Other Spaces" (1986), Michel Foucault focuses on the spatiality of cultural production, on the way cultural norms and social practices are revealed through space. In this sense, the space of the nursing home is narrated as a heterotopia of deviation, an example of

> those [spaces] in which individuals whose behavior is deviant in relation to the required mean or norm are placed. Cases of this are rest homes and psychiatric hospitals, and of course prisons; and one should perhaps add retirement homes that are, as it were, on the borderline between the heterotopia of crisis and the heterotopia of deviation since, after all, old age is a crisis, but is also a deviation since, in our society where leisure is the rule, idleness is a sort of deviation. (Foucault, "Of" 25)

Like the "vagabond" and "unproductive" people identified as political problems in seventeenth and eighteenth-century European societies addressed in Foucault's other work (Katz, *Disciplining* 19), Atwood's characters can hence be read as "excluded bodies" that are housed in the heterotopic site of the care home.

While the public in the story's radio show hotly debate the issue of the old as a social, financial and political danger, evidencing the normalization of "the old" as a "burdensome hazard" (Biggs and Powell 10), Ambrosia Manor's residents are slow to notice what is going on around them. They remain oblivious to the threatening developments, like the frog in the famous experiment where it sits in increasingly hot water, even when, unchallenged by the police, the mob outside the gate grows larger and louder every day. Atwood cleverly instils a doubt in readers' minds, suggesting that the repeated assertion that "help is on the way" (267) is a lie, while simultaneously making clear that resistance on the part of the residents will be futile. At the beginning of the story, incidents such as a laundry van or food delivery van being blocked by the increasingly aggressive group at the gates are received by the residents with curiosity rather than apprehension. Wilma, a widowed resident in her eighties, cannot "pinpoint exactly what it is that she's feeling. Not despair, not at all. And not hope. She only wants to see what will happen next. It certainly won't be the daily routine" (255). At least it gives the residents something to talk about over meals: "'They say they want us to make room. They want us to move over. Some of the signs say that: *Move Over.*' 'That means *die*, I suppose,' says Wilma. 'Are there any rolls today?' Sometimes there are the most delicious Parker House rolls, fresh from the oven" (244). Wilma observes that another inmate, Tobias, actually seems to be enjoying what is going on: "This turn of events has energized him; he is almost humming" (241). But he soon begins to be more concerned than anyone else in the residence, and, using Wilma's binoculars and her window as a lookout, keeps her informed about the latest developments. In sum, while some of the residents slowly begin to show signs of concern, others see Our Turn's gathering as a welcome change from their daily, boring routine. Living in the heterotopic world of the nursing home, where even Internet access is strictly limited (242), the residents have limited access to the developments happening outside.

The Burden Narrative of Old Age

The "burden narrative" of old age is not a recent phenomenon. The title of Andrea Charise's discussion of the "barely conscious figurative language that serves to construct perceptions of an aging population" (2), "Let the Reader Think of the Burden," is taken from Anthony Trollope's *The Fixed Period* (1882), the starting point for her account of the narrative from the nineteenth to the twenty-first century. Charise notes convincingly that metaphors such as "the silver tsunami" or the "rising tide" are part of a discourse that positions old age as a peculiar kind of "other:" "This ominous rhetoric of rising, swamping, tides, and disease – amplified by the authoritative tones of medical and health policy expertise – conceives of population aging as an imminent catastrophe. Conceived en masse, the elderly are naturalized as a liquid cataclysm whose volume exceeds the nation's ability to contain, or even guard against, an abstracted human burden" (Charise 3).

Stephen Katz has argued that the origins of this discourse of a "crisis of capacity" (Charise 1) can be found at the moment in the nineteenth century when "the elderly population was constituted as a subject of knowledge and politics through a discourse of alarmist demography" (Katz, *Disciplining* 127). According to Katz, "[t]he creation of the elderly as population must be seen against the historical background of demographic discourse itself. And demographic discourse is inseparable from the Malthusian-tinged, alarmist debates of the late nineteenth and twentieth centuries that accentuated the growing number, neediness, and poverty of elderly persons as a primary social problem" (Katz, *Disciplining* 72). This discourse of crisis and burden produces "the older population" as a distinct group that threatens social and economic stability.

Heike Hartung draws on the same novel to show how the burden narrative has both promoted and criticized "euthanasia and eugenics as possible solutions to the problem of old age" (Hartung, *Ageing* 35). In Trollope's satirical science-fiction novel, the law of the "Fixed Period" is introduced by the youthful Assembly of the fictive British colony of Britannula requiring that all citizens reaching the age of 65 move to an idyllic college called "Necropolis," where they are to spend one year of honorary retirement before being executed at the age of 67.5. As John Neverbend, the novel's first-person narrator, tells us, the Fixed Period law "consists altogether of the abolition of the miseries, weakness, and fainéant imbecility of old age, by the prearranged ceasing to live of those who would otherwise become old" (Trollope 9). Neverbend supports his argument with modern science:

> Statistics have told us that the sufficient sustenance of an old man is more costly than the feeding of a young one,—as is also the care, nourishment, and education of the as yet unprofitable child. Statistics also have told us that the unprofitable young and the no less unprofitable old form a third of the population. Let the reader think of the burden with which the labour of the world is thus saddled. [...] But for whose good are the old and effete to be maintained? (Trollope 10–11)

While the satire in *The Fixed Period* may be obvious to us, Hartung notes (*Ageing* 30) that it was not always so in the course of the development of early twentieth-century medical discourses on old age. According to her, in his influential study of old age, *Senescence* (1922), G. Stanley Hall treats the Fixed Period law "not from a readerly position of distance provided by satiric exaggeration or the temporal remove of the science-fiction setting but treats euthanasia as a possible future solution to the problem of old age" (Hartung, *Ageing* 30). Such an interpretation is only possible, Hartung observes, because the burden narrative of old age had become a normalized discourse in early gerontological literature.

This discourse continues to be prevalent in current anti-aging research. For instance, Aubrey de Grey, author of *Ending Aging*, explains that "it's very expensive indeed to be elderly. [...] [$200B/year is] how much it costs just in the USA alone for keeping the elderly going in the frail and decrepit state that a large proportion of them are in for that extra year or two" Grey n.p., 02:20–02:35). De Grey, whose radical ideas have provoked harsh opposition from critical gerontologists, has come to occupy a central position in the field of anti-ageing studies, as I have pointed out elsewhere (Kriebernegg 64). The costs de Grey presents (without quoting any sources) amount to a sum too large for a life not worth living, as he suggests. However appreciative he may be of the wisdom of the old (another commonplace), de Grey perpetuates the stereotype of the old as "parasites expensive to maintain" (Cruikshank, *Learning* 25). As opposed to a worthless life of decrepitude and frailty, a worthy life is one of youth and agility. As de Grey presents them, the old are threatening creatures, the "other" that stands outside of what he considers "normal" life; they embody decay, disease and death—conditions that need to be kept at bay as they evoke panic.

This discourse of old age as a social problem is central to "Torching the Dusties." As in *The Fixed Period*, there is a strong satirical undercurrent in Atwood's bitter and dystopic interpretation that portrays the possible consequences of ageism when old age is expressed in metaphors that link it to natural disasters such as the often-mentioned "silver tsunami," the "grey flood," the "agequake," or the "age wave," as Peter G. Peterson calls it in his book *Gray Dawn: How the Coming Age Wave will Transform America – and the World* (1999). Peterson, former CEO of Lehman Brothers, Secretary of Commerce and Chairman of the New York Federal Reserve Bank, worries about demographic change and equates the alleged threat of an ageing society to natural disasters: "Leaders have been willing to convene summits to discuss global warming. Why not global aging, which will hit us sooner and with greater certainty? (Peterson). He predicts a further chasm: "By the mid-2020s, will the contrast between North and South be better described as a contrast between Young and Old?" (Peterson). His reliance on the traditional burden narrative of old age is clear also when he claims that "'[g]lobal aging could trigger a crisis that engulfs the world economy. This crisis may even threaten democracy itself. [...] At the top of the list is the impact of the age wave on foreign policy and international security" (Peterson). Peterson does not offer a solution but warns of turmoil, disaster, and international social instability, fears that are at best exaggerated, as a 2011 study by the Canadian Institute for Health Information confirms.[7] Craig Karpel echoes these sentiments in *The Retirement Myth*, and in 1995 had already predicted that medical care would be rationed, which he terms "gerontocide." He stated that by 2015, homeless shelters would be filled with "dumpies" (destitute unprepared mature people (Karpel, qtd. in Parmelee 57), a term that resonates with Atwood's "dusties."

In Atwood's story, Peterson's predictions have become reality. Yet, the young group's aggression in "Torching the Dusties" is also motivated by their rage against the carelessness with which previous generations used to treat nature and natural resources. In an interview, Atwood explains,

> "It's a logical outcome of where our demographic is going. [...] Let us put it this way," she continues. "No life form can exist beyond its exhaustion of its food supply. No life form can exist beyond its exhaustion of its oxygen supply, and no life form can exist beyond its exhaustion of its fresh water supply, and all of those things are finite." At that point, she says, "Things usually get unpleasant." (Williams)

The ecological concerns even more inherent in Atwood's later dystopic, eco-critical work are prevalent also in this tale, where, exactly as Peterson has predicted, "the young" are pitted against "the old" in terms of resources. The old are positioned as scapegoats for the disastrous state of the world. As Tobias reports of Our Turn: "'They say it's their turn," says Tobias. [...] "Their turn at what?" "At life, they say. .... They say we've had our turn, those our age; they say we messed it up. Killing the planet with our own greed and so forth"' (Atwood 243–44). According to Tobias, the young activists wear baby masks to highlight their own innocence: "'Chubby, smiling babies. Some say Time to Go.' 'Time to go?' says Wilma. 'Babies? What does that mean? This isn't a maternity hospital.' About the opposite, she thinks caustically: it's an exit from life, not an entrance"

7 The 2011 report by the Canadian Institute for Health Information states that: "The common belief is that an aging population will lead to greater demands for health care services and accelerated growth in health spending. Contrary to common perception, population aging has been a very modest cost driver overall. Population aging contributed an annual average growth of only 0.8%" (vi).

(238), hinting at the spatiality of the life-course. The baby masks, impressively featured in Marlene Goldman's 2019 film adaptation (Marlene Goldman and McKee), serve to highlight the binary opposition between young and old that the story presents as another normalized discourse.

In contrast to the baby masks, which are put on voluntarily to emphasize the group's common identity as the "youth," Ambrosia Manor residents metaphorically wear what Mike Hepworth refers to as the "mask of old age" ("Images" 20), a mask created by a "subjective sense of distance between the inner or private self and the outer or physically observable social self" (20). This is a result, Hepworth argues, of the public imagery of old age as a social problem. He explains the "mask of old age" as follows:

> Coupled with the traditional Western belief in old age as a condition of geriatric disengagement from full active social life, the image of the physiognomic body creates a trap or prison that constitutes an effective barrier of communication with the wider world (Hepworth, 1991). This is the mask of old age: an image that reflects the subjective experience that many older people describe as being constrained by the expectations of others (often younger people) into wearing a mask or disguise of physical aging that, unlike the actor at the close of a theatrical performance of old age, they cannot remove and leave behind in the dressing room. [...] All of the world's a stage, but when it comes to old age, some roles are for real. ("Images" 20)

Soon Ambrosia Manor residents, who cannot take off their "masks," are made to feel that their roles are real. Our Turn begin to block access to and from the home and ask employees to leave, interpellating all inhabitants into their role of "the old"—the "other"—through an unfavorable "geriatric gaze" (Hepworth, "Images" 12), which literally traps them in the home. The contrast between young and old is established as a natural difference which manifests itself on the level of space:

> "They have blockaded the gate," Tobias announces. "They refuse to let anyone in." [...] "Are they letting anyone out?" [Wilma] asks Tobias. "Through the blockade." [...] "Only the staff," says Tobias. "They are more or less ordering them to go. Not the inhabitants. We have to stay. So they appear to have decreed." [...] "We could disguise ourselves," says Wilma. "To get out. As, well, as cleaners. Muslim cleaners, with our heads covered up. Or something." "I doubt very much that we would pass unchallenged, dear lady," Tobias says. "It is a question of the generations. Time leaves its markings." (253–255)

Old Age as a Liminal Stage Between Life and Death

The care home, Ambrosia Manor, serves as a heterotopic spatial metaphor that localizes the horrors of a life deprived of social and cultural recognition through the "othering" of old age. It represents the metaphorical "black hole of the fourth age," the "shadowlands of disability, diminishment, and death" (Gilleard and Higgs, "Aging" 121). The residents in "Torching the Dusties" are not only excluded from any social participation in their secluded heterotopic space, but are extremely vulnerable to violence, as the authorities have given up protecting the care homes from Our Turn. In this manner, Ambrosia Manor becomes a literal waiting room for death. The irony of the name is painful. Whereas in Greek mythology Ambrosia, as Abel notes, is "a celestial material exclusively the possession of the Olympian deities" and signifies "immortality" (15), the manor that bears its name instead marks a loss of identity. The association becomes more pointed when considering that Ambrosia is also the name of an invasive weed, a plant regarded as dangerous and therefore targeted for removal and destruction.[8] As a species that must be eradicated, it underscores the shift from divine nourishment to harmful weed, from value to devaluation. In this sense, the story resonates with what Agamben describes as "bare life" (4): a body stripped of personhood, excluded from political participation, subjected to sovereign violence, and ultimately "devoid of value" (88). Watching the aggressive mob gather in front of the gates puts the aged residents into a state between life and death. This liminal condition is depicted in the story with a certain cynicism when Atwood describes Wilma and Tobias watching a brace of paramedics hurrying in and out, and then exiting "at a more leisurely pace, wheeling a shape on a gurney. You can't tell from here, says Tobias as he peers through the binoculars, whether the body is alive or dead. 'Maybe you can't even tell from down there,' he's been known to add as a sepulchral joke" (235).

Tobias's supposedly humorous comment serves to emphasize the otherness of old age, where the body is anonymous ("a shape"), denied personhood and not even clearly alive or dead. The loss of identity in the fourth age is also illustrated by Wilma's increasing macular degeneration, which makes it difficult for her to see herself in the mirror: "The most worrisome item during her morning preparation is her face. She can scarcely make it out in the mirror: it's like one of those face-shaped blanks that once appeared on Internet accounts when you hadn't added your picture" (229). Small things such as putting on make-up

8 I am grateful to Miriam Haller who added this perspective in our discussion of the story.

have become a problem; misapplied lipstick, for instance, may have severe consequences: "if you look demented they're more likely to treat you as if you really are," and it would only be a short time until "you dwindle to nothing" (230). Wilma knows that he make-up, usually applied to conceal age, might make her look older than she is. She directs us as readers to look beyond the façade, also that of the care home. She is performing age deliberately, knowing how signs are being interpreted and knowing how she has to interpret the world of the care home.

Wilma experiences Charles Bonnet Syndrome, an eye condition characterized by visual hallucinations—in her case manifesting as what her eye doctor calls "Chuckies," tiny ornately dressed figures who parade through her room, accompanying her almost all day. These tiny mannequins converse among themselves but ignore Wilma entirely. Although Wilma, who is an excellent observer, recognizes that they are merely symptoms of her condition, the bizarre apparitions confront her with the harsh reality of losing both her vision and autonomy, as they appear unpredictably and beyond her control. The description of the characters wearing elaborately crafted "red velvet costumes, richly textured and patterned in gold" (266) performing an "airy dance" in which the men and women gracefully nod, curtsy, come together, and then move apart again (266) evokes imagery reminiscent of Renaissance court dances. This depiction can be interpreted as an intertextual reference to Elizabethan drama, particularly texts from that period addressing aging as a societal burden, such as the 17th century play *The Old Law* (Middleton et al.). In this tragicomedy, co-written by Shakespeare's contemporary Thomas Middleton, the title itself references the Elizabethan Poor Law of 1601. The play's edict mandates the execution of women at sixty, men at eighty, and anyone exhibiting "second infancy," a euphemism for cognitive decline or senility (Middleton et al. 1334), meaning "senility." These older characters are portrayed as burdensome and obsolete to society. In contrast, Thomas More explicitly rejected the idea of geronticide in his *Utopia* (1516), advocating instead for compassionate and dignified state-supported care, though he condoned voluntary euthanasia for those suffering severe pain or weakness. Middleton's play, influenced by More's earlier arguments (Schotland 161) can be read as satirical commentary—a critical stance also reflected in Atwood's text. The ruthless killing of old people in "Torching the Dusties" intensifies the clash between generations even more radically than in *The Old Law*, where older characters are ultimately spared (Kainradl and Kriebernegg).

Helen Snaith has an insightful explanation for Wilma's vision loss. She claims that "'[r]eading' the final tale through the failing eyes of Wilma also becomes critical in engaging with broader issues around an ageist society. [...] [I]t stands to reason that our understanding of the issues, much like Wilma's understanding, is limited. Therefore, Wilma's failing sight becomes analogous to our own limitations and ability to 'see' the potential failures of society in life outside of fiction" (Snaith 122). Despite the dystopian setting, she contends that Atwood's narrative strategy of the "persistent centering of Wilma's voice [...] as interpreter of events [...] [is a] deliberate subversion of narrative" (124) that counteracts the "double standard of aging" (Sontag). Goldman's movie adaptation can be read to highlight this, as she reverses the roles and has Tobias experience visual impairment while Wilma sees clearly. Yet, the film seems to center more strongly on presenting his perspective, which again underscores a more traditional narrative.

In the story, the narrative of decline, which reflects a common discourse on aging as lack, loss and decrepitude and makes aging entirely bodily (Gullette, *Aged* 7), is reinforced by olfactory imagery, such as the "acid, stale odour of aging bodies so noticeable when all the Ambrosiads are assembled in the dining room, their base note of slow decay and involuntary leakage papered over with applied layers of scent – delicate florals on the women, bracing spices on the men, the blooming rose or brusque pirate image inside each of them still fondly cherished" (Atwood, "Torching" 232). Wilma becomes aware of the fact that, as a human being, she cannot be separated from her body—a body that she feels is betraying her:

> You believed you could transcend the body as you aged, she tells herself. You believed you could rise above it, to a serene, nonphysical realm. But it's only through ecstasy you can do that, and ecstasy is achieved through the body itself. Without the bone and sinew of wings, no flight. Without that ecstasy you can only be dragged further down by the body, into its machinery. Its rusting, creaking, vengeful, brute machinery. (252)

Her aged body is giving up, experienced as the "other" of the mind, disloyal and letting her down. In addition, Wilma links her sense of having lost her physical and sexual attractiveness to her advanced age. This influences her relationship with Tobias, a suave Hungarian gentleman. Although he frequently compliments her on her looks, his boasts of earlier sexual adventures make her feel inferior. She secretly compares her old body with the beauties Tobias tells her about, and decides against a sexual relationship with him. Because of her visual disability, the heterotopic exclusion is even worse for Wilma, and Tobias is her last chance, even if a meagre one, to imagine at least a connection with a world outside:

> We have to be kind to one another in here, she tells herself. We're all we have left. The bottom line is that Tobias can still see. She can't afford to be annoyed by physical attractions of stale-dated stunners as long as Tobias can look out the window and tell her what's going on there in the grounds outside the imposing front door of Ambrosia Manor. She likes to be kept in the loop, insofar as there is one. (227)

At Ambrosia Manor, the residents are denied access to information from the outside world; they are forbidden to have private computers, and those in the Activity Centre have control software to limit access, "as for prepubescent children" (242). Through Wilma we become aware too of their lack of control over their time and, ultimately, their bodies, resonating with the concept of the "total institution." Residents are not treated as independent individuals but are deprived of their autonomy.

Wilma's distance from the world outside is not only due to Ambrosia Manor's heterotopic exclusion. The narration reveals that her two daughters and son do not count as a lifeline to the outer world, as her relationship to them is also distant. She complains that they are too busy to visit her, a procedure that would be tiresome anyway, as she convinces herself while observing the reluctance exhibited by other people, bearing a potted geranium, during their visits; they arrive "hauling a young, reluctant grand-child, summoning up false cheer, hoping to get this rich-old-relative thing over with as soon as possible" (235). She refers to only one of her daughters, Alyson, by name—the one who manages her ample funds—and barely remembers the time "back when she had family" (233). She only calls Alyson out of duty, finding these calls as tedious as her grandchildren, who are usually forced to say hello to her, must. Her other daughter and son are only mentioned as uncaring offspring; her daughter, because she keeps sending slippers of which Wilma now has "a glut" (234), and her son, because he still writes her postcards and "doesn't seem to grasp that she can no longer read his handwriting" (234). Their father, Wilma's late husband, is also only mentioned in passing and without a name, revealing her distance from the life she had before she entered Ambrosia Manor. Tobias is Wilma's only companion, and he helps her with her activities of daily living such as cooking breakfast or eating, as "she can no longer aim the spoon with accuracy" (233). Despite his devoted help, she does not trust him (nor anyone else in the residence for that matter). His answers seem sly and evasive, and he resembles the charming Eastern European trickster figure of Vitus Kovic in Leslie Larson's *Breaking Out of Bedlam*. Wilma "enjoys re-asking questions because the answers are sometimes the same, sometimes not. Tobias has had at least three birthplaces and has attended four universities, all at once. His passports are numerous" (248). Whoever Tobias was in his former life, he now seems to take good care of Wilma in Ambrosia Manor and is a loyal friend, and Wilma seems to appreciate this most of the time. The distance and caution expressed by her comments may stem simply from a sense of self-preservation. The representation of Wilma's distrust in "Torching the Dusties" illustrates the spatial and corporeal dispossession of nursing home inhabitants.

Ambrosia Manor is an upscale (and, as such, in its own way "exclusive") retirement facility with two wings, the "Early Assisted Living wing," which Wilma and Tobias inhabit, and the ironically named "Advanced Living" wing, where "things are different," but Wilma "hasn't wished to imagine exactly how different" (233). Wilma is afraid that she will soon be moved there against her will: "They don't really believe she's able to function on her own; they're just waiting for an excuse to slot her into Advanced Living and grab the rest of her furniture and her good china and silver, which they'll sell to support their profit margin. That's the deal, she signed it; it was the price of entry, the price of comfort, the price of safety. The price of not being a burden" (239). She is excluded and alienated from social participation and confined to the heterotopic parallel world of the home, but, even there, she is at risk of further spatial segregation because of perceived decline. Atwood draws attention to the commodification of care to further emphasize the heterotopian dimension of the nursing home, within which residents amount to social refuse produced by practices of spatial exclusion, as Radović argues in a different context (147). Wilma is aware that there are public care homes which do not offer the same hotel-like luxury she enjoys at Ambrosia Manor. She recognizes that: "Ambrosia Manor isn't cheap, and the relatives would not take kindly to ulcerating rashes on their loved ones. They want their money's worth, or so they'll claim. What they most likely want in truth is a rapid and blame-free finish for the old fossils. Then they can tidy up and collect the remnants of the net worth – the legacy, the leftovers, the remains – and tell themselves they deserve it" (238).

Old people are no longer chased out into the wilderness or put on ice floes as they may have been in the past; instead, "innovative services and goods are developing that seek to capitalize on the "silver dollar," as Anne Karpf (SR9) put it in her *New York Times* article on gerontophobia. Wilma knows that she is taken care of in a humane way because she pays large sums for it and keeps the nurses happy with little tips and presents. When the mob forces staff members to leave, her caregiver Katia comes into Wilma's room with a guilty conscience, weeping and apologizing because she needs to leave her. Ironically, it is Wilma who comforts Katia, telling her she will be all right and asking her to calm down. Wilma reacts to Katia's sobbing by giving her all the cash she has left in her purse, as well as her expensive wrapped floral-scented soaps. She still seems unaware of the threatening situation she is in herself. It seems more important to her to please and care for Katia, one of the few people she has at least some trust in. Knowing how comparatively fortunate she is, Wilma describes Ambrosia Manor as a surrogate home. However, the home's staff and its amenities, such as the silent hands at work behind the scenes who fold her nightgown and put chocolate on the pillow during dinner hour (253) do not provide her with the same feeling of comfort and extravagance she would enjoy in a hotel. Ambrosia Manor, a "shrine to past wealth" (Barry 154), has a "fountain with a replica of a famous Belgian statue, a naked angel-faced boy urinating into a stone basin" and a wall with "two ostentatious, depressed-looking stone lions" (234). While these decorative elements are, as she points out, fake, "the high brick wall, the imposing gateway with its overhead arch (234) are real, and remind her of a prison or hospital rather than a luxurious hotel. This duality highlights how "ruling metaphors (Braedley) converge in the story and are also expressed through Wilma's unhappiness in the luxury world. But, as Elizabeth Barry points out, Atwood's critique of capitalism remains ambiguous because the aging residents actively participate in this materialism. Barry notes, "The 'little world' of the residential home enshrines, memorialises and replicates a history of privilege, from the tiny feudal characters dancing at the edge of Wilma's eyeline (her visual hallucinations) to the figure of domestic service (explicitly costumed as Victorian in Marlene Goldman's film of the story)[9] to the fine-grained late capitalist differentiation of luxury foodstuffs" (153–54).

---

9 While Elizabeth Barry argues that the costumes are Victorian, Marlene Goldman asserted during a 2019 conference discussion about her film adaptation that she interpreted them as referencing the Newfoundland tradition of Mummering. As stated earlier, I contend that Atwood might employ intertextual references to the Renaissance play *The Old Law*.

The End of the Mansion

After all the staff have left the premises, as the more able residents are obliged to care for the less able, they begin to regain agency, assigning meaning to their lives and experiences and producing a new kind of institutional space for themselves. Some women take over the kitchen and make soup: "'Isn't this something?' [Noreen] says. 'Everyone's just rolling up their sleeves and pitching in! It's like summer camp! I suppose they thought we couldn't cope!'" (261). Once Our Turn takes over, however, there is no help for the people of the "fourth age" who are housed in "Advanced Living:" the connecting doors are locked, telephone lines cut, and computers and even TVs no longer work as they are consigned to their fate. Tobias has started to stock up on food and water for Wilma and himself, as part of his secret escape plan. But when a group of Ambrosia Manor inhabitants plan to march out the front door, claiming that the press has arrived, Tobias remains skeptical. He believes that even "with the world watching" the mob would never let them pass: "The whole world has an appetite for ringside seats at such events. Witch-burnings and public hangings were always well attended," he observes (262). Nonetheless, his fellow residents are not greatly concerned: "'I'm going to have a nap first,' says Noreen. 'Gather my strength. Before we march out. At least we don't have to do the dishes in that filthy kitchen, since we won't be here much longer'" (262). Noreen's plan, however, soon proves inoperable, and a violent incident occurs which causes the few courageous inhabitants who tried to march out to return to the house. In the meantime, the mob outside has begun to light fires in oil drums, and Wilma can hear them chanting, "*Time to Go. Fast Not Slow. Burn Baby Burn. It's Our Turn*" (265). It is clear that the agency and power briefly afforded to the residents as they take over the space of the home cannot last.

The conclusion of the story further emphasizes how difficult it is to challenge spatial segregation and the discourse of the old as burden. After dark, Tobias shows Wilma a way out through the storage area, which is populated by rats, and past the trash bins. In Marlene Goldman's film adaptation, they use a laundry bin to escape through the dark hallways, emphasizing the prison escape narrative, as Barry also points out (155). Wilma has to rely entirely on Tobias's guidance, and her narration once more reveals her loneliness and the difficult conditions of being helpless and dependent. She finds herself questioning her friend's motivation: "'What if he's a thrill killer', she asks herself, wondering if he 'has made everything up', and the chanting a recording or a student group he has hired" (266). Her panic only ebbs when he guides her to one of the gazebos in the garden where he has prepared blankets, food, coffee and her binoculars: "'Grandstand seats. We'll be quite comfortable here,' he says, feeding her peanuts just as Ambrosia Manor begins to burn" (266). Wilma's feelings of ambivalence about Tobias are underlined once more while she worries about the others who are still inside: "'There is nothing I can do for the others,' says Tobias. [...] 'It was always that way,' he says mournfully. 'Or is it coldly?'" (267). Throughout the story, he never fully gains her trust, and even after his attempt to rescue her, she finds it difficult to establish a trusting relationship with him. She can hardly trust herself, or her own body: "She's clutching – she notices – her own hands. They feel like somebody else" (267). Caught between dependence on Tobias and dependence on Ambrosia Manor, Wilma is left vulnerable and unable to connect not only with others, but also with her own body and sense of self. The story ends with Wilma and Tobias watching the bright flames consuming Ambrosia Manor. They wonder why there are no fire trucks and, hearing their fellow residents' fading screams, hope that they will have a quick death (268). Once more, Wilma, just as at the story's beginning, is accompanied by the "little people"—as grotesque as the murderers outside the gate—who blend in with the flames, "Look! Look! They are singing!" (268). As always, they show no compassion. Just like the general public, they seem to be enjoying the event. The little Chuckies can be read through Bakhtin's idea of the carnivalesque, where laughter mixes comedy with violence and turns death into a spectacle (cited in Russo 54). The residents are shown as disposable, their pain treated as entertainment. As Marta Dvorak points out, Atwood often uses grotesque humor in a "subversive carnivalesque tradition" that highlights cruelty rather than renewal (114). She notes that Atwood's "tall tale strategies generate the laughter that accompanies incongruity" (115), and the little Chuckies act like tall-tale figures—exaggerated, absurd, and out of place in such a dark scene. The mix of horror and play creates uneasy laughter. The story's "subdued carnival" (Atwood, "Torching" 247) becomes a parody of carnival, a bleak spectacle where laughter goes hand in hand with geronticide and old age is seen as disposable.

It remains open whether Tobias and Wilma will be able to escape after Our Turn has left the scene. Wilma and Tobias are tossed into a space beyond the heterotopia of the care home, they are the "living dead" who are no longer even discursively allocated a territory. What Andrea Charise has noted with regard to Anthony Trollope's *The Fixed Period* can also be applied to Margaret Atwood's tale. It "clarifies" for our day "how demographics and aesthetics conceive of older age as a potentially catastrophic force and, subsequently, how the rhetoric of capacity can be used to disaffiliate the aged from a privileged, non-old social body" (Charise 2). With nursing homes under attack, readers are left to wonder where Wilma and Tobias could go next, stuck in the liminal world between the care home and the city. Even the outside world is in "shambles, both economic and environmental" (257). "Torching the Dusties" lets "the reader think of the burden" (Trollope, 2008 [1882]: 10; Charise, 2012: 1)—but, as Barry contends, "images of ending can be enlivening. Atwood imagines in the Manor's destruction not the sweeping away a troublesome older generation but the putative end of an unequal system itself" (156) because, she observes, "the crisis is not located in the dystopian spaces of commercialised 'care,' but in the larger system that creates them" (160). "If these authors' stories reflect the dominance of the idea of looming closure as the defining chronotope of the contemporary short story, it is not so much that they have older characters as it is that the world they are writing about is facing the prospect of its own imminent ending. The older protagonists are simply waiting to see "what will happen next" (Atwood 255)" (Barry, "Glut" 161). As the smoke clears, Wilma and Tobias remain trapped within a heterochronotope, suspended between the displaced reality of the care home and the crumbling city outside, uncertain which version of the future—if any—they might enter next.

4 Fugitives and Escapees
Age, Gender, and the Spatiality of Resistance

Throughout history, Americans have tended to be infatuated with movement and fearful of settlement. Our mythology celebrates pilgrims, explorers, cowboys, prospectors, and pioneers, while it warns us against being trapped on a farm, in a hollow, in a puritanical village, or in a stifling city. We associate moving with adventure and freedom, while we associate staying put with confinement and backwardness.

— Philip B. Stafford, *Elderburbia*

You have brains in your head, you have feet in your shoes,
You can move yourself any direction you choose.
And you're on your own. And you know what you know.
And YOU are the guy who'll decide where to go.

— Dr. Seuss, *Oh, The Places You'll Go!*

This chapter is dedicated to "care home escape narratives," which are stories of fugitive mobility in which care home residents choose to break out and run away from their bleak institutional lives. In the texts presented in this part, older individuals transgress spatial boundaries, confront obstacles, and enacts forms of spatial resistance. Their agency challenges the pervasive notion that there are "fit surroundings" (Emerson 285) within which older individuals should safely be contained—a concept that continues to shape discursive formations with regard to the spatiality of old age and, in turn, informs our implicit understanding of institutional long-term care. As Doreen Massey argues, space is never neutral but inherently gendered, shaped by power relations that structure access, mobility, and agency. Care homes, as institutional spaces, reflect and reinforce these dynamics, often positioning older individuals—particularly women—as passive recipients of care rather than autonomous subjects. But what happens in this context, if the traditional matrix of "race, ethnicity, class, sex, gender, and able-bodiedness" is expanded to include age and examined through the lens of spatial analysis? While the literary motif of escape has been widely explored in various studies, a gendered reading of long-term care escape narratives that foregrounds aspects of spatial dynamics remains a largely unchartered area of inquiry.

The reasons why characters decide to run away from care homes differ among the stories. As will be shown, escape plans can be motivated by a mixture of push and pull factors. In all these stories, the care home serves as the starting point for a protagonist's journey, emphasizing the contrast between the limited world of the home and the freedom of the open road. As such, the figure of the care home presents a backdrop against which the road narrative can evolve, underlining the adventurous nature of the old characters, as well as their vigor and agency. While the characters presented in the previous chapter resisted their victimization from *within* the confining walls of the home, the protagonists presented in this chapter literally break out of the restraining structures and hit the road, enacting spatial resistance through mobility. The journeys they undertake are dual journeys, journeys of both the mind and body, physical and spiritual (Roberts 53), which often lead them to a new acceptance of themselves and to the reevaluation of their individual identities, a process that would not have been possible from within the confining contexts of the home.

Whereas the fictional space of the care home is usually not presented as a gendered space, the open road has traditionally been discursively constructed as a male realm. This chapter also offers a gendered reading of nursing home escape stories and examines the question of whether such stories can destabilize powerful regimes of age and gender, as well as of cultural and social differences. Using a variety of texts as touchstones and reading them through an intersectional perspective, I discuss escape as an act of resistance against the processes leading to homogenization, marginalization, and punishment of old age, and as an expression of the protagonists' wish for social participation.

The topic of escape is a foundational motif in American literature that can be traced as far back as the first immigrants escape from Europe (Bluefarb). It already played a role in late nineteenth century care home narratives such as Mary Wilkins Freeman's "A Mistaken Charity" (1887), in which two old sisters run away from an "Old Ladies' Home," since they feel like "two forlorn prisoners" in their genteel surroundings (Wilkins Freeman 244). In 1964, Margaret Laurence's *Stone Angel* most famously addressed the topic of escape again, but especially during the last two decades, a massive increase in the number of stories that feature older protagonists fleeing long-term institutional care has been observed. In the twenty-first century, the "escape narrative" seems to have developed into a very popular sub-genre of the care home novel. Old characters who refuse to obey institutional rules and claim the road for themselves feature more prominently in novels and films today than ever before, thus "conveying [a] shift from self-consciousness to self-empowerment" (Chivers, "On" 213). As Sally Chivers notes, "[c]ontemporary depictions of elderly characters on the road again do more than expand literary and film road genres; they reconfigure expectations of old age in a way that stands to make elderly mobility important enough to matter socially" (214).

A New Genre in the Making: The Care Home Escape Novel

In terms of genre, I argue that the "road novel" needs to be expanded to include older protagonists who flee from long-term institutional care. Individual texts that center on the care home as a place from which to escape follow the conventions and patterns of the escape narrative, road novel, quest story, or romance. Films and stories, therefore, can also be interpreted in terms of such genres. The aspect of age and the starting point of the nursing home add an additional dimension to the interpretation of such literature and films. For example, Chivers has observed that, in terms of nursing home escapes, the form of escape is important to consider: "[C]haracters seek to flee but often come up against perceptions of aging as comically incongruous, a time of boredom, or replete with ill health and abandonment" ("Blind" 135). Even if the protagonists' escapes are only temporary and end in confinement or even death, their journeys and explorations, as will be shown, affect their narratives of self and, thus, change them. From a reader's point of view, these circular texts point to the culturally and socially constructed nature of old age as a time of confinement and to the lack of alternative models of care, or even fantasies thereof.

The first part of this chapter is dedicated to an exploration of the question: why has the escape motif increasingly gained popularity in care home narratives? This theoretical introduction is followed by a brief discussion of the motif of the journey, the road narrative, and a gendered reading. The second part of this chapter discusses Oscar Casares's novel, *Amigoland* (2009), in which 91-year-old Don Fidencio leaves the nursing home to travel to Mexico in order to find peace. National borders are also crossed in the movie *Cloudburst* (2011), in which eighty-year-old Dot is institutionalized through trickery by her granddaughter, but then kidnapped from the home by her lover Stella. Because same-sex marriage is not yet legal in Maine, where they have been living together for more than thirty years, the lesbian couple travels across the border to Canada to get married, and thus prevent their separation. *Cloudburst* is compared and contrasted to Janet Hepburn's novel *Flee, Fly, Flown* (2013), in which the octogenarians Lillian and Audrey, two friends living with dementia, go on a holiday road-trip through Canada.

4.1 "Oh, The Places They'll Go!": When 90-Year-Old People Walk Out the Door and Disappear

> Acquiring mobility is often analogous to a struggle for acquiring new subjectivity.
>
> — Uteng and Cresswell, *Gendered Mobility*

In June 2014, WWII veteran Bernard Jordan made global headlines when he escaped from The Pines care home in East Sussex, England, to attend the 70th anniversary of D-Day. Wearing his war medals beneath his grey mac, he embarked on a cross-channel journey to France, defying the care home's restrictions. The Sussex Police's Twitter announcement captured the public's imagination: "Ninety-year-old veteran reported missing from care home. Turns out they'd said no to him going to #DDay70 but he went anyway. #fightingspirit" (Huffington Post n.p.). Jordan's story was immediately framed as an act of heroic defiance, with media reports portraying the care home as a site of confinement. The *Huffington Post Canada* wrote, "If the invasion of the Nazis couldn't take you down, chances are a nursing home's staff probably can't either" (Huffington Post n.p.). *The Daily Mail* dubbed his journey "The Great

Escape," drawing parallels to the famous 1963 war film[1] and reinforcing the idea of the care home is an oppressive space like the film's POW camps. Though administrators insisted Jordan had not been forbidden from attending, the media celebrated his breakout as an act of resistance, making him a symbol of autonomy and determination in old age. His story struck such a chord that within a day, a Facebook campaign (that is unfortunately no longer online) was launched to knight Jordan for his bravery, with supporters calling for his story to be made into a film. While many veterans of his age attended the commemorations in France, Jordan's escape captivated the public, revealing deep-seated anxieties about aging, autonomy, and the restrictive nature of institutional care.

The portrayal of the care home as an authoritarian space is reinforced by Jordan's own words in media interviews. Speaking to the *Daily Mail*, he acknowledged the significance of his journey, stating, "Being a veteran myself, this was important to me and it meant the world to be there. [...] I loved every minute. It was such an exciting experience." His remarks also suggest an underlying tension between personal autonomy and institutional control, as he added, "I will have to face the music at the care home now, but that is just one of those things in life." His playful confession, "I was naughty, but I had to be there" (Nicol and Craven) further amplifies the framing of his escape as an act of necessary rebellion, positioning the care home as a space where mobility and independence must be actively reclaimed (Dolan et al. n.p.).

Echoing John Urry's questions "why do people physically travel," and "why is there an increasing amount of physical, corporeal travel? Why bother with the risks, uncertainties and frustrations of corporeal movement?" (256), this section explores the growing popularity of care home escape stories. Their appeal can, in part, be understood through Urry's concept of social citizenship, which includes being "a full, active and engaged member of a society," and should "include socio-spatial access to participate within the main practices of one's society" (265). In long-term care facilities, such participation is often severely restricted. Institutional settings tend to limit not only physical mobility but also social and cultural engagement. Urry—even though not thinking about care homes specifically—claims that

1 In *The Great Escape*, starring Steve McQueen, James Garner, Charles Bronson, and Richard Attenborough, allied POWs try to dig a tunnel to flee the escape-proof camp.

> we could imagine that a "good society" would not limit, prohibit or re-direct the desire for such co-presence. The good society would seek to extend the possibilities of co-presence to every social group and regard infringements of this as involving undesirable social exclusion. [...] A socially inclusive society would elaborate and extend the possibilities of co-presence to all members. Significant inequalities with regard to access to such co-presence constitute undesirable social exclusion. A good society would minimize "coerced immobility" (as well as the many forms of "coerced mobility") and maximize the conditions for co-presence. (Urry 270)

Escape narratives push back against these limitations, against "coerced immobility," presenting protagonists who refuse to be confined by the spatial and symbolic constraints of institutional life.

Long-term care escape narratives can be read as constitutive of an activity narrative, which helps defeat the nursing home specter by promoting a new narrative of resistance. Their protagonists are "declining to decline" (Gullette, *Declining*) and take control of their own destiny. They position themselves as active and successful, and show readers that even nursing home residents still have hope. Such affirmative narratives of defiance and autonomy in old age help explain the widespread popularity of stories like *The Hundred-Year-Old Man Who Climbed Out of The Window and Disappeared* by Swedish author Jonas Jonasson. The 2009 novel, translated into 36 languages, and its 2013 film by Felix Herngren—screened in over 40 countries—became a cultural phenomenon, earning over $50 million in revenue, making it one of Sweden's the most successful Swedish films (Gustavsson, my translation). Despite its familiar plot, the novel's theme of an old man rejecting confinement and reclaiming agency resonated deeply with audiences. In France, Bernard Jordan was quickly labeled "The Ninety-Year-Old Man," drawing direct comparisons to Jonasson's fictional Allan Karlsson. As one commentator noted in the Huffington Post, "If you like this story, I recommend 'The 100-year-old man who climbed out of the window and disappeared.' It's a wonderful read! Great to hear a real-life version" (Cooper).

This merging of fact and fiction highlights the cultural appeal of escape narratives that challenge societal expectations of aging and celebrate the spirit of independence in later life. In a way that echoes Jean Baudrillard's concept of the hyperreal, "the generation by models of a real without origin or reality" (1), the media constructed Bernard Jordan as a "simulacrum" (1), aligning his real-life story with the fictional model of Jonasson's protagonist Allan Karlsson. To preserve Jonassonian escape narrative, key details of Jordan's story were subtly reshaped or omitted, such as the fact that he was actually never explicitly forbidden from leaving the care home and that his wife, also a resident there, was aware of his trip. These omissions transformed Jordan into a mythic figure of defiance, reinforcing the hyperreal image of the old escapee as an archetype rather than an individual.

Characters such as Bernard Jordan, as well as his fictional counterparts residing in long-term care facilities, are seen as voiceless victims while still in their roles as frail, old nursing home residents, but transform into picaresque heroes as soon as they attempt escape. As Pam Gravagne explains, "we secretly cheer for the elderly, for the success of those made less than human by an overarching narrative of decline" (47, also quoted in Chivers, "Blind" 139). Well-known literary examples of such escape stories are Sara Gruen's *Water for Elephants*[2] in which the 93-year-old protagonist, Jacob Jankowski, walks out the nursing home door one day and runs away with a circus, or Margaret Laurence's *The Stone Angel* (1964), in which Hagar Shipley runs away before her son and daughter-in-law can force her to move into the Silverthread nursing home. In Todd Johnson's *The Sweet By and By* (2009), Margaret and her friend Bernice escape from Ridgecrest, even if only to have dinner in a diner. In David Mitchell's *Cloud Atlas* (2004), a short break-out scene from the nursing home is added to one of the narrative threads. In Andrea Barrett's *The Forms of Water*, eighty-year old Brendan Auberon convinces his nephew to hijack the nursing home van to make a final visit to the only family estate remaining. In Gail Radley's *The Golden Days*,[3] Carlotta, an old lady who cannot stand the inhumane treatment she experiences in the nursing home and Cory, an eleven-year-old troubled foster child, become friends and run away to join a circus. Claire, in Janet Campbell Hale's short story by the same name (1999), dresses up as a man to flee the inhumane treatment she receives at Loma Vista and finds shelter with her relatives, and in the short film "The Greyed Escape" (Dehn)—the title, of course, alluding to the famous movie "The Great Escape" mentioned earlier—a nursing home inmate escapes in his late roommate's body bag in order to fulfil his dream of once more picking a couple of apples from a tree. Likewise, in "The Great Nursing Home Escape" (Hartswick), a simple stage play for lay actors, a group of seniors rethink their failed escape

2 The novel was adapted into a movie in 2011, starring Reese Witherspoon, Robert Pattinson, and Christoph Waltz.

3 John Sirmons's movie *The First of May* (1999) is based on Radley's 1991 novel.

attempt and hatch new plans, this time following the original story, digging a tunnel (27). A recent graphic novel, *Shadow Life* (2021) by Japanese-Canadian author Hiromi Goto "provides a new kind of queer aging" (Hess and Ullmann 131)" and focuses on Kumiko, a bisexual old woman who escapes a care home to reunite with her former lover, Alice.

There are several other "geriatric escape stories," as the genre has jokingly been called, and I will, after a brief exploration of the motif of each journey, offer a close reading of three of them: *Amigoland*, a novel by Oscar Casares; *Flee, Fly, Flown*, a novel by Janet Hepburn; and the movie *Cloudburst* by Thom Fitzgerald. The characters in these works gather all their strength and try to escape to resist interpellation (Althusser) into their roles as immobile, isolated, and inactive members of society—in short, "the old." In a Whitmanesque manner, they embark on journeys: Walt Whitman's "Song of the Open Road" from *Leaves of Grass* summarizes the fugitives' feelings: "Henceforth I whimper no more, postpone no more, need nothing / Done with indoor complaints, libraries, querulous criticisms / Strong and content I travel the open road" (Whitman 123). "You must not stay sleeping and dallying there in the house," Walt Whitman commands (131). The protagonists in the narratives that will be discussed seem to follow his advice and escape "out of the dark confinement" (131). Such narratives mirror and reinforce the powerful American myth of mobility, but, as will be shown in the following discussion, also reject it as an ideological construct, particularly with respect to gender and age.

The characters who escape confinement are struggling, as Uteng and Cresswell put it (2), to acquire a new kind of subjectivity. Their spiritual and physical journeys they undertake change them forever and challenge the notion of old age as being static and immobile. Thinking about the protagonists' physical and spiritual mobility is one way of theorizing the connections between age, gender, and spatiality. Kathleen Woodward underscores the significance of movement in shaping perceptions of aging, arguing that mobility is intrinsically linked to vitality, while "[l]ack of movement is characteristic of decrepit age," she argues. "If movement bespeaks life, immobility—lack of movement—is akin to death, and inertia verges dangerously on the inert" ("Instant" 53). From this perspective, escape narratives actively disrupt the myth of immobility in old age, celebrating the protagonists' defiance against the inertia imposed by institutional life. Whether these escape attempts can be considered "successful"—and by whose standards success is defined—will be a central focus of my analysis.

Care home narratives that culminate in escape include both old men and women who set out on their life-altering journeys as heroes and heroines. Thomas R. Cole analyzes the topos of the journey in his 1992 groundbreaking book *The Journey of Life: A Cultural History of Aging in America*, tracing it back to biblical traditions. In "The Aging Pilgrim's Progress in the New World," as chapter two is entitled (32–47): "The journey is among the most pervasive themes in world literature. Folk tales, poetry, drama, fiction, art, and religious teaching are filled with male heroes who set out from safe but constricting origins, undergo a series of adventures that transform them, and eventually reach or fail to reach a goal, or prize, or spiritual home," Cole states (xxxii). The journey narrative, which is often a quest narrative, is traditionally associated with a young man's experience of (self)discovery and liberation from social constraints, but as Gabriele Müller points out, an increasing number of narratives have been published that deal with post-retirement masculinity (and, I should add, also post-retirement femininity), use traveling as a motif (153), and challenge the master narrative of the young, white male going west.[4] In her study of late-life and institutional long-term care, Patricia Life asserts that by escaping the nursing home, "individuals exert agency over their surroundings, further enrich and expand their personal identities, and avoid application of the decline narrative to their own lives" (4). While I agree with her argument that "early twenty-first-century texts have begun to add a surprising new narrative where residents have acquired so much agency that they are able to walk away from the nursing home," (4) I would not go so far as to claim that they walk away "even from old age itself," as Life asserts (4). I would, however, argue that they have come to reevaluate what it means to be old and close to death. They finally begin to acknowledge the limitations their old age and/or the cultural assumptions connected to them bring about while—at least in some stories—a reevaluation of the life course takes place. Their journeys make them see their place in the world and their own aging differently. They allow protagonists to acquire new perspectives on themselves, on others, and their own lives. In other words, their journeys—always spiritual

4 In her essay, Gabriele Müller refers to Paul Mazursky's *Harry and Tonto* (1974), the story of a retired schoolteacher who travels with his cat across the USA, and contrasts it with more recent American movies, *About Schmidt* by Alexander Payne (2002), and David Lynch's *Straight Story* (1999), as well as European interpretations of the road movie, the German film *Schultze Gets the Blues* (2003) by Michael Schorr, and the Icelandic film *Children of Nature* by Fridrik Fridriksson (1992) (Müller 150).

as well as physical—change their lives, even if in spatial terms, they may end exactly where they began, often back in the care home, or, like in the case of *Cloudburst*, even in death.

At first glance, it may seem as if only few differences existed between old women and men with regard to the nature and outcome of their escapes from institutional care, an assumption which may be grounded in the incorrect and stereotypical notion that old age functions as a homogenizing factor. When taking a closer look at the structures of these individual escapes, however, it becomes clear that with regard to long-term care escape narratives and the protagonists' renegotiation of their identities, aspects of intersectionality cannot be ignored. Women's escapes differ significantly from those of men.

All fictional narratives discussed in this chapter use the journey as a motif and borrow narrative elements and generic conventions of the road novel or road movie. The genre's conventions, however, are turned upside down in these stories because older characters are positioned as heroes and heroines, a fact that highlights the importance of analyzing mobility with reference to space and age. With *Driving Visions* (2002), David Laderman has written an excellent book about the genre, but I absolutely disagree with his observation regarding older protagonists in road narratives. Suggesting that older characters diminish the genre's radical, countercultural edge, Laderman maintains:

> As we have seen throughout, the genre is born in and through the counterculture, and is driven essentially by *youthful* rebellion against stability, conformity, and tradition. More typically in the road movie, senior citizens signify such stability and tradition, epitomizing the law and home, both in terms of character (harking back to the "old days") and their physical limitations. Driving the genre with an elder senior, therefore, automatically inclines toward sanitizing its culturally critical core. As with road movies featuring children, such a perspective renders the genre more palatable, more family-oriented, more conventional—and less culturally critical. (Laderman 184)

I agree that traditionally, the road narrative (he refers exclusively to movies) is a genre that has been associated with young and usually male characters whose actions result in self-discovery and liberation from the constraints of social expectations. I also agree that it is a genre in which characters step outside the social and symbolic order to defamiliarize themselves from convention and conformity (Müller 153). I disagree, however, with his assumption that the perspective of older protagonists "sanitizes its culturally critical core." This assumption would mean that such movies are more conventional, less culturally critical, and less subversive. Here, he overlooks the radical potential of aging protagonists, particularly when they reject the social constraints of old age and resist narratives of decline. This also means accepting the binary of young and old and perpetuating the stereotype of the boring, conventional, homogeneous mass of old people, thereby also marginalizing them and denying their participation, not only in social and cultural life, but also in the criticism thereof. Laderman seems to define cultural critique solely through youthful rebellion against conventional norms. But age-based rebellion against societal constraints can be just as subversive. In recent years, old people, particularly also old women, have inscribed themselves into the genre without, however, rendering the genre more "palatable" or "conventional," as Laderman puts it. On the contrary, the inclusion of old men and women highlights crucial concerns, including the hotly debated issue of long-term care, self-determination in old age, and society's taboos about death. In addition, Laderman's argument treats old persons as monolithic, failing to consider how gender, race, class, and sexuality intersect with aging in road narratives.

Laderman is right when he argues that "driving the road movie with a senior can become a challenge to the genre itself. [...] Like that of women, gays, and people of color, this elder perspective becomes an outsider perspective within an outsider genre, a fresh revitalization of the typical young white male point of view of most classic road movies. [...] the genre gets fresh fuel from the new/'old' perspective behind the wheel" (Laderman 184). When older characters run away from the confinement of institutional care and hit the road, the genre's conventions are in fact challenged. Rather than diluting the rebellious core of the road movie, older protagonists often reframe and expand it. They do so with a different objective: Whereas young protagonists flee from conventions and break out of the familiar, the old protagonists attempt to reclaim the familiar, recover their place in society, and fight against the marginalized social role that has been assigned to them (Hartung and Maierhofer, "Introduction" 15). This, however, does not make the genre more palatable and conventional.

Heidi Slettedahl Macpherson's excellent feminist analysis in *Women's Movement. Escape as Transgression in North American Fiction* (2002) is a wonderful counterweight to Laderman's important book, as she focuses on gendered readings of escape narratives and points to crucial differences in terms of gender and mobility. Even if she, unfortunately, does not include aspects of aging and old age in her discussion, her work prepares the ground for such an intersectional reading.[5] She argues that "[t]o incorporate the female—especially the white, middle-class female—into a discourse of escape significantly alters the perception of the maneuver" (1). In addition to initiating a gendered reading of escape stories, Slettedahl Macpherson's study must be credited for widening the scope of the discussion by focusing on the importance of including spatial aspects. The gendered discursive space is integral to women's writing about escape, she maintains (6): "Seen as essentially voiceless and storyless while remaining in their prescribed gender roles, female characters undergo transformation when they take on the role of escaper. To escape is to transgress, and contemporary feminist fiction explores escape as an act of resistance to the status quo" (1). I argue that this transgression is also relevant for the aged male and female protagonists of care home narratives, whose voiceless and storyless existence while still institutional inmates can be contrasted with picaresque adventures or quest narratives that focus on their vigor and strength as soon as they plan to embark on their journeys. As the following analysis will show, however, women's spatial transgressions are met by more obstacles, and their escapes are less self-determined than those of men. Yet, they appear in novels as self-determined protagonists and voice their claims for "roads of their own."

In *Roads of Her Own: Gendered Space and Mobility in American Women's Road Narratives* (2009), Alexandra Ganser investigates American narratives of mobility from the perspective of transdifference, which she defines as "a category of analysis to describe the dissonant plurality of social and cultural affiliations as well as the narrative tensions produced by such pluralities" (11). She comes to the conclusion that women's road narratives "remap the road:"

> Female protagonists on the road—across media, national, and generational boundaries—have always confronted the limits of what is conceived as acceptable "feminine behavior" in certain spaces; both physical realities and

5 In terms of intersectionality, aspects such as class and ethnicity are equally important. It is interesting to note at this point that all of the primary texts that deal with the topic of long-term care present—with few exceptions such as Shani Mootoo's *Cereus Blooms at Night*—exclusively Caucasian care home residents; when Latinos and Latinas, African American or Black Canadian characters are present in the texts discussed, they are almost exclusively featured as care-givers. For a discussion of Thomas King's novel *Green Grass, Running Water* (1993) in the context of First Nation's and Native Americans' culture, see Patricia Life, *Long-Term Caring: Canadian Literary Narratives of Personal Agency and Identity in Late Life* (2014).

> ascriptions with which female bodies are confronted on the road have been imprinted on cultural representations of this spatial experience. Yet it is exactly in the act of facing these gendered spaces that women's road narratives remap the road: by questioning, subverting, and appropriating paradigms of mobility, they create transient, deterritorialized subjects and envision not "a road," but many "roads of their own." (311)

Road novels in which female protagonists claim their own spaces, as Ganser convincingly observes with reference to Virginia Woolf, constitute a way of deconstructing gender stereotypes; gender and narrative are established as fundamental for the production of space and mobility (311). With regard to road narratives that present old protagonists, the question of how such texts constitute a way of deconstructing *age* stereotypes arises. While, according to Ganser, women in road narratives usually flee domesticity ("On" 153), old women in care home narratives do not usually escape "from the hearth to the open road" (Waxman, *From*) but, just like their male counterparts, from the confines of institutional care. Although the nursing home specter is equally haunting for male and female fugitives, the literary construction of their escape stories is largely informed by generic conventions, and as such, by age and gender stereotypes.

Particularly in American, but also in Canadian literature and culture, the road has been one of the most preeminent tropes and is linked to notions such as Manifest Destiny, or the Puritan "errand into the wilderness:" "The specific dimension of North American ideas of mobility results from the foundational significance of a colonial settler mentality and a variety of journeys, migrations, and displacements" (*Roads* 15). As a literary genre, the road narrative goes back to the 1930s, Ganser argues with reference to Mikhail Bakhtin's essay "Forms of Time and Chronotope in the Novel" (1981/1937–38). Chance encounters and unexpected meetings, Bakhtin states, contribute to the dialogic quality of the road as a narrative space, where different lives intersect in meaningful ways. In John Urry's terms, this aligns with the concept of "co-presence"—the idea that human movement is often driven by the desire to share physical space with others (250). Notably, Bakhtin also acknowledges the role of age in shaping these encounters: "On the road [...] the spatial and temporal paths of the most varied people—representatives of all social classes, estates, religions, nationalities, ages—intersect at one spatial and temporal point. People who are normally kept separate by social and spatial distance can accidentally meet; any contrast may crop up, the most various fates may collide and interweave with one another" (243). He underlines how the road collapses social distance, allowing lives that would typically not intersect to intertwine:

> On the road the spatial and temporal series defining human fates and lives combine with one another in distinctive ways, even as they become more complex and more concrete by the collapse of *social distances*. The chronotope of the road is both a point of new departures and a place for events to find their denouement. Time, as it were, fuses together with space and flows in it (forming the road); this is the source of the rich metaphorical expansion on the image of the road as a course: "the course of a life," "to set out on a new course," "the course of history" and so on; varied and multi-leveled are the ways in which road is turned into a metaphor, but its fundamental pivot is the flow of time. (Bakhtin, "Forms" 243)

The road as a chronotope is juxtaposed to the nursing home, a place of stasis and death, a homogenizing place that transforms the most diverse individuals into "old people." As a literal and metaphorical space of transition and transgression, the road is a space "democratic, open to all and opposed to the closed" (Campbell 282, quoted in Ganser, *Roads* 38). The contrast between the static care home and the adventurous, liberating space of the road heightens the protagonists' longing to re-engage and participate in life, making their wish to escape understandable, even necessary. Their movement is not just a physical journey but an assertion of social participation and agency—a concept that aligns with John Urry's argument on the fundamental right to mobility (265). He stresses that participation in society is deeply tied to access to movement "In particular, participation involves issues of transportation and mobility – namely, how to facilitate widespread participation in society by all social groups, especially ensuring that divisions of class, gender, ethnicity, age, do not result in significant forms of socio-spatial exclusion, of 'mobility-exclusion'" (Urry 265).

Ganser builds on this idea, concluding that the road text functions as a means of shifting perspectives and challenging dominant assumptions: "The road text can be read as an articulation of the 'philosophical capacity to shift views and destabilize assumptions' (Campbell 284) and has therefore attracted emergent articulations by marginal social groups" (*Roads* 38). Among these marginalized voices are old people, especially old women, who navigate not only physical but also social and cultural restrictions on their movement. As Susan Sontag's "Double Standard of Aging" (1972) suggests, older women face heightened invisibility and stereotyping, making their representation in road narratives a powerful act of deconstruction and resistance in both literature and film.

4.2 The Idyllic Chronotope of Family Life: Oscar Casares's *Amigoland*

A man should be able to take a trip if he wants.

— Oscar Casares, *Amigoland*

Oscar Casares's first novel *Amigoland* (2009) chronicles the story of two estranged brothers, Don Fidencio and Don Celestino Rosales, as they reunite after not communicating with one another for many years, and embark on a road trip to Mexico. Don Fidencio, a grumpy 91-year-old retired postman, endures a miserable existence in Amigoland, a nursing home in Brownsville in the Rio Grande Valley, from where he repeatedly, but unsuccessfully, plots to escape. In contrast, his youngest brother, Don Celestino, a former hairdresser in his seventies, enjoys his comfortable retirement with Socorro, his much younger Mexican housekeeper and lover. The novel's third person narration shifts perspectives between these three characters, offering a triangular view of their journey and relationships.

Don Fidencio was forced into Amigoland by his daughter and son-in-law after falling in the yard and suffering an increasingly severe prostate problem, which causes occasional incontinence and unsettles him deeply. Feeling alienated and lonely, he sees the care home's name as ironic, as Don Fidencio does not have a single friend there: "Strangers, all strangers, they had taken everyone he knew and replaced them with strangers. This is where they had sent him to die, with strangers" (Casares 16). His greatest fear is not of death itself, but dying among strangers, disconnected from the world he once knew. His perspective serves as a cultural critique of institutionalized aging, contrasting the isolating nature of nursing homes with the preferred alternative of "aging in place," which preserves a sense of belonging and continuity.

Space theorist Yi-Fu Tuan has pointed out the importance of home as a "protected place," "a place that offers security, familiarity and nurture" (164). In *Space and Place*, he elaborates further on the notion of familiarity, an aspect Don Fidencio essentially lacks: "Familiarity is a characteristic of the past. The home provides an image of the past. Moreover in an ideal sense home lies at the center of one's life, and center (we have seen) connotes origin and beginning" (Tuan, *Space* 128). Amigoland is an unfamiliar space for Don Fidencio. He also criticizes the poor quality of care in the cold, impersonal environment of the nursing home. He longs to spend his final years without the interference of professional staff, whom he sees as indifferent caretakers who medicate him to keep him alive but not truly living. His frustration highlights the dehumanizing aspects of institutional care, where prolonging life takes precedence over preserving dignity and autonomy: "Tell me, why it is that nobody wants me, but nobody wants me to die either," he asks his brother (126). He desires a better way of living—and dying—and prays for it day by day: "It was just one more humble request added to the short but growing list of things he prayed for every night: [...] for him to find some way to escape from this prison where they kept him against his will; and for his freedom to come soon, even if it should cost him his life, so long as he didn't die here in this bed, surrounded by so many strange and unfamiliar faces" (10).

Like the novels discussed above, *Amigoland* illustrates what Bill Thomas identifies as the "three deadly plagues of the human spirit: Loneliness, Helplessness and Boredom" (The Eden Alternative 2). Don Fidencio knows these three plagues all too well. He feels no sense of home in Amigoland, which he repeatedly refers to as "the prison." As a form of resistance, he refuses to learn the names of either the nurses or the other residents, further emphasizing his detachment from the institution and its imposed social structure. He applies nicknames based on their characteristics, such as "The One With The Flat Face, The One With The Big Ones, The One With The Worried Face, ... The One With The Net On His Head" (26) or "The One Who Likes To Kiss Your Forehead" (37) when referring to staff, and "The One With The Hole In His Back" (31), "The One Who Always Looks Constipated" (10) "The One Who Cries Like a Dying Calf" (243) when referring to his fellow residents. With "the Turtles" (37), he collectively refers to the older female residents in the home. On the one hand, Don Fidencio's refusal to learn names reflects his lack of attachment and reinforces the impersonal, anonymous atmosphere of Amigoland. On the other hand, it serves as a coping mechanism, allowing him to hide his own memory lapses. He is aware that his recollection is slipping—his narration is interspersed with sudden flashbacks and dream sequences, signaling his growing confusion. This awareness deepens his cynicism and bitterness, rooted in his fear of losing all independence and becoming what he calls "The Useless One" (34). His fear of decline is also described on a spatial level, shaping his perception of the care home as a place of confinement, decline, and ultimately erasure.

Nowhere is this more evident than in his observation of the U-shaped table, where the most dependent residents are spoon-fed by aides:

> Alongside the window that looked onto the patio, one of the aides stood in the center of a U-shaped table and uncovered trays for the residents, all of them twitching in their reclining wheelchairs that were more like upright gurneys. She took a spoonful from the first tray [...] and then a second later the aide had to recover the yellowish dollop that had seeped onto the woman's chin. [...] How long could it be before they moved him over to the U-shaped table where the aides would be feeding him? (Casares 15–16)

As in many nursing home narratives, certain spaces and places within the institution signal a closer proximity to dependency, and ultimately death, than others. The U-shaped table where residents are spoon-fed, is one such space; another is the locked section of the building reserved for "The Ones Who Like to Wander Off" (42). These spaces serve as stark reminders of physical and cognitive declin7e, reinforcing Don Fidencio's fear of losing control over his own life. The nursing home itself becomes a symbol of his finitude, a place where he is confronted with the inevitable progression of aging. Ironically, despite repeatedly telling himself that he does not want to dwell on the past, its presence becomes unavoidable, intruding into his thoughts and forcing him to reflect on his life in ways he had resisted before: "The other reason he preferred to not look around was that he didn't like thinking about his life, how it used to be, how it was now, and what it would likely become, if God didn't do him the good favor of taking him soon. No matter how much he had lost, or they thought he had lost, he was still alert and understood what was happening to him" (16).

Childhood Memories Resurface

Ever since being placed in the nursing home, Don Fidencio finds himself dreaming about his childhood, particularly his grandfather. The nursing home itself functions as a *memento mori*—a constant reminder of his own mortality. Aware that his time is running out, he becomes increasingly preoccupied with clarifying a long-standing family myth about his grandfather's alleged kidnapping by Indigenous people. To uncover the truth, however, he must return to the place of his childhood, reconnecting with both his past and the roots of his ancestors. This idea holds particular significance for Don Fidencio, as uncovering the truth about their grandfather's disappearance could ultimately allow him to reconcile with his brother, Don Celestino. The two became estranged due to a decades-old argument over the true cause of their grandfather's disappearance, further strained by a minor disagreement in Don Celestino's barbershop years earlier. As Don Fidencio's memories resurface, so does his desire to reconnect with his brother, setting the stage for the journey that will unfold later in the story. His growing preoccupation with the past not only foreshadows the brothers' upcoming quest for answers but also suggests that their journey will be as much about healing familial wounds as uncovering historical truths:

> Of eight brothers and four sisters, only the two of them were left. At least he thought it was still the two of them. The youngest and the oldest, almost twenty years separating them. That the youngest was alive would make sense, he supposed, but what good reason could there be for the oldest to be alive and for the rest of his brothers and sisters to be gone? What sense did it make for him to be still walking around? For what? For him to be stuck here, waiting to die? At least if Celestino was alive he was probably out there living his life like a free man. *If...* They hadn't actually spoken in years. Why, though? (Casares 41)

A process of "life review" (Butler) is set in motion, which holds the possibility of coming to terms with past conflicts, to re-evaluate and re-narrate them in order to integrate them into a positive life course narrative. Don Fidencio feels "stuck" in the nursing home, while his brother, in contrast, remains a "free man." This growing sense of entrapment fuels his sudden urge to reach out to Don Celestino. However, with his faltering sense of time, he ends up calling him in the middle of the night—when Don Celestino, sleepy and disoriented, is too slow to answer. One day, however, Socorro persuades Don Celestino—who is also troubled by their old conflict—to visit his brother at Amigoland. When he arrives, Don Fidencio recognizes him almost instantly, referring to him as "The One With The White Hair," and without hesitation, pleads: "You should take me to live with you. Take your brother from this prison" (125). Though Don Celestino cannot grant this request, he continues to visit, becoming a vital lifeline—a connection that not only reintegrates Fidencio into the outside world but also rekindles the bond they both realize they need to mend. Determined to uncover the truth, Don Fidencio repeatedly begs his younger brother to take him on a road trip to the small Mexican village where their family once lived. For Don Celestino, their grandfather's alleged kidnapping seems like little more than a popular historical or folkloristic myth. But for Don Fidencio the story holds deeper significance: he sees it as the key to understanding his own existence (Sandick n.p.), a final chance to make sense of the past before time runs out. Don Celestino's visits spark a transformation in Don Fidencio, giving him a renewed sense of purpose. No longer resigned to his fate, he begins to (day)dream more vividly of his childhood home and past. The mental shift is mirrored in his physical rejuvenation; he stops using his walker, fights to reclaim his cane, and secretly practices walking without help. Each of these small acts signal his determination to regain control, preparing him for the journey he wants to take:

> They'd seen how much improvement he had made with his therapy and now they were scared that one of these days he would slip out and this time they wouldn't be able to catch up to him. One good, sturdy cane was all it would take. And soon, not even that. In the evenings he was still sweeping the floors with the dust mop, but now once he was out of sight of the nurses' station, he would lean the mop against the wall and continue on his own, staying close to the wooden railing, just in case. They probably thought he would never get anywhere without the walker. But that showed how much they knew Fidencio Rosales. (Casares 173)

The nursing home is seen as counterproductive to this progress, as the nurses keep taking away his canes and force him to use the walker in order to reduce the risk of falling. As in many care home novels, a fall serves as the catalyst for institutionalization, reinforcing the idea that physical instability marks the transition into dependency. Falling is seen as a metaphor for decline, a connection Stephen Katz explores in "Hold On! Falling, Embodiment, and the Materiality of Old Age" (198). He notes that while risk-taking is generally accepted as a natural part of younger life, fall prevention discourses reframe it as reckless and irresponsible in old age, reinforcing a medicalized model of care that prioritizes safety over autonomy:

> If falling embodies aging in ways that signify decline, then it is not surprising that aging individuals attribute falls to accidents, environmental hazards, and the contingencies of life, rather than to the failing or frailty of their bodies. Fall prevention discourses also frame any risk-taking, which is assumed to be a natural part of younger lives, as being dangerous and foolish in later life. (Katz, "Hold" 198)

By illustrating how the protagonist resists these constraints, the novel challenges the assumption that aging bodies must be strictly regulated, offering a critique of the disempowering institutional structures that equate care with control. The risks Don Fidencio will be taking on a road trip to Mexico provide a counter-narrative to the limitations and "risks" he experiences in the home.

Fidencio, meanwhile, also triggers a new interest in the past in Celestino, prompting him to confront his own mortality in the wake of his wife's passing six months earlier. As the estranged brothers tentatively reconnect, Celestino dusts off his old barbershop equipment and brings it to the nursing home, suggesting that he cut Fidencio's hair. This gesture not only revives a shared memory but also symbolically returns them to the moment that caused their rift—a childish fight in Celestino's former barbershop a decade ago. At first, Don Fidencio refuses the haircut, unwilling to sit in a wheelchair for the procedure, but when Celestino accommodates his request by fetching a regular chair, the small but meaningful act becomes a bridge to reconciliation, offering both brothers a chance to mend their fractured bond. "Don Fidencio stayed quiet for some time, looking into the mirror and watching his brother work, though later he seemed to be gazing at something more distant. [...] 'I can remember some of it.' 'Some of what?' Don Celestino asked, brushing the hair off his brother's shoulder" (135).

As Celestino meticulously cuts his brother's hair—a process described in vivid detail over four pages—they gradually slip into reminiscences of their childhood in the Rio Grande Valley, rediscovering their shared past through conversation and memory. Their physical closeness during the haircut—"Don Celestino [...] cupped his brother's chin and turned his head a few degrees to the left, then back toward the center, and then ever so slightly towards the right. The only thing left to do was snip some of the hairs along the rims of his ears, and growing out from his nostrils" (136)—becomes an intimate act of reconciliation, gradually dissolving the emotional distance that had separated them for years. Don Fidencio takes pleasure in this act of bodily care—a personal, familiar touch he has long missed. This intimate moment stands in stark contrast to the impersonal "bed-and-body work" (Gubrium, *Living* 123) typically associated with institutional care, highlighting the difference between affectionate, voluntary touch and the routine, clinical handling he experiences in the nursing home: "The showers and sponge baths didn't count as touching since the aides were wearing gloves and working so routinely that at times it felt as though he were going through a car wash with a half dozen other old men waiting in their wheelchairs behind him" (Casares 112). He usually resists all forms of bodily care and puts up a fight when nurses try to help him ("'How can we take care of you, Mr. Rosales, if you won't let us take care of you?' 'I don't need you or anybody taking care of me,'" 21). Don Celestino, however, manages to reach him. Once his haircut is complete, Don Fidencio is finally ready to reconnect with the past: "He turned toward the larger mirror again and kept gazing into it until he could see the faint traces of a face he had almost forgotten" (138). As in many literary texts on old age, the motif of the mirror also occurs in *Amigoland*. Whereas the texts discussed earlier depict the mirror as a site of alienation and disintegration of the self—"the mirror stage of old age" (Woodward, "Instant" 60; Life)—Don Fidencio's experience is different. Rather than feeling estranged from his reflection, he finds recognition in it. Through Don Celestino's care and attention, he does not see a fragmented or diminished self but instead glimpses the younger man he once was, ready to embark on a journey of rediscovery.

The rejuvenating effect of the haircut extends to Don Celestino who, despite having never imagined cutting hair again after selling his barbershop, "was surprised how nimble his fingers were" (133). This newfound energy in both brothers sets the stage for the journey ahead. A few days later, Don Fidencio's dreams intensify, revolving around two recurring themes: his desire to escape the nursing home (101–03) and the promise he once made to his grandfather to return to the ranchito in Linares: "Then he said to me, 'Tocayo,' because we were both Fidencio, but he hardly ever called me by my name. 'Tocayo, someday when you are older you should go back and see how things are now, what there is of my ranchito. Tell them I always wanted to go back'" (148).

While Don Celestino remains skeptical about the accuracy of Don Fidencio's kidnapping story, Socorro begins to take interest in the journey, not least because she wants to be closer to Don Celestino and, as she argues, to his only remaining family member, Don Fidencio. Having left her abusive husband in Mexico—a bold and liberating decision for which her mother and aunt have yet to forgive her—Socorro has embraced her independence by building a life for herself in the U.S., challenging traditional gender expectations along the way. Ultimately, it is Socorro who becomes the catalyst for the brothers' decision to embark on the journey, her determination and presence propelling them forward.

When the old story of their grandfather's kidnapping resurfaces, Socorro urges the brothers to finally travel to the *ranchito* near Linares to uncover the truth about their family history. Their plans come to an abrupt halt when Don Fidencio's daughter and legal guardian, Amalia, strictly forbids him from leaving the nursing home. "Don Fidencio tried to explain that the trip wouldn't take so long, a couple of days at most, but she wasn't listening. No was no" (192). This brief exchange underscores Don Fidencio's dependency, framing the moment as a reversal of traditional parent-child roles. Amalia's unwavering "No was no" mirrors the authoritative tone of a mother denying a young child permission to go out, reinforcing the infantilization often experienced by older adults in institutional settings. This interpretation is further supported by the brothers' ironic exchange that follows: "'Just because she said no this time doesn't mean anything. Maybe later she could change her mind.' 'You mean when I get a little older?'" (194), Don Fidencio responds cynically, highlighting the absurdity of his situation.

Don Fidencio cannot tolerate the constant infantilization he experiences in the nursing home, a theme that recurs throughout the novel. His struggle is evident when he vehemently resists the plastic bib he is forced to wear during meals (13–21), when he laments the lack of locks on bathroom doors and longs for privacy (31), when he dreads the discomfort of a plastic mattress lining (17), and when he fears the ultimate loss of dignity—being put in diapers (339). While such caregiving procedures may be deemed necessary for efficiency in a large institution, Don Fidencio perceives them as deeply humiliating, reinforcing his sense of powerlessness and eroding his autonomy. Such procedures, as Julia Twigg points out, are often considered embarrassing, because they emphasize the lack of control one has over bodily functions and are only directed at the body, not at the person. Such failures "return the person to babyhood and underpin the wider infantilization of clients in the care system," Twigg notes (66). This infantilization and the prison-like qualities of the home reinforce Don Fidencio's wish to leave.

As in most nursing home novels discussed in this chapter, a number of references and allusions are made to famous fictional escape narratives such as John Sturges's movie *The Great Escape*, Alexandre Dumas's novel *The Count of Monte Cristo*, or the movie *Runaway Train* (dir. Andrei Konchalovsky) that the care home "prisoners" seem to be familiar with when plotting escape. Usually, the old protagonists' escape plans mock these famous stories, and *Amigoland* is no exception. Don Fidencio also resorts to a movie as a template for a possible escape, but soon realizes the differences between a prison and a nursing home:

> A few nights ago he'd seen an old black and white about an innocent man who finally escaped prison by hiding inside a pile of dirty laundry that was later loaded into a delivery truck. When no one was looking Don Fidencio

> peeked inside the large container, then jerked away when he caught a whiff. What a way to die. They needed to drive it out into the country, burn whatever was inside there. (Casares 35–36)

Reclaiming Mobility

Don Fidencio's escape fantasies begin to consume him, and he constantly plots ways to break free. Twice, he tries to walk away from the care home, but is already apprehended at the first traffic light (34, 36). His subconscious anticipation of the journey ahead is reflected in his dreams, where his grandfather speaks to him, reinforcing his deep-seated desire to return to his roots. This longing suddenly takes shape when Don Celestino wakes him from a daydream: "'Andale, Fidencio,' 'Andale to where?' [...] 'I came to take you with me.' 'Remember I called you last night?' he said. 'I told you we were taking the trip to the other side, to Linares. The way Papá Grande wanted you to, remember?'" (201). Still sleepy, Fidencio complies, but vehemently refuses to take his walker with him, an act of defiance that underscores his determination to reclaim his independence.

The two brothers leave the nursing home in a taxi, joined by Socorro as they set off for Mexico. Notably, unlike traditional road narratives, their escape vehicle is not a Buick, Corvette, or Thunderbird (Soyka 29), but simply a taxi. While seemingly a minor detail, this choice subtly alters the conventional symbolism of the road trip, as the taxi—unlike a personally owned car—limits the characters' autonomy and self-realization. This departure from the classic road narrative framework highlights the constrained nature of their journey, both physically and symbolically. Mike Featherstone explores the implications of car-ownership and autonomy, explaining that "The term automobility works off the combination of autonomy, and mobility. In its broadest sense we can think of many automobilities—modes of autonomous, self-directed movement" (1). He further clarifies the origins of the word: "The auto in the term automobile initially referred to a self-propelled vehicle (a carriage without a horse). The autonomy was not just through the motor, but the capacity for independent motorized self-steering movement freed from the confines of a rail track" (1). The promise of automobility, he argues, is "self-steering autonomy and capacity to search out the open road or off-road, encapsulated in vehicles which afford not only speed and mobility, but act as comforting protected and enclosed private spaces" (2). Ultimately, the car represents "the capacity to go anywhere, to move and dwell without asking permission, the self-directed life free from the surveillance of the authorities" (Featherstone 2). This idea of freedom and control is elaborated on also by John Urry, who argues that "car-driving has become a central element of social citizenship" that counteract "socio-spatial exclusion" and "mobility exclusion" (Urry 265).

If the car is traditionally read as a status symbol and sign of masculinity and male mobility,[6] the taxi—still a car, but driven with the help of others—can be interpreted as symbolic of a loss of control and male power. The brothers are not in full control of their journey; they remain dependent on someone else to get them where they want to go, signaling a shift from the classic road narrative where the car represents autonomy and dominance.

This symbolic loss of agency extends beyond mobility and into the realm of virility. Don Fidencio's has difficulties to recall with whom and when he had last had sex with, "before women started treating him as if he were a harmless old creature and what he had once carried between his legs had now shriveled up and fallen off" (116). Similarly, Don Celestino discreetly stashes "little blue pills […] vitamins, if she [Socorro] had to know" (97) behind a hot water bottle in the medicine chest. The novel links the two old men's dependence on a taxi to their anxieties about their loss of virility, underlining how aging challenges traditional constructs of masculinity and independence.

Another adaptation of the traditional escape narrative lies in the nature of the "crime" that compels aged protagonists to flee. Unlike fugitives such as *Bonnie and Clyde*, they are not running from the law but from the confines of the nursing home. In addition, Don Fidencio's journey towards independence does not unfold in a high-speed car race but rather through a slow, deliberate reclaiming of mobility, quite literally, step-by-step. The walker he left behind at the home is replaced by a foldable walking stick that Socorro gets for Fidencio. While there is a clear progress narrative—moving from a wheelchair to a walker, then to a cane, and finally to a foldable walking stick—Fidencio's remobilization is not without setbacks. An embarrassing "accident" during the night delays their journey, forcing Socorro to find fresh clothes for him. This moment serves as a reminder that, despite his determination to regain control over his body and movement, the vulnerabilities of aging remain an unavoidable part of his escape.

After a two-day, adventure-filled taxi journey across the U.S.-Mexican border, the trio finally arrives in Linares. Initially, it seems they will be unable to locate their grandfather's Rancho Capote, but they soon learn that it was

6 "For nearly a century […] the auto has been identified with masculinity and male mobility" (Scharff 166, also quoted in Ganser, *Roads* 7)

renamed decades earlier and is now known as El Rancho De La Paz (308). This revelation allows them to find their way to the small ranch at last. Place names hold symbolic weight in the novel. Much like Amigoland, El Rancho De La Paz—literally The Ranch of Peace—is a meaningful name that foreshadows the novel's resolution. While Amigoland is a hybrid word blending English and Spanish—a linguistic mix that Don Fidencio resented at the nursing home—El Rancho De La Paz exists entirely in Spanish, the language in which he feels most at home. Unlike in the nursing home, where he had to "think of the right words before he could open his mouth" (18), here, he can speak freely, reclaiming not only his past but also his linguistic and cultural identity.

Upon arriving at the ranchito, the three travelers are welcomed by Carmen Rosales and her old, confused mother, Mamá Nene. The women immediately recognize the Rosales brothers as family and are overjoyed by their visit. "'We knew that with time you would find your way back. [...] We never stopped from hoping, always waiting for this day,' the old woman said, her voice quivering, [...] 'My father, he always told us that the boy would come back'" (317). In her confusion, she mistakes him for her long-lost uncle of the same name, who, as family lore recounts, was kidnapped by Indigenous people as a child. In an unexpected turn, Don Fidencio's version of the kidnapping story is confirmed through her fragmented memories. Though she and Don Celestino are in fact second cousins, Mamá Nene remains convinced that her uncle Fidencio has finally returned from his long-ago adventure. She clings to this belief, eagerly urging him to recount the details of his supposed past, further blurring the lines between history, memory, and identity. Don Fidencio plays along, telling her that nothing could have kept him from returning—which is true for him as well ("And this I told them from the beginning, that we needed to go, no matter what, that it was important, that I had made a promise to come back. If they'd let me, I would have walked all the way here," 314).

Don Fidencio complies with Mamá Nene's request, stepping into the role of his grandfather as he begins to recount the kidnapping story. Recognizing that it would be futile to correct her misconception, he closes his eyes and claims that more and more details are coming back to him. At this point, it becomes unclear what he genuinely remembers from his grandfather's narration and what he improvises along the way. When he describes how the boy was only released because he had wet his pants and smelled so bad, readers are prompted to question the accuracy of his account. At this stage in the story, the distinction between factual accuracy and "truth" becomes irrelevant for both Mamá Nene and Don Fidencio. Memories, wishes, dreams, and life review blend together: "He had made up so many things he couldn't say where the truth ended and the less-truthful parts began, so that with time it all became the same to him" (340). Through this act of storytelling, a deep bond forms between Don Fidencio and Mamá Nene, further solidifying his place in the family's history.

Closing the Life Cycle: Arriving in the Past

Moved by their reunion, Mamá Nene invites the travelers to stay overnight. While Don Celestino and Socorro prefer to return to their hotel, Don Fidencio—claiming that the trip back would be too exhausting—accepts her offer to spend the night at El Rancho De La Paz. His decision to stay reflects a deeper longing—not just for rest, but for a sense of belonging and permanence in a place that now feels like home. Don Fidencio's journey from the depersonalized, institutionalized care home in the U.S. to the small ranchito and his newfound "family" in Mexico can be understood through the lens of Thomas R. Cole's chapter "After the Life Cycle: The Moral Challenges of Later Life." Seen in this light, his journey is not merely physical but symbolic, leading him to a place where he can re-narrate his identity in a way that holds personal and cultural significance. Cole explores this shift by tracing the evolution from the pre-modern concept of the life cycle to the modern notion of the life course, explaining how these frameworks shape our understanding of aging and identity:

> During this transition to modernity, the cycle of life was effectively severed from the course of life. In pre-modern society, when generations of people lived on farms, in villages and small towns, local traditions of practice, belief, and behavior provided external moral norms as each generation visibly cycled into the next; the problem of identity as we know it did not arise. [...] "The idea of the 'life cycle,'" writes Anthony Giddens "[...] makes very little sense once the connections between the individual life and the interchange of the generations have been broken." In a modern, mobile society stages of life are disembedded from place; the individual "is more and more freed from externalities associated with pre-established ties to family, individuals, and groups." [7] (Cole, "After" 142)

Cole's insight underscores the significance of Don Fidencio's transformation. Don Fidencio's journey—which is not really a return, because he had never

7 Cole here cites Giddens, Anthony. *Modernity and Self-Identity: Self and Society in the Late Modern Age*. Stanford UP, 1991, p. 147.

in his life visited the ranch before—is narrated as a closing of the life cycle. His identity merges with that of his grandfather, and generations also meet through his connection to Mamá Nene. The pre-modern, familiar Mexican space of the ranch is juxtaposed against the modern and alienating nursing home. In his new environment, he can redefine himself, not only as a needy patient, "The Useless One," a self-definition that he had come to accept due to his isolation, but as a person who is needed by others. This, as Thomas Cole observes in a different context, is crucial for a person's sense of self: "My point is that the dominant social identities available to older people have been narrowly confined to the roles of patients, pensioners, and consumers. [...] Falling into purposelessness is not only a matter of individual will and character but also a matter of culture and public policy. Older people—like all people—need to be needed" (Cole, "After" 148). Cole notes with reference to Charles Taylor that meaningful relationships are crucial: "We become full, self-aware, and responsible human persons by engaging with others. Our identities must be confirmed or recognized in dialogue and negotiated with others. Self-definition is not possible in isolation, apart from social forms of expression and the expectations, needs, and values of others" ("After" 145). Mamá Nene not only validates Fidencio's identity but also gives him a renewed sense of being needed and connected. John Urry expands on this idea when he explains why people travel, emphasizing the importance of "co-presence" in maintaining social bonds: "Such intense moments of co-presence are necessary to sustain normal patterns of social life often organized on the basis of extensive time–space distanciation with lengthy periods of distance and solitude (Urry 261). Through her presence, Mamá Nene but also his brother Don Celestino, provide Fidencio with the kind of meaningful connection that bridges the isolation of his nursing home existence, reaffirming his place in the world.

Don Fidencio's experience offers a direct answer to John Urry's question of why people travel (Urry 256). For Fidencio, returning to his childhood landscape is not just about movement—it is about reclaiming a lost sense of self and belonging. Urry argues that "To be there for oneself is critical. Many places need to be seen 'for oneself', to be experienced directly: to meet at a particular house, say, of one's childhood or ... walk along a certain river valley or ... feel one's hands touching a rock-face and so on. It is only then that we know what a place is really like" (261). For Fidencio, this journey fulfills precisely that need—to physically return, to see, feel, and inhabit the spaces of his past in order to truly know them again. His travel reconnects him to memory, identity, and the sensory experience of place, reinforcing Urry's idea that some places must be lived firsthand to hold meaning.

Awakening the next morning, Don Fidencio feels an unfamiliar sense of peace. For the first time in a long while, he has not wet the bed, and unlike in the nursing home, he is free to smoke in the bathroom without restriction. Most importantly, he feels at home. As Carmen brings him a cup of coffee in the garden, he soaks in his surroundings, realizing that El Rancho De La Paz is where he truly belongs. The physical and emotional comfort he experiences stands in stark contrast to the confinement of the nursing home, reinforcing his longing for a space that offers both autonomy and connection:

> Earlier the granddaughter had made him some huevos a la mexicana with just enough chiles and spices that he realized he had forgotten what a real breakfast was supposed to taste like. She wasn't his granddaughter, he realized, but her name had gotten away from him again, and in any case, she treated him like he imagined a granddaughter might treat a grandfather. Just yesterday evening when they had already left the store, it had occurred to her to turn the truck around and go back so she could buy him a pack of cigarettes, just in case he ran out in the middle of the night. And this morning after his breakfast, she had brought the coffee to where he was sitting outside, smoking. (Casares 350–51)

Although Carmen's name escapes him, she does not become just another "The One Who"-figures; instead, he instinctively claims her as family. This contrasts sharply with his life in the nursing home, where every moment was dictated by routine and restriction. There, he had to wait for someone to unlock the patio just to smoke, followed by another wait to enter the mess hall, where the same monotonous breakfast was served every day: "Monday, oatmeal and raisins. Tuesday, oatmeal and raisins. Wednesday, oatmeal and raisins. On and on that way" (25). Surrounded by pastel paintings on pastel walls (33), forced to wear diapers at night and a bib at meals, his autonomy had been stripped away. Now, in contrast, he is free—free to walk whenever and wherever he pleases, to smoke in the bathroom, and to sit outside in the morning, savoring his coffee while gazing up at the vast sky: "Looking up past the first forty feet of the trunk, as the branches became more dense and entangled, eventually blocking out most of the rising sun and leaving only a narrow passageway to see where the sky opened up" (351). Like the protagonist in Waltner-Toews' short story "A Sunny Day in Canada," Fidencio senses a newfound openness, a symbolic pathway to the sky, where confinement gives way to possibility and release. The next day, when Don Celestino returns to pick him up, Don Fidencio refuses to leave. His journey has been successful in three crucial ways: he has fulfilled his promise to his grandfather to return to Mexico, he has escaped institutional confinement, and he has found a new home where he can spend his final days in peace.

Janice P. Stout, in *The Journey Narrative in American Literature*, identifies several key patterns in American quest narratives, all of which resonate with Don Fidencio's experience. His story follows the "journey home" pattern and the "home-founding journey" (41), in which travel leads to the creation of a new home, while also incorporating the "exploration and escape" (245) pattern. In a way, Fidencio's escape has brought him full circle—he has not only left a place of confinement but arrived at a place of belonging. When Carmen and Mamá Nene invite him to stay with them forever, he happily accepts, marking the true end of his journey—not just an escape from the past, but a return to the sense of home he had long been missing.

Why Carmen agrees to care for someone she barely knows remains ambiguous. The narrative offers no clear explanation—there is no indication of altruism on her part, nor any mention of financial compensation that might justify her decision. Instead, her openness is framed as a cultural contrast to the capitalist, individualistic values of the U.S., where care is often institutionalized. Even if Carmen accepts Don Fidencio's deeply human desire to die in peace, not among strangers but with family, this resolution is sentimentalized and elevated to a near-mythical level. The irony is that he does not actually know the Rosales family with whom he now chooses to stay. His sense of homecoming, then, is not rooted in personal history but rather in a romanticized ideal of belonging and familial connection, raising questions about how cultural narratives of kinship and care shape the story's resolution.

The Idyllic Chronotope of El Rancho de la Paz

The ranch, an idyllic space where past and present converge, can be interpreted through Mikhail Bakhtin's concept of "The Idyllic Chronotope in the Novel." This framework helps explain the story's otherwise improbable conclusion, in which Don Fidencio, despite his old age and need for care, finds a seemingly effortless new home. Bakhtin's idyllic chronotope idealizes time and space, erasing the complexities of daily life in favor of a harmonious, timeless present: "Strictly speaking, the idyll does not know the trivial details of everyday life" (Bakhtin, "Forms" 226). Bakhtin, by introducing the term "chronotope," refers to a convergence of time and space, or, as Heike Hartung precisely puts it, "translates spatial simultaneity into temporal sequence, thus localising time in concrete space" (*Narrating* 8). Reading *Amigoland* through this Bakhtinian lens, El Rancho De La Paz embodies the essence of the idyllic chronotope. Bakhtin describes the idyll as a world where life is deeply rooted in a specific place, binding generations together: "Idyllic life and its events are inseparable from this concrete, spatial corner of the world where the fathers and grandfathers lived and where one's children and their children will live. This little spatial world is limited and sufficient unto itself, not linked in any intrinsic way with other places, with the rest of the world" (225). In this closed, self-sustaining world, generations are bound to place rather than time, blurring the distinctions between past, present, and future:

> This unity of place in the life of generations weakens and renders less distinct all the temporal boundaries between individual lives and between various phases of one and the same life. The unity of place brings together and even fuses the cradle and the grave (the same little corner, the same earth) and brings together as well childhood and old age (the same grove, stream, the same lime trees, the same house) the life of the various generations who had also lived in that same place, under the same conditions, and who had seen the same things. This blurring of all the temporal boundaries made possible by a unity of place also contributes in an essential way to the creation of the cyclic rhythmicalness of time so characteristic of the idyll. (Bakhtin, "Forms" 225)

El Rancho De La Paz functions not just as a physical refuge for Don Fidencio but as a mythic, eternal home, where the anxieties of aging and displacement are replaced by a sense of belonging that transcends time. Employing Bakhtin's perspective, Casares's ending appears both plausible and inevitable, as it aligns with the long tradition of the idyllic family novel. Through this lens, El Rancho De La Paz serves as the natural resolution to Don Fidencio's journey, offering a space where generations symbolically reunite and time loses its linear constraints. What emerges is that Casares, in crafting his novel, draws not only from familiar narratives of the nursing home as a prison but also from the structural narrative conventions of the novel itself. As Bakhtin's historical analysis of the genre reveals, such idyllic endings are not simply narrative choices but well-established literary patterns—ones that shape the ways in which stories of home, belonging, and escape are told.

In the end, Don Fidencio firmly asserts his decision to stay in Mexico. When he informs Amalia, she argues with him and promises that he can live with her and her husband. As he does not trust that her promise will hold, he tells Don Celestino that he will not return to the U.S. "Suddenly I have so many places to live—everybody wants me for themselves," he remarks cynically (354). Don Celestino tries to persuade him, but Don Fidencio offers a simple, resolute response: "'Why are you doing this, Fidencio?' 'Just to live in peace'" (254). Realizing that he cannot change his brother's mind, Don Celestino prepares to leave, needing to catch up with Socorro, who had returned home earlier that morning after an argument. As the brothers say goodbye, Don Celestino discovers a plastic bag left behind in the taxi: "But when Don Celestino looked inside the bag, the pill dispenser was still packed and the extra vials hadn't been opened. Everything was the same as it was when they left the pharmacy five days earlier" (357). Not only has Don Fidencio left his walker behind, but he has also abandoned his medication, symbolizing his rejection of medicalized aging and institutional care. The novel ends without absolute closure, but it strongly suggests that Don Fidencio's journey—both physical and existential—has reached its conclusion. Having completed his "life review," he waves as Don Celestino's taxi disappears down the road: "'Nobody,' Don Fidencio said, and then he waved. 'Nobody forgot anything'" (357).

Amigoland is not only a quest narrative, but also a *Vollendungsroman*, a novel of completion, of "winding up," as Constance Rooke calls it in her essay "Old Age in Contemporary Fiction. A New Paradigm of Hope" (245). This genre focuses on the final stages of life, which entail letting go and finding "some kind of affirmation in the face of loss" (248). The life review is one of the most common themes of the *Vollendungsroman*. Don Fidencio engages in just such a life review, undertaking a journey not only to recover his family's history but also to assert his autonomy and dignity in old age. Andrew Achenbaum, with reference to Robert N. Butler, describes the process as follows:

> Some of the positive results of a life review can be the righting of old wrongs, making up with enemies, coming to accept one's own mortality, gaining a sense of serenity, pride in accomplishment and a feeling of having done one's best. Life review gives people an opportunity to decide what to do with the time left to them and work out emotional and material legacies. People become ready to die. (204)

Don Fidencio's quest is successful in that it aligns with the aspects addressed by Andrew Achenbaum. He reclaims what he considers essential at the end of life and embarks on a journey to restore his dignity. The road trip serves as both a return to his past and a step toward the future, embodying what Bakhtin describes as the "blurring of all the temporal boundaries" (225). By retracing his roots, Don Fidencio seeks closure and belonging, making the journey a necessary step in bringing his life to a meaningful conclusion—even if in a somewhat folkloristic manner, in the home of his ancestors. Heather Gardiner further explains the importance of returning to one's origins as follows:

> Through retrospect, the wheel of life is turned back to youth and childhood and in many instances, but not all, new pathways are opened towards a different kind of homecoming. The old person ends the journey of life where he or she began it, seeing its full span with a perspective which is only possible when age restricts the physical momentum of life and the journey comes "full circle" in some yet "untrodden" pathways of the mind. (59–60)

Don Fidencio's journey comes full circle, returning him to the place his grandfather—or, in his own version of the story, a fusion of his grandfather's identity and his own—had once left behind. By merging past and present, he creates a unified narrative of his life, finding a sense of wholeness and completion. He has fulfilled his goals, kept his promise, and secured a place of peace—the idyllic Rancho De La Paz—where he will be cared for until the end of his days by those he now considers family. His escape from the nightmarish institution leads not just to freedom but to a fairy tale-like resolution, transforming his story into a "happily ever after" ending.

As previously discussed, protagonists who experience confinement, isolation, and entrapment in old age often respond by turning inward, "initiating an exploration of distant memories," as Gardiner metaphorically describes it, "in the attic of the mind" (57). Don Fidencio's journeys—both the physical journey from Texas to Mexico and the imaginary journey undertaken in his grandfather's name—serve not only his own need for closure but also bring peace to Mamá Nene, who can finally stop waiting for the return of "her uncle." Beyond fulfilling a family myth, these journeys facilitate Don Fidencio's life review, allowing him to re-narrate his own story, reconcile with his Mexican-American identity, and bring the journey of his life to a meaningful and positive conclusion.

Socorro: The Border of Tradition and Modernity

Questions of space and place in the novel extend beyond individual experience, shaping a larger cultural and ideological landscape. By contrasting Mexico with the U.S. and family with institutional care, the narrative reinforces the idea that "blood is thicker than water"—implicitly endorsing the problematic notion that ethnicity is rooted in blood and soil. The novel draws on the common trope that Mexican culture remains pre-modern, where families, rather than institutions, are expected to care for their elders until the end of their lives. This romanticized view ignores the realities of social and demographic change. While eldercare in Mexico has traditionally been the responsibility of families—particularly women caregivers—shifting economic and demographic factors indicate that institutional care will soon become a necessity. As Robledo et al. highlight in their article "The State of Elder Care in Mexico" (2012), this transformation has already been recognized by social scientists and policymakers, raising important questions about the future of aging and care in Mexican society:

> Currently, the majority of the older population lives at home with their spouse or partner, children, grandchildren or other close relatives. Here, most of the long-term care they need is provided to them and within this pool of family members, mostly by women. Nevertheless, reduced fertility rates, constant rural-urban migration within Mexico and international migration, women's increasing participation in the labor force and activities outside the home, among other factors, have changed family size and composition and pose future challenges to the availability of household care and support. (187)

This binary opposition between family-based eldercare in Mexico and institutional care in the U.S. is not only embodied by Carmen Rosales and Mamá Nene, but also by Socorro, who lives across the border in Matamoros, where she cares for her mother and aunt. Her daily routine revolves around household duties and caregiving, as she continues "cooking and cleaning and shopping and going to the pharmacy for these pills or that salve that her mother might need" (Casares, *Amigoland* 81). Her mother and aunt, both older women themselves, fear that if Socorro marries the "old American," they will lose their primary caregiver. Their concerns reveal the deeply ingrained expectation that eldercare remains a familial—and specifically female—responsibility. In response, they urge her to distance herself from Don Celestino, advising her to find another house to clean and stop seeing him, reinforcing the gendered burden of care within traditional Mexican households.

> "You worry because you think I would go away." "Bah, now she thinks we cannot live without her." Her aunt laughed. The wheelchair squeaked as her mother adjusted herself. "You think your poor tía hasn't sacrificed to be here with us?" "And where else was she going to go?" Socorro said. "If before this she was living with her mother?" "Taking care of her." Her aunt stepped off the bed and went to stand behind the wheelchair. "Until God needed her." (174)

Socorro's mother and aunt make it clear that they expect Socorro to adhere to a normative femininity defined by with home, hearth, family, and traditional patterns of caregiving. Socorro, a woman of the borderlands, disrupts these expectations. Moving fluidly between Mexico and the U.S., she embodies a more independent and transgressive identity, breaking with traditional gender roles. Yet, despite this independence, Socorro still performs acts of caregiving, particularly for Don Fidencio. When he soils his bed at their stopover, she compassionately removes the sheets, provides him with fresh clothes, and helps him shower and dress. These moments highlight how caregiving remains an ingrained part of her identity, even as she resists the rigid structures imposed on her. Marrying Don Celestino, a man thirty years her senior, could eventually mean assuming caregiving responsibilities for him as well. While she may have left behind the traditional Mexican gender roles expected by her family, her future in the United States may still lead her back into a similar role, suggesting that care work remains an inescapable expectation for women, regardless of cultural or geographical boundaries.

The novel presents an ambivalent stance on the tension between tradition and modernity, yet it can be interpreted as a passionate indictment of the institutionalization of older adults. *Amigoland* lays bare the deficiencies of institutional care, vividly depicting the fears and anxieties experienced by its residents. In doing so, the novel echoes critical perspectives found in well-known nursing home ethnographies, which have long exposed the depersonalization, loss of autonomy, and emotional toll of institutional aging. Among these influential works are Jaber F. Gubrium's *Living and Dying at Murray Manor* (1975) and *Speaking of Life* (1993), in Timothy Diamond's *Making Gray Gold* (1992), in *The Culture of Long Term Care* (1995) edited by J. Neil Henderson and Maria D. Vesperi, or in *Gray Areas: Ethnographic Encounters with Nursing Home Culture* edited by Philip

B. Stafford. As Oscar Casares states in an interview, the story is based on his personal experience with his ninety year-old father, who fell and broke his hip, and spent the last three years of his life in a nursing home, an experience that was "possibly one of the most difficult for [his] family" (Casares 8).

Despite its idyllic and, at times, sentimental overtones, the novel also offers a meaningful exploration of what good end-of-life care entails. By centering Don Fidencio's perspective, *Amigoland* invites readers to experience empathy, potentially leading to "changed attitudes, improved motives, and better care and justice," as Susan Keen suggests in "A Theory of Narrative Empathy" (208). Aspects such as privacy, intimacy, friendship, community, and warmth are absent in the nursing home but are instead found in Mexico, where care is provided by a "family member" rather than institutional staff. Carmen and El Rancho De La Paz serve as the binary opposite of Amigoland, which fails to provide relationship-centered care. In this regard, Casares's novel does not reimagine institutional care in a way that redeems it, nor does it offer a vision for reform. Instead, the nursing home is portrayed as a place to be avoided at all costs—a sentiment made explicit by Don Fidencio's desperate nightly prayers: "It was just one more humble request added to the short but growing list of things he prayed for every night [...] for his freedom to come soon, even if it should cost him his life" (10). While the nursing home setting evokes isolation, dependency, infantilization, boredom, frailty, and confinement, the concept of travel represents its antithesis—implying movement, transformation, independence, agency, freedom, and choice.

Amigoland illustrates Don Fidencio's journey to freedom, which grants him dignity at the end of his days. By finding a place where he feels at home and at peace despite his physical ailments, he does not exemplify what is commonly seen as "successful aging," but what Wendy Lustbader terms "successful frailty" (Lustbader 15, also qtd. in Cole, "After" 152). She argues that "the alchemy of successful frailty" depends on "[t]urning the 'nothing' of empty time into the 'something' of good days" and the "insults of illness into privileges of being" (Lustbader 15, qtd. in Cole, "After" 152).

Like other nursing home escape novels, such as Sara Gruen's *Water for Elephants* or Jonas Jonasson's *The Hundred-Year-Old Man Who Climbed Out Of The Window And Disappeared* that feature male protagonists, Don Fidencio's journey is successful: his need for care, his dependence, but also his connection with Mamá Nene and the stories he tells her contribute to his "successful frailty" at *El Rancho De La Paz*. Successful frailty, I argue, is a defining feature of the *Vollendungsroman*, a genre concerned with closure and reconciliation in old age.

As Rooke describes, this stage entails "leaving the social stage" (245), yet the *Vollendungsroman* seeks to offer both its protagonist and its readers "some kind of affirmation in the face of loss" (248). Don Fidencio's journey fulfills this function, allowing him to find peace and dignity as he approaches the end of his life.

4.3 Women on the Run: Thom Fitzgerald's *Cloudburst* and Janet Hepburn's *Flee, Fly, Flown*

While *Amigoland* is an example of a road narrative that portrays escape as necessary and, most importantly, successful in terms of fulfilling the quest for the spiritual and cultural redefinition of the male protagonist's identity, Janet Hepburn's first novel *Flee, Fly, Flown* (2013) and Thom Fitzgerald' movie *Cloudburst* (2011) end on a sadder note. Both of the stories portray old women who escape long-term care facilities and embrace the space of the open road. In *Flee, Fly, Flown,* Lillian and Audrey, two nursing home residents living with dementia, decide that they have had enough of their boring lives in the home and that it is time for a holiday. They escape the lock-down unit of Ottawa's Tranquil Meadows Nursing Home, steal a car, and drive west to see the Rockies of British Columbia. Unfortunately, their short vacation ends before they reach their final destination and they are taken back to the care home. In *Cloudburst,* Dot and Stella travel north from Maine in the U.S. to Canada. The lesbian couple had been separated after Dot's granddaughter assigned her to a nursing home in order to take over Dot's house, which would leave Stella homeless. Stella kidnaps Dot from the home, and they flee to Canada, where same-sex marriage is legal, with the hope of finally marrying, but before they can officially wed, Dot falls severely ill and dies in Stella's arms in their car.

Unlike Don Fidencio and Don Celestino, who are never concerned about the police chasing them, the runaway women in both *Flee, Fly, Flown* and *Cloudburst* meet many obstacles, must disguise themselves, use false names, and hide from the police, their families, and the nursing home administrators who are frantically looking for them. In addition, each of the stories includes a young man without whose help and, more importantly, without whose protection the old women would not be able to undertake their journeys. While Socorro, the young woman in *Amigoland,* also travels with the two old protagonists, her function in the story is a different one. She is the catalyst that initiates the journey, but throughout the narration, she is merely configured as Don Celestino's lover rather than as an indispensable helpmate. Once on the road, however, the two men are able to reach *El Rancho De La Paz* without Socorro's support, whereas the young, male characters of Rayne in *Flee, Fly, Flown* and Prentice in *Cloudburst* literally become lifesavers.

In both cases, and in contrast to Don Fidencio, the women travelers ultimately find themselves denied a place where they can truly be at home. While one might argue that this outcome aligns with the conventions of traditional road novels—where characters set out not to establish a new home but to escape confinement—this discussion will demonstrate that their continued displacement is also deeply tied to their age, gender, and sexuality. The nursing home is contrasted in both narratives with the free and open space of the road; in fact, the two spaces are configured as binary opposites. While the nursing home, despite its bleak perspective, is represented as a safe place, the open road becomes a life-threatening space that forces the women to accept the limits of their own very existence in the end.

As Alexandra Ganser argues in her analysis of road narratives, the road is a gendered space, constructed differently for women on the run than for men. She highlights how Ronald Primeau's *Romance of the Road: The Literature of the American Highway* (1996) relegates women's experiences on the road to a single section—one of eight—grouped alongside "other minorities" (107) including African American and (male) Native American writers (Ganser, "On" 156). This marginalization reflects a broader tendency to overlook or diminish the distinct challenges women face in road narratives. She further explains that:

> Drawing on recent remappings in cultural geography, the "open road" appears as a dangerous frontier—in which women's physical and emotional well-being is always at perilous stake—rather than as an adventurous playground. In women's road stories, the American [and Canadian] highway does not maintain its mythical, iconic status, signifying freedom and the heroic quest for identity, which has been ascribed to it at least since the legendary accounts of the flight from domesticity by Jack Kerouac and his fellow (anti-)heroes of the Beat generation. (Ganser, "On" 153)

In this framework, the road is not a site of self-discovery and liberation for women but a perilous space that reinforces their vulnerability. In the two narratives discussed in the following section, the road is anything but "fit surroundings" for frail old women. My discussion examines intersectionality through the lenses of gender, sexuality, age, and illness/disability, analyzing how the protagonists' experiences in both the nursing home and on the road are represented. If, as Ganser argues, "these stories reflect a gendered economy of space that creates the road as all but the 'right(ful)' place for a woman" (Ganser, "On" 160), how do factors such as old age, homosexuality, frailty, and dementia intersect in these narratives? How do these additional layers of identity and vulnerability further complicate the protagonists' relationship to space and mobility?

4.3.1 "So Much Space Is Disconcerting": Janet Hepburn's *Flee, Fly, Flown*

> You can get so confused that you'll start in to race
> Down long wiggled roads at a break-necking pace
> And grind on for miles across weirdish wild space,
> Headed, I fear, towards the most useless place.
> The Waiting Place.
>
> — Dr. Seuss. *Oh, The Places You'll Go!*

Janet Hepburn's novel, much like Oscar Casares's *Amigoland*, is also based on the author's personal experience, as she witnessed a frail parent's treatment in a long-term care facility. The novel, as she states in a video interview, was inspired by the wish that her mother would have had the opportunity to make choices for herself:

> I had to write a story about how a person in that position could be free, how they could be more in charge of their own destiny, of how they could live more like they wanted to live, because it's so regimented in there, everything is about safety of care, while there's really nothing about what a person needs or wants psychologically. (Hepburn, "Janet" 2)

In the interview, Hepburn reflects on her experiences as both a daughter and caregiver, expressing her concerns about placing her mother in institutional long-term care. She contrasts the nursing home—depicted as a space of confinement and loss of autonomy—with an imagined space where freedom, control, and independence could be reclaimed. In her novel, she attempts to construct such an alternative world for her protagonists, sending them on a road trip across Canada, from their nursing home in Ottawa to the Canadian West. However, by the journey's end, the adventure proves too dangerous and exhausting for the two women, ultimately leading to their re-institutionalization.

In the following discussion, I examine the genre crossover in *Flee, Fly, Flown*, where Hepburn blends elements of the nursing home novel, dementia narrative, and road narrative. This analysis explores how the story is shaped by the intersection of gender, age, dementia/disability, and space. Specifically, how does the "gendered space of the open road" that Alexandra Ganser analyzes manifest for Lillian and Audrey, the two aging, forgetful *pícaras*? How do their experiences on the road challenge or reinforce the limitations imposed by their identities?

A reviewer has described *Flee, Fly, Flown* as a "*Thelma & Louise* for the Canadian geriatric set" (Quill and Quire n.p.). The reviewer's comparison with *Thelma & Louise* is not surprising given the similarities in plot and the novels' intertextual references, elements that have become integral to road movies and narratives over the past decades (Mayer 371). That *Flee, Fly, Flown* firmly belongs to the road narrative genre is evident from its opening, when Hepburn has Lillian declare, "We'll be like Jack Whatisname. You know, *On the Road*? Or Bob Hope and Bing Crosby in *The Road to*...wherever? We'll just see where we end up" (30). But the reviewer also cautions against dismissing the novel as merely a geriatric escape story, noting that "the novel's subtle nod to issues involving the treatment of persons with dementia infuses the story with a surprising complexity" (Quill and Quire n.p.). On the one hand, the novel employs dementia as an end-of-life-narrative to justify the protagonists' reinstitutionalization. As Heike Hartung explains, "[dementia narratives] may define the limits of development by narrating the end of memory and consciousness. In approaching the dissolution of the autonomous subject, these stories are concerned with loss and crisis" (Hartung, *Narrating* 277). On the other hand, Hartung further states:

> Dementia narratives also question the boundaries of life stories by contesting notions such as development, autonomy and personhood. Narratives of Alzheimer's and other age-related dementias depict old age in both its negative and positive aspects. This involves a discourse of crisis, in which Alzheimer's becomes a metaphor for the fears of ageing and a new "burden narrative" of old age for the twenty-first century. But it also enables a counter-discourse of "heroic helplessness" (Scott-Maxwell 17), in which dementia is represented as part of a relational process of development that

> moves beyond Cartesian subjectivity to embrace a prospective ending of life. (*Ageing* 172)

In line with Hartung's argument, *Flee, Fly, Flown* challenges the assumption that memory loss can be equated with the loss of autonomous subjectivity and personhood. While the journey west traditionally symbolizes progress and self-discovery, the protagonists ultimately never reach their destination and are instead forced to return. This raises a crucial question: what does adequate and responsible caregiving for individuals with memory loss truly look like? In the following discussion, I explore how the spatiality of old age, frailty, and subjectivity are renegotiated on the open road.

Flee, Fly, Flown opens with Lillian, the novel's first-person narrator, and her friend Audrey lamenting the unappetizing meals served at Tranquil Meadows—"tasteless mush" (3) and "rubbery cubes" (4). As Lillian surveys her surroundings, she describes a sterile, depersonalized environment: "Pastel uniforms with white sneakers perch on stools, spooning food into random open mouths [...] They write on clipboards, recording how much we eat, how much we leave behind. [...] A mint-green uniform stops at our table and takes away my untouched dinner" (4). In this depiction, residents are reduced to fragmented bodies, their "mouths" serving as a *pars pro toto* for their existence, while caregivers remain nameless, synecdochically identified only by their uniforms—"'Are you cold,' the uniform asks" (4). This erasure of individuality mirrors the institutional dehumanization seen in *Amigoland*, where care is defined by efficiency rather than meaningful relationships. As Lillian, Audrey, and their fellow residents become "institutional bodies"—measured, observed, and charted (Wiersma and Dupuis)—they lose their personhood, reinforcing the novel's critique of long-term care as a space of confinement rather than dignity.

On the level of space and time, the institution imposes rigid structures that dictate residents' lives. The nursing home is portrayed as a monotonous, pastel-colored environment where daily routines revolve around bingo, meals, and "silly games and repetitive sing-songs" (11), reducing time to an indistinguishable blur: "[d]ays and months are no longer distinguishable, one from the other in this place" (11). The dominance of institutional control over space and time has been widely discussed, as Elaine Wiersma highlights in "Conceptualizing Time in Older Age" (75). She points out that while much research has focused on institutional routines and the experiences of medical staff, far less attention has been given to how residents themselves perceive and experience time in long-term care settings (75). Existing analyses primarily emphasize the institutional culture of "time and task" (Henderson 42), a reality vividly illustrated through Lillian's frustrations: "And everything is timed, you know, like a timetable. I eat when they tell me, sleep when they tell me, play bingo when they tell me. Jeez, I even have a poop when they tell me. I could never poop on demand before. I don't know why I have to start now" (Hepburn, *Flee* 20). As in many care-home novels, the home's sterile atmosphere, meaningless yet rigid schedules, and severe limitations on personal agency reminds of the "total institution." The nursing home represents inertia and motionlessness, where individuality is suppressed, and change or self-determination becomes virtually impossible.

Because both Audrey and Lillian have been diagnosed with dementia, they reside in the locked ward of Tranquil Meadows. Early on, it becomes clear to the reader that Lillian's narration is unreliable. For instance, she complains that her family rarely visits, but when her daughter Carol arrives from Toronto to take her on a planned shopping trip, Lillian fails to recognize her and has evidently forgotten their arrangement (12–13). Her first-person narration is fragmented by flashbacks and dream-like sequences, signaling her confusion over words, people, events, places, and times. The same is true for Audrey, but unlike the reader, Lillian is not always aware of these lapses. What remains evident is that regardless of their cognitive decline, both women experience persistent boredom, loneliness, and isolation—a triad of afflictions that, as mentioned earlier, Thomas refers to as the "three deadly plagues of the human spirit" (The Eden Alternative 2). These emotions underscore the novel's critique of institutional life, where residents, despite their diagnoses, are denied meaningful engagement and autonomy, further deepening their sense of disconnection.

One day, "a uniform" questions why Lillian is cold despite the summer heat, prompting Lillian to recall that August is a "holiday month." Inspired by this realization, she decides that she and Audrey also deserve a vacation. To ensure they do not forget their plan, they share the responsibility of remembering, "I wipe my eyes with my sleeve and pull a pen from my sweater pocket. On a napkin, I scribble the word vacation. Twice. I tear the napkin in two and give one piece to Audrey. I fold the other and place it carefully in my pocket beside the pen. 'So we don't forget,' I say. 'This is important'" (Hepburn, *Flee* 6). Despite their memory loss and physical frailty, the two women prove remarkably resourceful in outwitting those around them—people who tend to underestimate them as "sweet old ladies." Each step of their escape is carefully orchestrated. Lillian keeps track of details in a small notepad, persuades her daughter to buy her sneakers and a backpack, and keenly observes her to learn how to withdraw money from the bank. Their ingenuity extends to signing up for a crafts class to obtain scissors, which they use to cut off their electronic SafeChip wristbands—devices that trigger an alarm if a resident leaves the building.

Their escape culminates in a series of opportunistic but calculated moves. Audrey, discovering car keys in her handbag, remembers selling her blue Oldsmobile Intrigue to her neighbors' son. Seizing the moment, they trick a taxi driver into unlocking the nursing home door from the outside, allowing them to slip away under the false assumption that he had been summoned. Audrey, in a moment of lucidity, recalls that her home address is written on her expired driver's license. The duo takes the cab there, steals what was once Audrey's car from her neighbor's driveway, and—despite their precarious driving—manages to reach the bank to withdraw Lillian's money. In front of the bank, Audrey struggles to park the car. Ever flirtatious, she enlists the help of Rayne, a young man sitting nearby with a guitar case, backpack, and sleeping bag. This encounter, which recalls *Thelma & Louise*, raises initial doubts about Rayne's intentions—prompting the reader to wonder whether he will exploit the women as J.D. did in the road movie, stealing all of Thelma and Louise's money. As Audrey strikes up a conversation, Lillian, in a moment of confusion, mistakes Rayne for her son Tom. But Rayne, rather than correcting her, seems unbothered by the misidentification. The women invite him to join them as a driver, and in doing so, relinquish control over their destination. Lillian and Audrey, having no clear sense of where they want to go, allow Rayne to determine their course—he eagerly seizes the chance to visit his father in British Columbia. By surrendering their roles as drivers and choosing instead to be passengers, the women subvert one of the defining conventions of the traditional road narrative: the car as a symbol of autonomy and self-determination. Much like *Amigoland*, *Flee, Fly, Flown* reconfigures this central trope, emphasizing not independence but interdependence—further complicating the relationship between agency, mobility, and aging.

As their journey progresses, the travelers adopt a stray dog, which they name Shadow and take along with them. At this stage, Rayne remains unaware that he is driving two nursing home fugitives and car thieves. Unlike "the uniforms" at the nursing home, he treats the women with genuine respect. He establishes clear boundaries while maintaining a sense of equality, telling them: "I'm just setting up my own rules for the trip. If we're gonna be traveling together, we need to be equals. No acting like my guardian, telling me what I can and can't do. You treat me with respect and I'll do the same for you. How's that sound?" (53–54). His patience further sets him apart from the institutional caregivers they left behind. When the women repeatedly ask, "Where are we going?" (171, 172), he responds calmly each time, demonstrating a level of understanding and kindness that contrasts sharply with their previous experiences of infantilization and control.

While Lillian and Audrey never seem to mistrust Rayne, readers may approach him with a degree of skepticism. Although he establishes early on that they are equals, it remains unclear whether or not he intends to take advantage of the two women. This suspicion is reinforced during a scene at a casino, where the women, eager to experience the thrill of gambling, ask Rayne to take them to the slot machines. Overwhelmed by the flashing lights and complex buttons, they rely on his guidance. Lillian, despite not fully understanding the game, ends up winning a significant amount with Rayne's help:

> Players at nearby terminals watch the attendant return with the money. She counts it out into Rayne's palm, but with all the confusion, I can't see or hear the amount. He tucks it into his pocket. We follow Rayne out through the maze of machines and past the man in the lobby. Inside the van, Rayne hands each of us fifty dollars. "Congratulations," he says. "That's it?" I ask. "With all the lights and bells, it seemed like we won millions." [...] "Yeah, we all won." (Hepburn, *Flee* 187–88)

Readers suspicions about Rayne's honesty deepen when they learn that he is, in many ways, a subdued version of *Thelma & Louise*'s J.D.—"a homeless guy with nothing in his pockets and a record showing a couple of petty charges and vagrancy" (94). The casino scene further highlights the women's financial dependence, a theme that echoes *Thelma & Louise*, where, as Dowell observes, the protagonists—"like countless fictional women ... can't hold on to their cash" (Dowell 29, qtd. in Soyka 60). Unlike Thelma and Louise, Lillian and Audrey are entirely reliant on Rayne, who serves not only as their driver and treasurer but also as their guardian and surrogate memory. Here, the novel underlines aspects of interdependency. As Patricia Life maintains, Rayne's role is multifaceted:

> Rayne's role in the story is complex. Hepburn presents him as a son figure in need of guidance, a handsome chivalric prince who sweeps in to rescue the damsels from the distress of living in a nursing home, and also as a Byronic "bad boy" who encourages the ladies in their wild adventures. For example,

> despite their obvious health limitations, he goes camping with them by a lake and shares some marijuana with Lillian. (171)

While the women trust Rayne unreservedly, he begins to have doubts about their trustworthiness. Upon learning about the background of their "vacation," Rayne is afraid that kidnapping and car theft will be added to his less than impeccable police record. He advises the women to turn themselves in to the police and abandons them, taking the stray dog, Shadow, with him.

Rayne's absence immediately exposes Lillian and Audrey's vulnerability. When they stop at a supermarket to buy chips, Lillian absentmindedly forgets to pay at the cash register and is accused of shoplifting. Ironically, the cashier does not believe her confusion is genuine, instead suspecting her of feigning forgetfulness. The situation escalates as the manager arrives and insists that the women follow him to his office. Lillian, however, resists, putting up a fight until the "baby-faced young man" (100) becomes embarrassed and ultimately lets them go. Outside, their helplessness becomes even more pronounced. Lillian, overwhelmed by pain and exhaustion, struggles to find their car in the parking lot. Meanwhile, Audrey attempts to seek assistance from two young men, only to become a victim of violence—when she extends her hand in greeting, the "hoodlums" (102) seize her purse and shove her to the ground. The situation nearly brings their journey to an abrupt end. A passing young mother intervenes, offering to call an ambulance and the police. Recognizing their frailty and confusion, she hesitates, torn between her instinct to help and her crying toddler's demands. Ultimately, her child's distress distracts her from following through with a 911 call, and instead, she reluctantly helps them locate their car. Linda McDowell's analysis of the intersection of gender and space offers a crucial lens through which to examine this scene. She highlights how gender divisions shape experiences of public space, reinforcing women's vulnerability:

> When we turn to public spaces we clearly see the effect of the associations of the public/private divide with gender divisions. Because of the strong associations between women and the home, those interior spaces of domesticity, feminist investigations of public spaces have often focused on the problems and dangers that women experience 'outside' compared with an assumption that men may take for granted their freedom in and dominance of these spaces. (McDowell 148)

McDowell further discusses how women's presence in public spaces is often marked by fear, anxiety, and exposure to violence:

> Thus there is a significant literature about the ways in which women experience fear and anxiety, as well as physical danger, harassment and attack in streets and open spaces. [...] [W]omen who did not conform or keep to their place were constructed as wicked or fallen, subjected to abuse or vulnerable to physical danger, forcing them to reconsider their decision to participate in the public sphere. (148–49)

In this context, Lillian and Audrey's experience in the parking lot is not just an unfortunate mishap but a reflection of broader gendered anxieties surrounding mobility and public space. Their physical vulnerability, coupled with their age and cognitive impairment, makes them easy targets—further reinforcing the idea that for women, especially older women, public spaces can be sites of exclusion, risk, and instability. Without Rayne, the two women are left defenseless in an unfamiliar world. Still, Lillian and Audrey manage to get back on the road, but Lillian realizes that she is too shaken to continue driving: "My head is spinning, fogging up so that I have to pull over in the lot and turn off the car. I can't drive. I need time to sort out all that has happened" (Hepburn, *Flee* 103). Disoriented and exhausted, they have lost all sense of time and place—uncertain of where they are, how long they have been traveling, or even where they are going. Audrey, overwhelmed, pleads with Lillian: "Please take me home now" (104). At this point, time and space have become ungraspable concepts for them. Lillian, unable to make sense of her surroundings, longs for comfort and familiarity. She finds herself unsettled by the vastness of the open road: "So much space is disconcerting," she thinks (171). Yet, rather than comparing the road to the structured confinement of the nursing home, she contrasts it with her childhood home—a place where space was limited but where she felt a deep sense of belonging: "At home it's crowded but I don't mind. I share a bedroom with my sisters, and space at the table is always cramped. My brothers take up more room than they should with sharp elbows and big feet" (171).

Audrey desperately wants to return to the nursing home, which, in contrast to the open road, is represented as a place of safety and stability. At this moment, the novel reinforces a binary ideological construction: the (care) home as a protected space versus public space as dangerous and unpredictable. This opposition is mirrored in the portrayal of gender and age dynamics—where young men, like Rayne, are depicted as powerful and in control, while older women, like Lillian and Audrey, are shown as fragile and vulnerable. Their age and memory loss further compound this vulnerability, making their experience of the road even more precarious than that of younger women in narratives like *Thelma & Louise*. Despite these limitations, Lillian resists the notion that returning to the nursing home is their only option. Instead, she insists on continuing their journey: "We're not going home. We're going back onto the highway and we're getting away from this place and all the places we live. [...] You signed up, and now you're stuck with me. Lucy and Ethel on the move" (104). Lillian's reference to Lucy and Ethel—a comedic female duo known for their misadventures—reinforces the theme of two women navigating an unpredictable world together. Her repeated exclamation, "Jeez Louise," further evokes *Thelma & Louise*, subtly aligning their journey with the famous road film. Moreover, Lillian's determination to press forward resonates with Thelma's climactic command: "Let's not get caught. Let's keep going! Go!" (Scott 01:59:00, qtd. in Soyka 66). By echoing this moment, *Flee, Fly, Flown* situates itself within the tradition of women's road narratives while simultaneously reconfiguring it through the lens of aging, disability, and interdependence.

Shaken and disoriented, the two women continue driving through the pouring rain, only to nearly run over Rayne and the dog. The downpour compels Rayne to get back into the car, but his decision is also fueled by guilt: "Okay, maybe you're right. I couldn't stop thinking that my grandma would kick my ass if she knew I'd abandoned you, too" (107). Recognizing the need to dispose of the stolen car, Rayne rents a van, and their journey westward resumes. They make stops at grocery stores, diners, and cheap motels, while also camping outdoors—an experience the women surprisingly enjoy, despite their physical limitations and incontinence. To manage, they rely on adult diapers, a fact Audrey shares with an unusual sense of pride: "'We shouldn't need to stop again for a while,' Audrey says, a proud look spreading across her face." "'Please don't explain,' Rayne interrupts. 'I don't need to know everything'" (Hepburn, *Flee* 110). Unlike Socorro in *Amigoland*, who assumes a caregiving role by cleaning up after Don Fidencio and ensuring he has fresh clothes—reinforcing traditional gender expectations—Rayne's role remains strictly that of a more detached driver. As "helper characters" (Soyka 35), both Socorro and Rayne fulfill roles that align with the conventions of the road novel genre. But their functions in the narrative also reveal a clear adherence to traditional gender stereotypes.

Both Audrey and Lillian experience frequent cognitive slips, and the narration often highlights the absurdity of their conversations. Lillian repeatedly mistakes Rayne for Audrey's boyfriend, her own son Tom, or her late husband Albert, while Audrey insists she must return home to her husband Terry. Lillian also struggles to decipher notes meant to aid her memory, and Audrey frequently loses her sense of direction. Despite these disorientations, Rayne accepts them as they are, in contrast to institutional caregivers and family members who primarily see them as dementia patients. Unbothered by their lapses, he embraces them as a surrogate family: "You two are more like my grandmother than I first thought" (Hepburn, *Flee* 61). Rayne even invites them to meet his father and stay at his house. As Patricia Life observes, Rayne "sees no problem with letting them use his memory as an extension of their own, and thus considers that it is reasonable for them to have left the dementia unit. When he eventually has to take Lillian to the hospital, he explains to the "uniform" that "she may need help remembering" (231). Significantly, he does not say that she does not remember, merely that she "may need help to remember" (169).

The novel highlights the significance of intergenerational relationships in shaping identity for both the older women and the young man. Initially, Rayne perceives Lillian and Audrey as entirely different from himself, reinforcing a binary opposition between youth and old age. But as he comes to understand their shared desires—for a caring family, a sense of belonging, and a place to call home—he begins to identify with them, recognizing their mutual interdependence. Rayne's acceptance of their differences ultimately leads to a deeper acknowledgment of their individuality. This recognition aligns with Maierhofer's argument that an awareness of difference can facilitate "an acceptance of the other in the self" ("Crossing" 255–256). One night, as Rayne takes out his guitar and plays songs he learned from his grandfather, the dynamic of care momentarily shifts—this time, it is he who needs Audrey's help. While Rayne remembers the chords and the familiar words of the chorus, Audrey recalls the full lyrics. Together, they reconstruct the music from their respective childhoods and youth (Hepburn, *Flee* 214), illustrating how intergenerational connections bridge past and present, memory and identity.

Their holiday is once again jeopardized when the police stop them for speeding, revealing that Rayne is actually Wayne Carpenter, a man with "a few minor brushes with the law" (161). Lillian and Audrey's use of the fake names "Lucy and Ethel" only heightens the officer's suspicions, leading to their detention at the police station. Although it is quickly established that "Lucy and Ethel" are in fact Lillian Gorsen and Audrey Clark—the two missing women from the nursing home—the police are unable to force their return. Despite their Alzheimer's diagnoses, they are legally adults and free to travel

(166). Stunned by this unexpected confirmation of their autonomy, the women agree to let the officer notify the nursing home that they are safe, on the condition that their location remains undisclosed. This newfound freedom is reinforced through spatial imagery: "Outside, an ocean of brilliant golden-yellow blooms stretches north across a field. It takes my breath away" (169). Lillian, unfamiliar with the flowers, asks what they are. Rayne explains they are sunflowers, picking one for each woman "to celebrate four days on the road" (169). The scene transforms their legal independence into a symbolic moment of liberation, where the vast, sunlit landscape mirrors the openness of possibility. A moment later, Lillian again enjoys the free space and the colors of nature: "The colors outside are as vivid as acrylic paint in the mid-morning sun. I imagine myself walking to the horizon in my navy pants and pale blue shirt; picture the trek as color wading through color.' [...] 'It looks like a postcard,' I say" (181–82). The strong natural colors are contrasted with the pastel nursing home colors and the open landscape, with the confined space of the care home. Lillian's immersion into nature resembles Walt Whitman's "Song of the Open Road" when he writes, "The earth expanding right hand and left hand / The picture alive, every part in its best light" (125). Here, the novel partakes in the discourse and myth of mobility and freedom and emphasizes the open road's connotation of individualism, independence, and control for the old women, which can be read as "a textual intervention into normative spatialities," as Ganser observes in another context (*Roads* 14). Even if the novel is ambivalent at times with regard to its representation of the women's needs, it emphasizes their rights to maintain their agency and freedom and indicates that these are more important than their physical safety. Sitting around a fire pit near a forest one night, Lillian and Audrey have reached a level of individual independence: "I can't stop smiling. 'This is a grand adventure!' 'You said it.' Audrey drops down onto the log. 'I can die happy now.' [...] I say, 'It's funny; I'm not afraid of dying anymore. I don't know when that changed for me'" (Hepburn, *Flee* 116). The act of passing through the Canadian wilderness, and the transformations this enacts, functions as a rite of passage for the women.

The old women's newly won feelings of freedom are soon stifled. When the three travelers reach Saskatchewan, Rayne reminds Lillian and Audrey that after they meet his dad, they should begin to consider returning. The women do not want to hear any of this, and Lillian immediately feels sick to her stomach (174). After a while, Rayne convinces them to phone the home as well as Audrey's niece, Teresa, and Lillian's children, Carol and Tom: "I also know what it feels like to have a mom leave and not know where she's gone. You're not gonna want to hear this, Lillian, but even though your kids are adults now, it's still gotta be tough on them. For me, that's hard to reconcile" (174). The responsibility of taking care of Lillian and Audrey begins to become a burden to Rayne as soon as he realizes that he will need to continue to be responsible for them even after reaching his home.

Their phone calls tether them back to the confined world of their families and the nursing home, acting as a spatial trap that threatens their newfound freedom. The telephone becomes an instrument of control, pinpointing their exact location for Carol, who orders Lillian to wait for her at the motel. When Lillian tentatively asks if she could live with Carol and her husband, the response is definitive—Carol refuses, promising instead to find a nursing home for her closer to Toronto. Lillian immediately understands that this conversation marks the end of their journey: "'No. That's not what I want.' I hang up the phone and stare at the metal-framed print on the wall—a snow-capped mountain scene with a lake beyond. It's so ordinary, so unexceptional and yet I can't take my eyes off of it" (220). The mountains she had longed to see in person remain out of reach, reduced to an image on the wall—static, confined, and symbolic of the unfulfilled adventure. In this moment, Lillian realizes that her journey will not take her as far as the Rockies; her escape, like the landscape before her, is now merely a surrogate reality.

At dawn, Lillian quietly slips out of the motel with Shadow. In the park, she imagines her late husband, Albert, seducing her: "Albert brushes past. He ducks inside a tent and opens the flap, calls to me, 'Come see the surprise I have for you, sexy lady.' He flashes his buck-naked body at me, all pink and erect, ready" (221). Her imagined sexual encounter in the wilderness reinforces a stark contrast—being fully alive in nature versus the slow decline of institutional confinement. As she searches for Albert, she wanders deeper into the woods, toward the river, believing she has arrived in Algonquin Park. Overcome by desperation, she steps into the cold water, momentarily paralyzed by the weight of reality: "A heaviness settles back over me. It feels all wrong. I am my own person now with new friends, making my own choices, and it's good. I'm on my own adventure, and Carol's call, her coming here to get me, is going to bring it all crashing down" (222). This moment encapsulates Lillian's internal conflict—her fleeting sense of independence threatened by the looming return to institutional life:

> I don't want to go back there—nurses wearing surgical gloves, scrubbing my armpits and privates with a scratchy washcloth, rinsing me off with a hose,

> a bed with railings, and Jell-O and pudding and green beans every day, and I don't want to go somewhere new.
> The sky is getting brighter. The air is still. The water is clear despite its churning motion, the riverbank along the edge a scree of stones and rocks, gray and brown with flecks of deep red and gold. It looks like the bottom drops off near the middle, partially hidden by swirls and reflections. (Hepburn, *Flee* 222–23)

Lillian takes in the beauty of nature—the cold water on her feet, the warmth of Shadow's fur. Her immersion in nature and water is ambiguous. In Canadian literature, water is often portrayed as both life-giving and dangerous, an "ambivalent image" that represents "both the (female) source of life [...] and purification and the cause of death" (Hutcheon 224). For Lillian, it nearly becomes the latter. Whether she intends to end her life remains unclear. She secures Shadow's leash to a root, removes her shoes, and steps further into the river. The novel's second section, "Fly," ends here, giving way to "Flown"—a shift in tense that suggests the journey's most unrestrained phase is over.

Lillian hears Albert calling for her, though it is likely Rayne searching for her. Just as she resolves to leave the water and "stop acting like a child, a defeated, compulsive child" (227), her feet cramp, and she is swept away by the current. The river hurls her over rocks and branches until she becomes entangled in a tree. Rayne rushes to pull her out. The fragmented first-person narration suggests Lillian loses consciousness, and she awakens only in the motel, where Audrey—mistaking her injuries as the work of her abusive husband, Terry—tries to help her out of the bathtub. While Audrey remains trapped in past fears, Lillian refuses to give in: "We're on the road, honey. That's where we are. We're going somewhere" (230). At this point, Rayne's decisions become reckless. Instead of insisting they seek medical help, he assures them that their journey will continue: "By mid-afternoon, we'll be passing by Calgary. Keep watching and you'll see the city skyline. I want you to look just beyond that" (230). They get Lillian back into the van, but as her pain intensifies, she loses consciousness again. When she wakes, she is in a hospital, where her disoriented narration and Audrey's confusion immediately expose their cognitive decline.

When Lillian wakes, Carol has already arrived to take her and Audrey back home. Rayne, having ensured their safety, has informed Carol of their whereabouts and left for British Columbia. Before departing, he leaves them a note and an envelope filled with the casino winnings he had been holding onto. The novel concludes in Ottawa, with Carol driving Audrey and Lillian from the airport back to the nursing home. Their westward journey—symbolic of freedom and progress—is starkly contrasted with the rapid plane ride east, a return to confinement. While Audrey will likely remain at the facility, Carol has decided to relocate Lillian to an even more secure institution, one where she cannot escape. The looming separation of the two friends raises questions about their well-being, but Carol refuses to engage in any discussion about her mother's future. The final sentence hints at Lillian's defiance: "I pat the envelope that bulges in my pocket, search through my pack for my pen and pad. I need to make a note. So I don't forget" (237). Despite her determination, her frail health and Carol's resolve make another escape seem unlikely. The novel closes with a tension between Lillian's enduring desire for autonomy and the inescapable realities of institutional control.

The novel's ending remains highly ambivalent. As Patricia Life points out, *Flee, Fly, Flown* "asks readers to weigh the relative merits of freedom and safety in the lives of aging adults. How much risk is appropriate, and at what point does someone lose the right to assume that risk?" (174). The book urges reflection on responsibility, independence, and self-determination, as well as on the need for better models of caregiving. While one reading suggests that Lillian and Audrey's return to Tranquil Meadows is for their own good, this interpretation is far from definitive. Viewed through the lens of the road novel, the women's journey highlights spatial transgressions. Road narratives often center on escape, expressing "the fury and suffering at the extremities of civilized life, and giv[ing] their restless protagonists the false hope of a one-way ticket to nowhere" (Atkinson 16, quoted in Soyka 10). Here, the narrative adheres to gender and age conventions in such a way that Rayne—despite his initial defiance—ultimately has no choice but to return the women to institutional care. Lillian and Audrey, as Tim Cresswell's concept of being "out of place" suggests, have violated the spatial and social norms assigned to them: "[S]pace and place are used to structure a normative landscape—the way in which ideas about what is right, just, and appropriate are transmitted through space and place" (Cresswell 8). Clearly, Lillian and Audrey have transgressed the limits of the space and place assigned to them, exposing the gendered ageism they experience. In contrast to the male characters in *Amigoland*, *Water for Elephants*, and *The Forms of Water*, whose journeys normalize escape and desertion, the old women's mobility is framed as deviant or even reckless (Slettedahl Macpherson 231). As Heidi Slettedahl Macpherson argues,

> Of those female escapes which entail a physical journey, most end either with a nod to home, or an actual return; those that do not, attempt to envision a space outside of patriarchal ideology. That space may be the wilderness, as it is for many feminist novels of the 1970s, or it may be marginality, a more common site of escape in the 1980s. Regardless of the ending of these narratives, they are clearly involved in questioning the roles of women, and their "traditional" placement within the domestic sphere. (231)

In this regard, *Flee, Fly, Flown* resembles *Thelma & Louise*, which also underscores the impossibility of escaping social and spatial constraints. As Ganser writes, such narratives express "the wish for a better place [but are] frustrated by the realization that moving beyond or stepping outside the social and symbolic order altogether is indeed impossible" (*Roads* 87). Read intertextually, Lillian and Audrey's forced return to the nursing home functions as a symbolic death—similar to *Thelma & Louise*, whose protagonists evade capture by driving off a cliff. In the road movie/novel tradition, death is a conventional endpoint, but its meaning differs by gender: male protagonists often die as heroes, while female protagonists rarely receive such recognition. *Thelma & Louise* complicates this genre convention, reframing their final act not as heroic, but as punishment for transgressing gendered and spatial boundaries (Soyka 67).

For Lillian and Audrey, this punishment takes the form of forced reinstitutionalization—an act that not only strips them of their autonomy but also signals their potential descent into the oblivion of death. Despite their return to institutional care, Hepburn's "Thelma & Louise for the Canadian geriatric set" (Quill and Quire n.p.) actively challenges the conventions of both the road novel and the nursing home novel. By blending these genres, the narrative disrupts entrenched dichotomies of space, gender, and age, exposing how such categories are both naturalized and internalized. As Doreen Massey writes, "[o]ne gender-disturbing message might be—in terms of both identity and space—keep moving! The challenge is to achieve this whilst at the same time recognizing one's necessary locatedness and embeddedness/embodiedness, and taking responsibility for it" (Massey 11). In this sense, while the novel acknowledges the constraints imposed on aging women, it also suggests a form of resistance: movement—whether physical, psychological, or symbolic—remains an act of defiance against the structures that seek to contain them. Yet the negative ending also signals the limits of such resistance: for authors (and perhaps for our culture at large), it may still be unimaginable to allow aging female protagonists genuine and sustained agency.

4.3.2 "Ain't Life Sweet When You're Not Afraid to Care": Thom Fitzgerald's *Cloudburst*

Like *Flee, Fly, Flown,* the Canadian movie *Cloudburst* also features two old women on the run from institutional care. "There are considerable pleasures in Thom Fitzgerald's geriatric romantic comedy *Cloudburst*, which is a sort of Thelma & Louise on a pension," a reviewer writes (National Post), again referring to the two women who have come to epitomize the female road-movie since the early 1990s. Indeed, *Cloudburst* contains several intertextual references and quotations that link it to *Thelma & Louise*, positioning Stella and Dot within the legacy of female road narratives while reconfiguring the genre through the lens of aging and same-sex relationships. *Cloudburst* is "a romance catalyzed by the threat of long-term residential care (Chivers, "Blind" 136), demonstrating "the pervasiveness of institutional care as failure and the power of the fantasy of continually fulfilled desire the pervasiveness of institutional care as failure and the power of the fantasy of continually fulfilled desire" (136). The use of the term "geriatric" (which is often used to signify "old," thereby conflating "old" and "sick") points out the latent ageism that films about older women have to face.

Thom Fitzgerald originally wrote *Cloudburst* as a stage play, which premiered in Halifax, Canada, in 2010 before being adapted into a successful, award-winning film. The movie stars Olympia Dukakis and Brenda Fricker as Stella and Dot, an octogenarian butch/femme couple who have lived together for over 31 years in Dot's home, a small coastal village in Maine. Stella is feisty and unapologetically bold, with short gray hair, jeans, lumberjack shirts, plaid jackets, and a cowboy hat. She swears freely, drinks tequila straight from the bottle, and refuses to conform to societal expectations. In contrast, Dot is gentle, clumsy, and plump, with curly gray hair and a warm, caring nature. She has a sharp sense of humor and a quick tongue, but she is also nearly blind and struggles with mobility. One night, while watching a lesbian porn movie—"Imagine. You can now buy lesbian porn at the gas station!"—Stella playfully teases Dotty with a vibrator. Though not in a sexual way, but in a way that suggests that they had had fun in the past, the moment triggers a fit of laughter that sends Dot tumbling out of bed. She "sprains her ass" (00:06:00) and ends up hospitalized, setting off a chain of events that will challenge their autonomy and relationship.

Her prudish granddaughter, Molly, who is more interested in Dot's house than in her granny's well-being, takes advantage of this opportunity and reserves a place for Dot in a nursing home in Bangor. She informs Stella of this plan ("I am her only living family. [...] Nonna is coming with me, and she is going to live where people with more training can take care of her," 00:11:27) and tells Stella that she will eventually need to move out of Dot's house. Stella does not want to hear any of this, defending their relationship, their home, and her ability to be Dot's care-giver, and violently kicks Molly out. Unfortunately, Molly returns when Stella is out of the house and tricks her grandmother into signing over a power of attorney. As soon as Dot has signed the papers, the camera moves outside and frames Dot, using a low-angle shot of the wooden window, trapping her behind what looks like prison bars (00:09:38). Soon after, Molly shows up with her boyfriend, a local policeman, with a court order in hand to take Dot away. Dot, defenseless, still unsuspecting, surprised, and overwhelmed, complies, while Stella is absolutely furious. Stella physically and verbally confronts Molly and the policeman, who initially refuses to intervene. When he realizes that the women genuinely do not want to be separated—and that Molly is oblivious to their relationship—his stance wavers: "'They're lesbians, Mol, hello!' 'Oh Tommy, listen to yourself, Nonna is my grandmother. She gave birth to my mother by heterosexual means, she is not a lesbian, Einstein. [Pause] But... that would color Stella's opposition! You might be right about Stella'" (00:12:56), Molly's disbelief exposes her refusal to see Dot and Stella as anything more than "best friends" rather than a committed couple. By emotionally manipulating the officer—questioning his loyalty and their future marriage—she convinces him to comply. Together, they forcibly remove Dot from her home. "She's taking you to an old folks home, to cremate you," Stella warns Dot, as she is led to the car by Molly (00:14:03). "'You're going to cremate me?,' Dot gullibly asks her granddaughter. 'Um, not right away,'" Molly answers in a surprised tone and closes the car door, revealing her emotional coldness (00:14:16). The nursing home specter looms large as an existential threat over the couple's heads.

Devastated but determined, Stella hatches a plan, tequila bottle in hand. That night, she parks her red pickup outside Dot's care facility—an uninspiring square brick building—and disguises herself as an "old lady" by throwing a nightie over her shirt and jeans. Masquerading with a headscarf, slippers, and a cane, she performs age and gender in a deliberately exaggerated way (Woodward, "Performing"). The contrast between "the old lady" and Stella's butch identity not only reinforces the performative nature of the scene but also serves as a critique of stereotypical depictions of aging. She knocks on the locked entrance door and is scolded by the night nurse, who sits behind the admittance desk, for being outside after 8:30 p.m. Her fake institutionalization is successful: she "passes" for an "old woman." "It's like being nine years old all over again," she complains to the nurse, who answers, "Hey, I don't make the rules!" "That's what Joseph Goebbels said," Stella's vents her anger, pressing the elevator button with her cane and leaving the night nurse speechless (00:17:20). Her statement, although "low and sitcom dull" (Groen), yet again establishes a link between the home and a "total institution." The number of prohibitory signs and its architecture underline the home's identity as "panopticon" (Foucault, *Discipline* 205): when Stella has to hide from the night nurse during her inspection round, the "institutional gaze" (205) of the home is highlighted. To maintain surveillance, all doors remain wide open, despite the large, wired glass windows already allowing constant monitoring of the double rooms. This creates a tension between private and public space, where residents are visible at all times yet deprived of autonomy. The dimly lit linoleum floors and austere hallways—filmed in near darkness, illuminated only by emergency lights and an exit sign—reinforce the institution's hospital-like atmosphere, where control takes precedence over privacy. As in many other texts and films, the nursing home is depicted as a space of confinement and decline. As Sally Chivers aptly observes, it serves as "a figurative repository of cultural fears of aging as a dead-end" ("Blind" 137). The bleak, institutional nightly world of the home is contrasted with the beautiful landscape, sea, and scenic sunsets seen in the women's home town on the coast of Maine and in Nova Scotia.

Stella finally finds Dot, who is whimpering in her sleep. A close-up frames Stella's face as she peers through the wired glass window, the harsh lighting emphasizing the grid between them—a visual marker of their temporary separation. When Stella enters, Dot wakes in confusion: "Did they get you, too?" (00:18:50). Dot shares the room with Wilma, a heavily sedated woman with dementia—"a druggie" who has been put to sleep "with a horse tranquilizer, she'll never wake up" (00:18:59), as Dot explains. To create a diversion, they place the unconscious Wilma in a wheelchair and send her down to the reception area via the elevator. While the night nurse rushes to return Wilma to her room, Stella and Dot slip out through the stairwell and into the parking lot. Stella sheds her disguise, leaving it discarded in the street, and reclaims her brash, cursing self as she climbs into the truck. With laughter and exhilaration, the two women speed off in their red pickup, trading the confining walls of the nursing home for the open road and the freedom of their own journey. Sally Chivers analyzes this scene as follows:

> There is a self-mocking hilarity to these older characters' liberation, reinforced by their choices not to conform to the appearances expected of them, slippers, nighties and so on. This humor foregrounds not the infantilization of these seniors but rather the ridiculousness of how they are viewed from the perspective of the facilities and the people who think they can only safely reside there. The comic tone emphasizes the ingenuity of their escapes as well as the enjoyment they glean from regaining their relative freedom. ("Blind" 138)

As soon as they have calmed down, Dot becomes hungry. As in many road movies, diners also play a decisive role in *Cloudburst*; Dotty and Stella have breakfast in a diner and think about their further escape plans:

> STELLA: You know, I saw this TV show, Rosie O'Donnell took a bunch of dykes on a cruise to Nova Scotia. Then this flock of lesbians got married there.
> DOT: Flock?
> STELLA: Well, that's what they call us when we're in a group. You know, a gaggle of gays, a flock of lesbians, like in nature.
> DOT: Stella, are you proposing to me?
> STELLA: Maybe.
> DOT: Are you down on one knee?
> STELLA: Yeah.
> DOT: I don't believe in marriage. I was married, remember, and that was like having a brain clot.
> STELLA: I loved you for thirty-one years, I loved you when you got fat, I loved you when you went blind. I'm gonna love you forever.
> [...]
> DOT: [...] Thirty one years. Well, I have lived with you for thirty-one years, I suppose I put up with you for another thirty-one.
> STELLA: Thirty-one year trial commitment. That's a deal.
> [They shake hands over the table]
> DOT: That's a deal. And then we can see other people.
> [...]
> STELLA: We'll drive to Canada to get legally married, and then no one can separate us.
> DOT: Great.
> *(00:21:11—00:23:10)*

Stella's marriage proposal is pragmatic, rather than romantic, and Dot, having already experienced heterosexual marriage, reacts with ambivalence. The film engages with the highly debated issue of same-sex marriage in the U.S., highlighting the legal and social challenges many LGBTQIA+ elders face in a heteronormative society,[8] particularly when navigating long-term care.[9] Stella and Dot embark on their journey to Canada, where same-sex marriage is legal,[10] not just as an act of love but as a necessity. Their decision to marry is about securing legal protections—ensuring that Stella has the right to care for Dot, with the hope that such rights might one day be recognized in the U.S. as well.

The next day, as the women drive through a picturesque landscape, Stella spots a young hitchhiker. They decide to pick him up, reasoning that adding a third traveler "will confuse anyone looking for two old broads" (00:25:02). The hitchhiker, Prentice (played by Ryan Doucette), is a strikingly handsome young man who confidently flaunts his half-naked, athletic body. However, Stella quickly shuts down any attempt at seduction: "Pull up your pants, kid," she quips. "You're humping the wrong fire hydrant" (00:25:25). Amused by Stella's bluntness, Prentice reveals himself to be a struggling modern dancer and occasional stripper, heading home to Canada to care for his terminally ill mother—trapped in a loveless marriage and financial hardship. His presence starkly contrasts youth and age, further reinforcing one of the film's central themes. According to director Thom Fitzgerald, Prentice also serves a strategic function, making the "geriatric lesbian road movie" more accessible to a broader audience.

Beyond rejecting the discrimination implicit in Fitzgerald's argument—based on sex, age, gender, and able-bodiedness—I also challenge his claim that Prentice influences Stella and Dot as much as they influence him. His inclusion in the film adheres to a conventional narrative structure: he serves as yet another "helper character" (Soyka 35). Unlike the male antagonists in *Thelma &*

8 As a recent study shows, LGBTQIA+ elders have "a tougher time securing health care, affordable housing, and economic security due to institutionalized heterosexism in the Federalized programs and policies governing these service arenas" (Scheidt 516).

9 The issue of long-term care for LGBTQIA+ seniors is addressed in the award-winning 2010 documentary film, *Gen Silent Maddux*, which follows the lives of six LGBTQIA+ seniors living in the Boston area, showing "the disparity in the quality of paid caregiving from mainstream care facilities committed making their LGBTQIA+ residents safe and happy, to places where LGBTQIA+ elders face discrimination by staff and bullying by other seniors" (Programsforelderly).

10 Same-sex marriage became legal by popular vote in Maine on December 29, 2012, after the film was shot. In Canada, it was legalized country-wide in 2005.

Louise, both Rayne in *Flee, Fly, Flown* and Prentice in *Cloudburst* function as binary opposites to the aging, vulnerable women, reinforcing the idea that they cannot travel independently. Rayne acts as their external memory and driver, while Prentice—added as "eye candy"—serves both as a distraction for viewers and a means of misleading law enforcement searching for the fugitives. Like Rayne, Prentice learns mid-journey that the women are on the run. Unlike Rayne, however, he finds this revelation exhilarating: "Awesome!" (00:30:12), he exclaims upon hearing that there's already an all-points bulletin out for them. His enthusiastic reaction underscores his role as a conventional sidekick, reinforcing rather than disrupting traditional road movie dynamics.

When analyzing aspects of space and place in *Cloudburst*, it is interesting to observe that the women's journey across the Canadian border is not initially driven by their marriage plans, which only take shape once they are already on the road. Instead, their escape unfolds as a resistance to forced separation, underscoring the film's tension between movement and restriction. The narrative plays with two competing stereotypes—old age as static and immobile versus queerness as inherently fluid. As Daniel Mudie Cunningham, drawing on Eve Sedgwick, argues, queerness is "always 'on the go'—both as a concept and as a lived experience:

> Eve Sedgwick once claimed that "queer" is movement, not only in the sense that it refers to a community, collective, or even a cinematic movement, but because it moves in the literal sense. Sedgwick writes: "The word 'queer' itself means across [...] The immemorial current that queer represents is antiseparatist as it is anti-assimilationist. Keenly, it is relational and strange." (xii)

Cunningham further explores how this sense of movement is central to queer cinema: "One of the consistent features of New Queer Cinema is that queerness is continually represented in terms of 'movement'. Queerness is always 'on the go'. The ability to move and a general resistance against standing still is a strong, identifiable trope in much queer cinema" (1). In many queer films, this "movability" is symbolized through the road movie:

> The "movability" of queer is often expressed in queer cinema through the recurring motif of the road. The idea that queer moves across things is evocative because in some queer films, its subjects don't inhabit any one specific place for too long. Instead, such characters keep moving across the landscape, forever passing through and between places, identities, things. For ex-

> ample, some of the most notable films of the New Queer Cinema were road movies about young, free-floating characters who hustle their way through life. (Cunningham 1)

By placing *Cloudburst* within this framework, its road narrative can be understood not just as an escape from institutionalization, but as an embodiment of queer resistance—where movement itself becomes an act of defiance against restrictive social and spatial norms. Stella and Dot are old and usually not free-floating, but rather settled characters, who are forced out of their long-term home by Maine's heteronormative legislation. The only reason for them to become *picaras* "on the go" is because they are marked as "different" in terms of their sexual orientation—and they embrace the risk of the open road.

Their marginalization is further underscored by Prentice, the embodiment of everything they are not: young, heterosexual, healthy, and free-floating. His physicality—highlighted during the eponymous cloudburst scene where he strips to do laundry on the beach, and later, when a high-angle shot captures him naked, thumb-sucking, and curled up like a baby in the truck bed—stands in stark contrast to Dot's aging, overweight, and immobile body. Throughout the film, Dot is visually framed as out of place and incapable of independent survival, both at home and on the road. Indoors, she is always seen lying in bed or sitting in a chair, reinforcing her physical limitations. The juxtaposition of her constrained movement with Prentice's effortless mobility highlights the gendered and ageist structures that define who gets to be free on the road.

When the trio arrives at Prentice's parents' house, his mother—a frail, broken woman—is relieved to see him but warns that his father will not tolerate his stay. After a series of slapstick moments, including Prentice's naked father furiously chasing them from the house after Dot accidentally falls asleep in his bed, it becomes clear that Prentice no longer has a home. Recognizing his predicament, Stella and Dot take him with them—not just as a companion, but as their best man, reinforcing their unconventional yet chosen family dynamic.

Adopting Prentice proves life-saving. While walking along the beach, Stella—empty tequila bottle in hand—realizes too late that the tide is rising, cutting them off from the shore. As in many scenes, the characters' liminality is reinforced through their spatial positioning—frequently depicted at the water's edge. This recurring motif emphasizes their in-betweenness, symbolizing both transition and uncertainty, as they navigate the boundaries between freedom and confinement, past and future, life and death. Stranded on what is quickly becoming an island, she urges Dot to hurry, but as during their nursing home escape, Dot cannot move as fast as Stella wants. This time, Dot falls into the water and cannot get up on her own. Stella tries to lift her, but she isn't strong enough. Panic sets in as the waves rise around them. From a distance, Prentice—once again half-naked, lounging on the hood of their car—hears their cries and sprints to their aid. Together, he and Stella manage to pull Dot to safety. An extreme long shot captures their tiny figures against the vast ocean, visually emphasizing their vulnerability. The moment exposes Dot's physical frailty and, more painfully, Stella's growing realization that she may no longer be able to care for her. Later, at the hotel, Stella voices her doubts to Prentice: "I can't do it. [...] Taking Dotty on this trip, I nearly killed us both. Watching her almost drown... I couldn't—I couldn't—she's my life! If you hadn't been there, we'd both be dead. Molly's right. I can't take care of Dotty anymore. That's it. That's it!" (01:13:30–01:14:19). As a result, Stella withdraws her marriage proposal—but Dot refuses to accept it:

> DOT: No, no, you promised me, Stella. You can't break your promise now.
> STELLA: It's not gonna change anything, Dotty. It's not gonna make us younger. It's not gonna mean we can live together. You still have to go to that special care home. And I don't need special care, so I can't go with you. I mean, it's not gonna mean anything to Molly, and it's sure as hell not going to mean anything to that damn judge.
> DOT: It's not going to not change anything. It's going to change everything. [...] If I'm going to die in some nursing home somewhere alone, I want to die there as your wife.
> *(01:14:35—01:16:55)*

Although she had been the one skeptical of marriage, she now makes it clear to Stella that there is "a romantic and a political element to her transformed desire for matrimony" (Chivers, "Blind" 139). Because marriage is the only possibility that will allow them to reach a decision about who will take care of Dot together, they strike a deal with Prentice: he will join them to live in Dot's house in Maine and "will do the driving and all the heavy lifting" (01:22:32).

Just as Stella and Dot are about to be married, their ceremony is abruptly interrupted by Molly and her policeman boyfriend, who storm in and attempt to handcuff Dot. But Dot convinces the registrar that she was deceived by her granddaughter. The ceremony is postponed, and instead, Molly is the one led away in handcuffs. At the police station, Dot speaks with Molly, revealing more about their family history and pleading for forgiveness for leaving her husband—Molly's grandfather—decades earlier. In a moment of reconciliation, she promises to have Molly released on the condition that she agrees to be her bridesmaid. With tensions momentarily resolved, the group sets out once more to complete the wedding.

As they drive through the countryside, Stella basks in the beauty of the open road, feeling a sense of relief: "Nothing but blue, blue skies, blue water. Open. Nothing in the way" (01:23:15). It seems all obstacles have finally been cleared. But suddenly, Dot falls violently ill in the car. They are forced to stop, and with her last reserves of strength, Dot begs Prentice to marry them on the spot. Despite Molly's protests, he complies, performing an impromptu ceremony and pronouncing them "women and wives" (01:25:09) just before Dot dies in Stella's arms. By the film's end, it remains uncertain whether Stella will be allowed to stay in Dot's home. The final scene shows Prentice and Stella standing at the shore, gazing at the ocean as the sun sets—silent, remembering Dot. The Soundtrack (Penny Lang) that played at the beginning of their road trip is repeated: "Ain't life sweet, when we know what we're doing. Ain't life sweet, when we're not afraid to care" (01:29:30).

Dot's death replicates the conventions of traditional escape movies. The protagonist's death highlights the search for individual freedom and identity and the social conflicts that precede an escape. In this sense, the film advocates aging in place, as Sally Chivers also writes, "while appearing to embrace, if not ultimately enact, alternative care arrangements" ("Blind" 139). *Cloudburst* invites fantasies of what such alternatives could look like, as its heroines escape the nursing home specter, even if they only escape it to enjoy freedom for a short while and their marriage does not even last a day ("best fucking day in my life," as Stella calls it (01:29:33)), it is an empowering journey on more than one level.

Conclusion

> We are old, we are young, we are in this together
> Vagabonds and children, prisoners forever
> With pulses a-raging and eyes full of wonder
> Kicking out behind us again
>
> — New Model Army, *"Vagabonds"*

This book has examined how literary and cinematic portrayals of care homes in contemporary anglophone Canadian and U.S. contexts construct, contest, and complicate dominant cultural narratives about aging. My primary aim has been to explore how these fictionalized spaces—designed to house the "oldest old"—reflect and shape broader societal understandings of later life, and how they both produce and are produced by narratives of age, identity, and spatial belonging. The texts and films analyzed here vary significantly in genre, plot, style, and tone, yet they share a common approach in constructing aging identities: They "put age in its place." That phrase, which serves as the title of this book, captures both the literal inscription of older adults into institutional settings and the symbolic work that care homes perform as cultural metaphors. At the same time, some of the works under discussion refuse to reduce old age to a singular or homogenous phase of life, challenging the assumption—famously articulated by Ralph Waldo Emerson and critically echoed by Glenda Laws—that old age "requires fit surroundings" (Emerson 285; Laws, "Spatiality" 90). Instead, they ask what "fit surroundings" might mean, and for whom.

Care Homes as Cultural Constructs

Throughout the preceding chapters, I have discussed how care homes operate as complex spatial and discursive constructs—what Michel Foucault would call heterotopias—that simultaneously reveal and conceal structures of age-based marginalization. These institutional settings are never just neutral backdrops for narratives of aging and old age; instead, they actively participate in the storytelling process. Whether depicted as hotels, hospitals, prisons, sanctuaries, liminal spaces, or contested zones of agency, care homes are narrative devices that echo, reinforce, and at times destabilize cultural scripts about what it means to grow old. Analyzing the setting of the care home through the lens of spatial theory illuminates how physical environments are entangled with the social and symbolic meanings of old age, and how those meanings are continually re-negotiated in cultural representation.

The institutionalization of North American eldercare, with its roots in the poorhouse system, has seen major transformations across the twentieth and twenty-first century; however, the fear of transitioning to a care home remains ingrained in the public imagination. Today, anxieties around long-term care are about bodily decline but also concern the spatial and symbolic displacement of older adults from familiar social worlds. The Spatial Turn in cultural gerontology has drawn attention to the ways in which space and place shape identities in later life. Henri Lefebvre's spatial triad—conceived, perceived, and lived space—helps illuminate how care homes are socially constructed environments that both reflect and reinforce cultural narratives of aging. Michel Foucault's concept of heterotopia underscores their function as spaces of exclusion and regulation. Nursing homes, as Jaber Gubrium and James Holstein argue, operate as "discursive anchors" that frame old age in terms of bodily decline, reinforcing the distinction between the imaginary of the "third age" of activity and autonomy, and the "fourth age" of frailty and dependency (519). These theoretical frameworks elicit how spatial configurations within care homes both shape and constrain the lived experiences, determining the degrees of autonomy, agency, and belonging available to older adults.

From "Horrible Homes" to Ambivalent Resistance

Despite the predominance of negative portrayals, some recent texts and films complicate the dominant narrative of the "horrible home." The emergence of the care home novel as a distinct genre in the late twentieth and early twenty-first centuries has introduced diverse representations of aging, often blending elements of detective fiction, comedy, horror, and even escape narrative. Works such as May Sarton's *As We Are Now* or Janet Hepburn's *Flee, Fly, Flown* depict aging protagonists who resist institutional confinement and subvert ageist stereotypes. Films like *Cloudburst* offer alternative visions of late-life care, focusing on communal living and self-determination, even if only fleetingly. Authors such as Margaret Atwood in "Torching the Dusties" use satire to expose the ageism and social segregation underpinning the rhetoric of demographic crisis, while Shani Mootoo's *Cereus Blooms at Night* opens imaginative space for care homes as sites of nurturing, tenderness, and queer kinship.

These evolving representations are not free of ambivalence. Many texts introduce moments of resistance or acts of defiance but struggle to sustain them through to radical potential. Narrative closure often forecloses transformation, re-asserting order and constraint. In such cases, later life, especially in institutional care, is depicted as linear and finite, leaving little room for reinvention. Still, some texts do offer glimpses of aging as a dynamic process: unfinished, relational, and politically resonant. Together, these works expand the imaginative horizon of what institutional care can mean, even as they remain tethered to dominant cultural anxieties about decline.

Exclusions, Neoliberal Frames, and Structural Conditions

A critical question remains: who gains visibility in these stories, and who is left out? Fictional and cinematic depictions of care homes tend to focus on relatively privileged, independent, and cognitively healthy residents. The frailest members of society—those with advanced dementia or severe disability—are often marginalized or erased. Likewise, issues of race, gender, and class are frequently underdeveloped, despite the reality that caregiving is performed largely by low-wage migrant workers, many of them women from the Global South. These silences are significant and reflect broader cultural patterns of neglect and invisibility.

Moreover, neoliberal logics shape how value in old age is narratively assigned. Protagonists remain meaningful primarily insofar as they are active, resourceful, or narratively useful, while dependency and vulnerability are displaced to the margins. This reinforces a conditional model of worth, one that privileges productivity and autonomy over interdependence and care. Many texts even mobilize assisted dying, like in *Exit Lines*, or suicide, like in *As We Are Now*, as narrative "solutions" to dependency. Caro Spencer, for instance, enacts her ultimate protest through self-chosen death, writing her story as legacy. While powerful as an act of resistance—and open to feminist readings that recuperate its agency—such stories might risk naturalizing death as the only dignified escape from prolonged dependence.[1] *Half Life* offers an example

1 Chie Hayakawa's film *Plan 75* (2022) is a prime example of such a kind of geronticide: a state-managed, voluntary program promotes euthanasia for anyone older than 75

of this logic when Agnes dismisses Mrs. O'Neill's passing with the sardonic remark, "At least she doesn't have to do crafts anymore" (Mighton 44)—a line that reduces death to a welcome release from the trivial indignities of institutional life. In such cultural scripts, the care home is imagined more as a terminal site framing mortality as the inevitable resolution to dependency than as a space for rethinking care. In this way, systemic shortcomings are obscured: rather than envisioning improved models of care, such stories conclude through the erasure of the dependent subject altogether. Such endings align closely with neoliberal discourses of cost containment, where the "fourth age" subject is cast not as someone to be supported but as a burden to be relieved—or even eliminated as abject.

However, as I also tried to show, some of the protagonists discussed in this book embody resilience in their own ways, but their acts of defiance do more than assert individual agency: they illuminate the structural conditions that shape late-life experience. From Stella and Dot in *Cloudburst* to Mala Ramchandin in *Cereus Blooms at Night*, from Sylvia Lodge in *Exit Lines* to Cora Sledge in *Breaking Out of Bedlam*, these characters resist being "put in their place." In reclaiming space through imagination, escape, or subversion and opposition, they expose how cultural narratives of aging are entwined with gendered ageism, systemic inequalities, and neoliberal pressures. These ambivalent depictions of care homes point to a broader cultural unease with dependency and vulnerability in later life. Reflecting on human relationships as relationships of care opens up the possibility of overcoming "the aversion to 'dependency' in modern industrialized societies that still give prime value to individual agency" (Puig de la Bellacasa 4). Engagement with literary texts that describe the end of life makes it clear that the dominant, idealized paradigm of successful and active aging—conceived as a counter-model to the bleak social imaginaries of the so-called fourth age—perpetuates neoliberal narratives of progress. Dystopian fiction highlights this by placing questions of responsibility and connectedness at the center. At the same time, old age is often reduced to narratives of catastrophe and burden, while an idealized image of independent, high-performing individuals is simultaneously constructed.

---

years, regardless of health or fitness. It "critiques the dehumanizing narratives that frame aging as an economic and social burden [...] By exposing the state's role in assigning value to human lives based on productive futurity assumed solely based on age, the film challenges the moral and emotional toll of policies that treat older people as waste" (Kriebernegg and Danely 2025).

Old Age as a Spatial and Temporal Construct

All these readings suggest that old age is both a temporal and a spatial construct. Care homes, as sites of spatial-temporal liminality between life and death, highlight the paradox of being simultaneously dependent and independent, finite and unfinished, confined and yet capable of creativity. They reveal how the young/old binary is culturally constructed and how power dynamics in aging are shaped and reinforced by spatial structures. While it is important to challenge the decline narrative by portraying old age as a time of agency and self-determination, fictional care home narratives go even further. According to Bakhtin's concept of the chronotope, they enable us to see how the past, present, and future all merge into a single narrative space. The protagonists in a number of the texts under discussion are physically confined in institutional settings that restrict their autonomy, and they experience time non-linearly—alternating between memories of their youth and their current realities. They are heterotopias in Foucault's sense: they exist simultaneously inside and outside society as sites of exclusion and contestation. The reason existential questions are staged there with such intensity is because they represent the lack of a future. Since the care facility is culturally coded as a final station, unlike a hotel or cruise ship, it is ideal for examining the circumstances of finitude, dependency, and meaning in later life.

Additionally, these texts show how ageist dichotomies—young versus old, agency versus decline, and autonomy versus dependence—are reproduced by spatial structures. Yet they also show how such binaries can be unsettled, even if only temporarily. Road narratives like *Flee, Fly, Flown* or *Amigoland* reimagine mobility as an intergenerational and late-life possibility, challenging assumptions that movement and freedom belong solely to the young. Other narratives depict smaller but still significant forms of resistance within institutional walls, such as reclaiming memory, establishing new forms of community, or asserting dignity. In all these cases, space and time are relational and connected to the cultural imagination of aging.

Responsibility and Future Directions

Representations of aging in literature and film are never merely descriptive; they actively shape cultural expectations, policies, and social realities. The stories we tell about care homes matter because they influence how societies imagine the boundaries of age, dependency, and care itself. Taking responsibility as readers and scholars means acknowledging our own ambivalences toward aging, resisting interpretations that naturalize decline, and questioning the persistent assumption that "aging in place" is always preferable to institutional care. It also requires interrogating silences around race, class, frailty, and care labor, and insisting that cultural analyses of aging account for those most often left invisible in dominant narratives. Only by interpreting the care home in such narratives as a space for self-determination and agency can we understand experiences of old age as meaningful at all times in all places.

The New Model Army lyric that frames this conclusion underlines the importance of intergenerational solidarity: "we are young, we are old, we are in this together." Breaking down binaries between youth and old age is not only a scholarly endeavor but also a cultural and political imperative. Care home narratives, with their ambivalences and contradictions, provide a vital space for imagining how aging might be lived otherwise. They remind us that agency in later life need not be tied exclusively to autonomy or productivity, but can also emerge through interdependence, vulnerability, and collective forms of living. Having agency in old age should not be undermined by established genre conventions or conventional interpretations that are guided by preconceived and stereotypical notions of age and aging as decline. Interpretations of care home novels as disempowering often reflect ageist readings that portray frail, old people as victims. What remains is the challenge of understanding representations of the "fourth age," and the spaces associated with it, not as "black holes" only relevant to those experiencing it, but for us all, and to redefine them as meaningful to understand our existence throughout the life course. As the spatiality of age relations is socially and culturally constructed, the way we narrate and interpret old age is always determined by our own position as readers.

Putting age in its place, then, means interpreting texts with the narrative power they hold while making conscious our own ambivalences about aging. It also means recognizing age's spatial, temporal, and cultural power to reshape how we imagine care, community, and our collective futures of aging.

Works Cited

AARP. "Boomers Turning 65, Boomer Voices, Baby Boom Generation." *Carolina Demography*, 2014, carolinademography.cpc.unc.edu/2015/05/14/nc-in-focus-population-proportion-65-and-older-2010-2035/. Accessed 23 Mar. 2025.

Abel, Ernest L. *Intoxication in Mythology: A Worldwide Dictionary of Gods, Rites, Intoxicants and Places*. McFarland, 2006.

Achenbaum, Andrew W. "Risk, Rights, and Responsibility." *What Does It Mean to Grow Old? Reflections from the Humanities*, edited by Thomas R. Cole and Sally A. Gadow, Duke UP, 1986, pp. 63–100.

—. *Robert N. Butler, MD: Visionary of Healthy Aging*. Columbia UP, 2013.

Adams, Annmarie, and Sally Chivers. "Home Pages: Domesticity and Duplicity in Images of Architecture for Ageing." *Seachange*, 2013, pp. 80–102.

—. "Architecture and Aging: The Depiction of Home in Sarah Polley's *Away from Her*." *Age, Culture, Humanities: An Interdisciplinary Journal, no.* 2, 2015, ageculturehumanities.org/WP/architecture-and-aging-the-depiction-of-home-in-sarah-polleys-away-from-her/.

Agamben, Giorgio. *Homo Sacer: Sovereign Power and Bare Life*. Stanford UP, 1998.

Age, Culture, Humanities: An Interdisciplinary Journal. Royal Danish Library, eISSN 2373–5481, *Age, Culture, Humanities*, https://tidsskrift.dk/ageculturehumanities/index. Accessed 24 Aug. 2025.

Alford, Edna. *A Sleep Full of Dreams*. Oolichan Books, 1981.

—. "Fear of the Novel." *Writing Saskatchewan: 20 Critical Essays*, edited by Kenneth G. Probert, 1st ed., Canadian Plains Research Center, U of Regina, 1989, pp. 173–79.

Althusser, Louis. "Ideology and Ideological State Apparatuses." *Marxists Internet Archive*, 12 Sep. 2009, https://www.marxists.org/reference/archive/althusser/1970/ideology.htm. Accessed 23 Mar. 2025.

Andrews, Gavin J. "Residential Homes: From Distributions in Space to the Elements of Place." *Ageing and Place: Perspectives, Policy, Practice*, edited by Gavin J. Andrews and David R. Phillips, Routledge, 2005, pp. 61–78.

—, et al. "'Airplanes Are Flying Nursing Homes': Geographies in the Concepts and Locales of Gerontological Nursing Practice." *Journal of Clinical Nursing*, vol. 14, 2005, pp. 109–20. Wiley Online Library, https://doi.org/10.1111/j.1365-2702.2005.01276.x.

—, and David R. Phillips. "Changing Local Geographies of Private Residential Care for Older People 1983–1999: Lessons for Social Policy in England and Wales." *Social Science & Medicine*, vol. 55, 2002, pp. 63–78.

—, editors. *Ageing and Place: Perspectives, Policy, Practice*. Routledge, 2005.

Angelou, Maya. *All God's Children Need Traveling Shoes.* 1st Random House ed. Random House, 1986.

Arber, Sara, and Maria Evandrou, editors. *Ageing, Independence, and the Life Course.* Jessica Kingsley in association with the British Society of Gerontology, 1993.

Arber, Sara, and Jay Ginn. "Class, Caring and the Life Course." *Ageing, Independence, and the Life Course*, edited by Sara Arber and Maria Evandrou, Jessica Kingsley in association with the British Society of Gerontology, 1993, pp. 149–68.

Armstrong, Hugh. "Piercing the Corporate Veil: Nursing Home Ownership in Turbulent Times." In *Care Homes in a Turbulent Era: Do They Have a Future?*, edited by Pat Armstrong and Susan Braedley, Edward Elgar, 2023, pp. 19–33.

Armstrong, Pat, and Susan Braedley, editors. *Care Homes in a Turbulent Era: Do They Have a Future?*. Edward Elgar, 2023. In a Turbulent Era Series.

—. "Care Homes in Crisis: Promising Ways Forward." In *Care Homes in a Turbulent Era: Do They Have a Future?*, edited by Pat Armstrong and Susan Braedley, Edward Elgar, 2023, pp. 1–18.

Ashworth, Rebecca. "Reading Through Shame: Shani Mootoo's *Cereus Blooms at Night*." *Journal of West Indian Literature*, vol. 19, no. 2, 2011, pp. 34–51.

Atkinson, Michael. "Crossing the Frontiers." *Sight and Sound*, vol. 1, no. 1, 1994, pp. 14–17.

Atwood, Margaret. "King Lear in Respite Care." *Morning in the Burned House*, Houghton Mifflin, 1995, pp. 85–87.

—. "Alphinland." *Stone Mattress: Nine Tales*, Nan A. Talese / Doubleday, 2014, pp. 1–34.

—. *Stone Mattress: Nine Tales*. Nan A. Talese / Doubleday, 2014.

—. "Torching the Dusties." *Stone Mattress: Nine Tales*, Nan A. Talese / Doubleday, 2014, pp. 225–68.

Auden, W. H. "Old People's Home." *Collected Poems*, edited by Edward Mendelson, First Vintage International edition, 1991, p. 860. Vintage International.

Augé, Marc. *An Anthropology for Contemporaneous Worlds*. Stanford UP, 1999. Mestizo Spaces.

Bachelard, Gaston. *The Poetics of Space*. Beacon, 1994.

Bachmann, Andreas. "Harald Friedl: '24-Stunden-Pflegerinnen Sind Leistungsträgerinnen.'" *Moment.at*, 2024, https://www.moment.at/story/harald-friedl-24-stunden-pflegerinnen-leistungstraegerinnen/. Accessed 8 Mar. 2025.

Bakhtin, Mikhail Mikhailovich. "Forms of Time and Chronotope in the Novel. Notes Toward a Historical Poetics." *The Dialogic Imagination: Four Essays*, edited by Michael Holquist, U of Texas P, 1981 (1937–38), pp. 84–258. U of Texas P Slavic Series 1.

—. *Rabelais and His World*, trans. Helene Iswolsky. Indiana UP, 1984.

Banerjee, Albert. *An Overview of Long-Term Care in Canada and Selected Provinces and Territories*. 2007. https://www.womenandhealthcarereform.ca/publications/banerjee_overviewLTC.pdf. Accessed 23 Mar. 2025.

Barfoot, Joan. *Exit Lines*. Vintage Canada, 2009 [2008].

—. *Duet for Three*. Women's Press, 1986.

Barnett, Michael L., and David C. Grabowski. "Nursing Homes Are Ground Zero for COVID-19 Pandemic." *JAMA Health Forum*, vol. 1, no. 3, 2020, e200369-e200369. https://doi.org/10.1001/jamahealthforum.2020.0369. Accessed 31 Aug 2025.

Barrett, Andrea. *The Forms of Water*. Washington Square, 2002.

Barry, Elizabeth. "A Glut of Slippers: The Chronotope of Older Age in the Contemporary North American Short Story." *Contemporary Narratives of Ageing, Illness, Care*, edited by Katsura Sako and Sarah Falcus, Routledge, 2022, pp. 144–62. Routledge Interdisciplinary Perspectives on Literature.

Basting, Anne Davis, et al. *The Penelope Project: An Arts-Based Odyssey to Change Elder Care*. U of Iowa P, 2016. Humanities and Public Life.

Baudrillard, Jean. *Simulacra and Simulation*. Translated by Sheila Faria Glaser, U of Michigan P, 1994.

Bayley, John. *Elegy for Iris: A Memoir.* 1st Picador USA pbk. ed. Picador USA, 2000 [1999].

—. *Iris: A Memoir of Iris Murdoch*. Abacus, 2000 [1998].

Beauvoir, Simone de. *The Coming of Age*. Translated by Patrick O'Brian, W.W. Norton & Company, 1996.

Bedard, Michael. *Redwork*. 1st ed. Atheneum, 1990.

Befeler, Mike. *Retirement Homes Are Murder.* Five Star, 2007. Paul Jacobson Geezer-Lit Mystery Series 1.

—. *Living with Your Kids Is Murder*. Five Star, 2009. Paul Jacobson Geezer-Lit Mystery Series 2.

—. *Senior Moments Are Murder*. Five Star, 2011. Paul Jacobson Geezer-Lit Mystery Series 3.

—. *Cruising in Your Eighties Is Murder*. Five Star, 2012. Paul Jacobson Geezer-Lit Mystery Series 4.

—. *Care Homes Are Murder.* Five Star, 2013. Paul Jacobson Geezer-Lit Mystery Series 5.

—. *The Back Wing*. Courtney Literary, 2013.

—. *Nursing Homes Are Murder*. Five Star, 2014. Paul Jacobson Geezer-Lit Mystery Series 6.

Bender, John. *Imagining the Penitentiary: Fiction and the Architecture of Mind in Eighteenth-Century England*. U of Chicago P, 1987.

Bhabha, Homi K. *The Location of Culture*. Routledge, 1994.

Biggs, Simon, and Jason L. Powell. "A Foucauldian Analysis of Old Age and the Power of Social Welfare." *Journal of Aging and Social Policy*, vol. 12, no. 2, 2001, pp. 1–20.

Blaikie, Andrew. *Ageing and Popular Culture*. Cambridge UP, 1999.

—. "Imagined Landscapes of Age and Identity." In *Ageing and Place: Perspectives, Policy, Practice*, edited by Gavin J. Andrews and David R. Phillips, Routledge, 2005, pp. 164–75.

Bluefarb, Sam. *The Escape Motif in the American Novel: Mark Twain to Richard Wright*. Ohio State UP, 1972.

Börjesson, Ulrika, and Joy Cristina Torgé. "'They Say This Is a Home': The Challenge of 'Home' in Residential Care Settings for Old and Young." *Journal of Housing and the Built Environment*, vol. 37, 2021, pp. 1093–108.

Braedley, Susan. "Reinventing the Nursing Home: Metaphors That Design Care." In Katz, *Ageing in Everyday Life*, pp. 45–62.

Burger, Robert E. "Who Cares for the Aged?" *Saturday Review*, no. 25, 1969, pp. 14–17. https://www.unz.com/Pub/SaturdayRev-1969jan25-00014/?View=PDFPages. Accessed 31 Aug. 2025.

Burns, Lorna. "Politicising Paradise: Sites of Resistance in *Cereus Blooms at Night*." *Journal of West Indian Literature*, vol. 19, no. 2, 2011, p. 52.

Buse, Christina, et al. "Imagined Bodies: Architects and Their Constructions of Later Life." *Ageing & Society*, vol. 37, 2017, pp. 1435–57. https://doi.org/10.1017/S0144686X16000362. Accessed 25 Aug. 2025.

Butler, Robert N. "The Life Review: An Interpretation of Reminiscence in the Aged." *New Thoughts on Old Age*, edited by Robert Kastenbaum, Springer, 1964, pp. 265–80.

Calasanti, Toni. "Gender and Ageing in the Context of Globalisation." *The Sage Handbook of Social Gerontology*, edited by Dale Dannefer and Chris Phillipson, Sage, 2010, pp. 137–49.

Campbell, Neil. "Road Narratives and Western Identity." *Western American Literature*, vol. 36, no. 3, 2001, pp. 279–90.

Caouette, Elaine. "The Image of Nursing Homes and Its Impact on the Meaning of Home for Elders." In Rowles and Chaudhury, *Home and Identity in Late Life*, Springer, 2005, pp. 251–75.

Carleton, William McKendree. "Over the Hill to the Poorhouse." In *Famous Poems from Bygone Days*, edited by Martin Gardner, Dover Publications, 1995, pp. 30–32.

Carrington, Leonora. *The Hearing Trumpet*. Introduction by Helen Byatt, Exact Change, 1996 [1974].

—. *The Hearing Trumpet*. Introduction by Ali Smith, Penguin, 2003 [1974].

Casares, Oscar. *Amigoland*. Back Bay Books, 2009.

Casteel, Sarah Phillips. "New World Pastoral: The Caribbean Garden and Emplacement in Gisèle Pineau and Shani Mootoo." *Interventions*, vol. 5, no. 1, 2003, pp. 12–28. https://doi.org/10.1080/1369803200004977O. Accessed 31 Aug. 2025.

Caudell, William A. *The Psychiatric Hospital as a Small Society*. Harvard UP, 1958.

Certeau, Michel de. *The Practice of Everyday Life*. U of California P, 1984.

Charcot, Jean Martin. *Clinical Lectures on the Diseases of Old Age*. Translated by Leigh H. Hunt; contributed to by Alfred L. Loomis, William Wood & Company, 1881. *Internet Archive*, https://archive.org/details/clinicallecturesooch ar. Accessed 24 Aug. 2025.

Charise, Andrea. "'Let the Reader Think of the Burden': Old Age and the Crisis of Capacity." *Occasion: Interdisciplinary Studies in the Humanities*, no. 4, 31 May 2012, pp. 1–16. https://shc.stanford.edu/sites/default/files/2012-06/OCCASION_v04_Charise_053112_0.pdf. Accessed 31 Aug. 2025.

Chast, Roz. *Can't We Talk About Something More Pleasant?* First United States edition. Bloomsbury, 2014.

Chivers, Sally. *From Old Woman to Older Women: Contemporary Culture and Women's Narratives*. Ohio State UP, 2003.

—. "On the Road Again: Aritha Van Herk's *No Fixed Address* and Suzette Mayr's *The Widows*." In Perrakis, *Adventures of the Spirit*, Ohio State UP, 2007, pp. 200–15.

—. "Reimagining Care: Images of Aging and Creativity in *House Calls* and *a Year at Sherbrooke*." *International Journal of Ageing and Later Life*, vol. 7, no. 2, 2012, pp. 53–71. https://doi.org/10.3384/ijal.1652-8670.1272a3. Accessed 31 Aug. 2025.

—. "'Blind People Don't Run': Escaping the 'Nursing Home Specter' in *Children of Nature* and *Cloudburst*." *Journal of Aging Studies*, vol. 34, 2015, pp. 134–41. https://doi.org/10.1016/j.jaging.2015.06.001. Accessed 31 Aug. 2025.

—. "What's Exotic About the Best Exotic Marigold Hotel? Cinema, Everyday Life and the Materialisation of Ageing." In Katz, *Ageing in Everyday Life*, pp. 83–98.

—, and Ulla Kriebernegg, editors. *Care Home Stories: Aging, Disability, and Long-Term Residential Care*. transcript, 2017. Aging Studies 14.

Clendinen, Dudley. *A Place Called Canterbury: Tales of the New Old Age in America*. Viking, 2008.

Cole, Thomas R. *The Journey of Life: A Cultural History of Aging in America*. Cambridge UP, 1992.

—. "After the Life Cycle: The Moral Challenges of Later Life." In Cutter, *Midrash & Medicine: Healing Body and Soul in the Jewish Interpretive Tradition*, Jewish Lights, 2011, pp. 137–59.

—, and Sally A. Gadow, editors. *What Does It Mean to Grow Old?: Reflections from the Humanities*. Duke UP, 1986.

—, Ruth Ray, and Robert Kastenbaum, editors. *A Guide to Humanistic Studies in Aging: What Does It Mean to Grow Old?*. Johns Hopkins UP, 2010.

Cooper, Ann. *Ladies and Gentlemen, Bernard Jordan. The Huffington Post Canada*, Facebook Post, 2014. https://www.facebook.com/HuffPostCanada/posts/751697564850425. Accessed 18 Aug. 2014.

Cresswell, Tim. *In Place/Out of Place: Geography, Ideology, and Transgression*. U of Minnesota P, 1996.

Cruikshank, Margaret. *Learning to Be Old: Gender, Culture, and Aging*. Rowman & Littlefield, 2003.

—. *Successful Aging?*. Silver Century Foundation, 2015. Accessed 20 Jan. 2015.

Cruz, Mariana. "Of Cats and Crones: Hope and Ecofeminist Utopianism in Leonora Carrington's *The Hearing Trumpet*." *Anglo Saxonica*, vol. 20, no. 1, 2022, pp. 1–11. https://doi.org/10.5334/as.87.

Cunningham, Daniel Mudie. "Driving into the 'Dustless Highway' of Queer Cinema." [*Film Journal*, vol. 1, no. 5, 2003], currently only available on https://danmudcun.com/criticism/the-dustless-highway. Accessed 05 Nov. 2025.

Dalmer, Nicole, and Lucia Cedeira Serantes. "Ageing and the Media: Imag(In)Ing Ageing Futures in Comics and Graphic Novels." *International Perspectives*, edited by Virpi Ylänne, Policy Press, 2022, pp. 133–54.

Davies, Megan J. "Renovating the Canadian Old Age Home: The Evolution of Residential Care Facilities in B.C., 1930–1960." *Journal of the Canadian Historical Association*, vol. 12, no. 1, 2001, p. 155. https://doi.org/10.7202/031146ar. Accessed 24 Aug. 2025.

—. *Into the House of Old: A History of Residential Care in British Columbia*. McGill-Queen's UP, 2004.

DeFalco, Amelia. "Graphic Somatography: Life Writing, Comics, and the Ethics of Care." *Journal of Medical Humanities*, vol. 37, no. 3, 2016, pp. 223–40. https://doi.org/10.1007/s10912-015-9360-6. Accessed 24 Aug. 2025.

Dekkers, Wim. "Dwelling, House and Home: Towards a Home-Led Perspective on Dementia Care." *Medicine, Health Care, and Philosophy*, vol. 14, no. 3, 2011, pp. 291–300. https://doi.org/10.1007/s11019-011-9307-2. Accessed 24 Aug. 2025.

Derrida, Jacques. "Structure, Sign, and Play in the Discourse of the Human Sciences." *Writing and Difference*. U of Chicago P, 1978, pp. 278–94.

Diamond, Timothy. "Nursing Homes as Trouble." *Journal of Contemporary Ethnography*, vol. 12, no. 3, 1983, pp. 269–86. https://doi.org/10.1177/0098303983012003003. Accessed 24 Aug. 2025.

—. *Making Gray Gold: Narratives of Nursing Home Care*. U of Chicago P, 1992.

Dolan, Andy, et al. "'I Loved Every Minute... I'd Do It Again Tomorrow!'" *Daily Mail Online*, 6 June 2014, https://www.dailymail.co.uk/news/article-2650882/ Accessed 23 Mar. 2025.

Dowell, Pat. "The Impotence of Women." *Cineaste*, vol. 18, no. 4, 91, pp. 28–30.

Dowling, Emma. *The Care Crisis: What Caused It and How Can We End It?* First edition paperback. Verso, 2021.

Dumas, Alexandre. *The Count of Monte Cristo*. Wordsworth Editions, 1997. Wordsworth Classics.

Du Toit, Catherine. "Ageing in the Twenty-First Century." *Readings in Twenty-First-Century European Literatures*, edited by Michael Gratzke et al., Peter Lang, 2013, pp. 279–301.

Dvorak, Marta. "Margaret Atwood's Humor." *The Cambridge Companion to Margaret Atwood*, edited by Coral Ann Howells, Cambridge UP, 2006, pp. 114–29. Cambridge Companions to Literature.

Dyck, Isabel, et al. "The Home as a Site for Long-Term Care: Meanings and Management of Bodies and Spaces." *Health & Place*, vol. 11, no. 2, 2005, pp. 173–85. https://doi.org/10.1016/j.healthplace.2004.06.001. Accessed 24 Aug. 2025.

Edgerton, Clyde. *Lunch at the Piccadilly: A Novel.* 1st ed. Ballantine Books, 2004.

Eiby, May Bjerre. *May Bjerre Eiby. Dagmarsminde.* https://www.maybjerreeiby.dk/ Accessed 24 Aug. 2025.

—, and Dorthe Boss Kyhn. *Living Normally with Dementia: One Care Home's Story and How to Make It Yours*. Health Professions Press, 2023.

Elden, Stuart. *Understanding Henri Lefebvre: Theory and the Possible*. Continuum, 2004. Continuum Studies in Philosophy.

ElderWeb. *1950–1980: Nursing Home Fires: Award-Winning Online Eldercare Sourcebook*. 2015, https://www.elderweb.com/book/appendix/1950-1980-nursing-home-fires. Accessed 22 Apr. 2015.

Emerson, Caryl, and Michael Holquist, transl. *The Dialogic Imagination: Four Essays.* By Mikhail Mikhailovich Bakhtin. Edited by Michael Holquist. U of Texas P, 1981 (1937–38). U of Texas P Slavic Series, 1.

Emerson, Ralph Waldo. "Old Age." *Society and Solitude. Twelve Chapters.* Fields, Osgood & Co, 1870, pp. 279–300.

Enßle-Reinhardt, Friederike, and Ilse Helbrecht. "'That Is When You Realize Your Age'—A Spatial Approach to Age(Ing)." *Canadian Geographies / Géographies canadiennes*, vol. 66, no. 1, 2022, pp. 172–83. https://doi.org/10.1111/cag.12727. Accessed 24 Aug. 2025.

Essig, Rolf-Bernhard. *Der offene Brief: Geschichte und Funktion einer publizistischen Form von Isokrates bis Günter Grass*. Könighausen & Neumann, 2000. Epistemata. Reihe Literaturwissenschaft 267.

Falcus, Sarah, Heike Hartung, and Raquel Medina, editors. *The Bloomsbury Handbook to Ageing in Contemporary Literature and Film*. Bloomsbury Academic, 2023. Bloomsbury Handbooks.

Farrell, Chris. *Could This Idea Help Fix America's Shortage of Home Care Workers? How the AARP Foundation Aims to Improve Home Care Pay and Benefits*. Next Avenue. 2017. Accessed 23 Mar. 2025.

Fay, Roger, and Ceridwen Owen. "'Home' in the Aged Care Institution: Authentic or Ersatz." *Procedia – Social and Behavioral Sciences*, vol. 35, 2012, pp. 33–43. https://doi.org/10.1016/j.sbspro.2012.02.060. Accessed 24 Aug. 2025.

Featherstone, Mike. "Automobilities: An Introduction." *Theory, Culture & Society*, vol. 21, 4–5, 2004, pp. 1–24. https://doi.org/10.1177/0263276404046058. Accessed 24 Aug. 2025.

—, and Mike Hepworth. "Images of Positive Aging: A Case Study of *Retirement Choice Magazine*." *Images of Aging: Cultural Representations of Later Life*, edited by Mike Featherstone and Andrew Wernick, Routledge, 1995, pp. 29–47.

—, and Andrew Wernick, editors. *Images of Aging: Cultural Representations of Later Life*. Routledge, 1995.

Felman, Shoshana. "Education and Crisis, or the Vicissitudes of Teaching." *Testimony: Crises of Witnessing in Literature, Psychoanalysis, and History*, edited by Shoshana Felman and Dori Laub, Routledge, 1991, pp. 1–56.

Feng, Zhanlian, et al. "The Care Span: Growth of Racial and Ethnic Minorities in US Nursing Homes Driven by Demographics and Possible Disparities in Options." *Health affairs (Project Hope)*, vol. 30, no. 7, 2011, pp. 1–10. https://doi.org/10.1377/hlthaff.2011.0126. Accessed 24 Aug. 2025.

Fetterley, Judith. *The Resisting Reader: A Feminist Approach to American Fiction*. Indiana UP, 1978.

Fisher, Berenice, and Joan C. Tronto. "Toward a Feminist Theory of Caring." *Circles of Care: Work and Identity in Women's Lives*, edited by Emily Abel and Margaret Nelson, State University of New York Press, 1990, pp. 35–61.

Fleming, Anne M., et al. "Care Homes: The Developing Ideology of a Homelike Place to Live." *Maturitas*, vol. 99, 2017, pp. 92–97. https://doi.org/10.1016/j.maturitas.2017.02.013. Accessed 05 Nov. 2025.

Foucault, Michel. *Power/Knowledge. Selected Interviews and Other Writings 1972–77*. Edited by Colin Gordon. Pantheon Books, 1980.

—. "Of Other Spaces." *Diacritics: A Review of Contemporary Criticism*, vol. 16, no. 1, 1986, pp. 22–27.

—. "Technologies of the Self." *Technologies of the Self: A Seminar with Michel Foucault*, edited by Luther H. Martin et al., U of Massachusetts P, 1988, pp. 16–49.

—. *The Birth of the Clinic: An Archaeology of Medical Perception*. Vintage, 1994 [1963].

—. *Discipline and Punish: The Birth of the Prison*. Random House, 1995.

—. *Security, Territory, Population: Lectures at the Collège de France, 1977 – 1978*. Palgrave Macmillan, 2009.

Foundation Aiding the Elderly (FATE). *The History of Nursing Homes*. n.d., https://www.4fate.org/history.html. Accessed 22 July 2013.

Fox, Linda Chris. "The Paradise Alms House: Siting Literary Thirdspace in Shani Mootoo's *Cereus Blooms at Night*." *Canadian Literature*, Summer, no. 205, 2010, pp. 70–84.

Friedan, Betty. *The Fountain of Age*. Simon & Schuster, 1993.

Friedman, Susan Stanford. *Mappings: Feminism and the Cultural Geographies of Encounter*. Princeton UP, 1998.

Fulk, Mark K. *Understanding May Sarton*. U of South Carolina P, 2001.

Ganser, Alexandra. "On the Asphalt Frontier: American Women's Road Narratives, Spatiality, and Transgression." *Journal of International Women's Studies*, vol. 7, no. 4, 2006, pp. 153–67.

—. *Roads of Her Own: Gendered Space and Mobility in American Women's Road Narratives, 1970–2000*. Rodopi, 2009.

__, et al. "Bakhtin's Chronotope on the Road: Space, Time, and Place in Road Movies Since the 1970s." *Facta Universitatis. Linguistics and Literature*, vol. 4, no. 1, 2006, pp. 1–17.

Gardiner, Heather. *The Portrayal of Old Age in English-Canadian Fiction*. PhD dissertation, University of Toronto, 1998.

Garvin, Richard M., and Robert E. Burger. *Where They Go to Die: The Tragedy of America's Aged*. Delacorte Press, 1968.

Gass, Thomas Edward, and Bruce C. Vladeck. *Nobody's Home: Candid Reflections of a Nursing Home Aide*. ILR Press, 2004.

Gaugler, Joseph E. "Innovations in Long-Term Care." *Handbook of Aging and the Social Sciences*, edited by Linda K. George et al., Eighth edition, Elsevier, 2016, pp. 419–40. Handbooks of Aging.

Genova, Lisa. *Still Alice*. Pocket Books, 2009.

Giddens, Anthony. *Modernity and Self-Identity: Self and Society in the Late Modern Age*. Stanford UP, 1991.

Gilbert, Sandra M., and Susan Gubar. *The Madwoman in the Attic: The Woman Writer and the Nineteenth-Century Literary Imagination*. 2nd ed. Yale UP, 2000 [1979].

Gilleard, Chris, and Paul Higgs. *Cultures of Ageing*. Prentice Hall-Pearson Education, 2000.

—. "Aging Without Agency: Theorizing the Fourth Age." *Aging & Mental Health*, vol. 14, no. 2, 2010, pp. 121–28. https://doi.org/10.1080/13607860903228762. Accessed 24 Aug. 2025.

—. "Ageing Abjection and Embodiment in the Fourth Age." *Journal of Aging Studies*, vol. 25, no. 2, 2011, pp. 135–42. https://doi.org/10.1016/j.jaging.2010.08.018. Accessed 24 Aug. 2025.

—. "The Fourth Age and the Concept of a 'Social Imaginary': A Theoretical Excursus." *Journal of Aging Studies*, vol. 27, no. 4, 2013, pp. 368–76. https://doi.org/10.1016/j.jaging.2013.08.004. Accessed 24 Aug. 2025.

Give World War 2 Veteran Bernard Jordan a Knighthood. Facebook. 2014, https://www.facebook.com/BernardJordanKnighthood. Accessed 13 Aug. 2014.

Goffman, Erving. *Asylums: Essays on the Social Situation of Mental Patients and Other Inmates*. 1st ed. Anchor Books, 1961.

—. *Stigma: Notes on the Management of Spoiled Identity*. Simon & Schuster, 1986 [1963].

Goldman, Marlene. "'Their Dark Cells': Transference, Memory, and Postmemory in John Mighton's *Half Life*." *Canadian Literature and Cultural Memory*, edited by Eleanor Rose Ty and Cynthia Conchita Sugars, Oxford UP, 2014, pp. 118–33.

Gratton, Brian. *Urban Elders: Family, Work, and Welfare among Boston's Aged, 1890–1950*. Temple UP, 1986.

Gravagne, Pamela H. *The Becoming of Age: Cinematic Visions of Mind, Body and Identity in Later Life*. McFarland, 2013.

Green Kuhn, Meredith Anne. *The Eye of Beauty: Creating a Place for Elite and Aging Elders*. PhD Dissertation, University of Arizona, 2007, arizona.openrepository.com/arizona/bitstreaUPm/10150/193736/1/azu_etd_2700_sip1_m.pdf. Accessed 23 Mar. 2025.

Grenier, Amanda. *Transitions and the Lifecourse: Challenging the Constructions of 'Growing Old'*. Policy Press, 2012. Ageing and the Lifecourse.

Grey, Aubrey D. N. J. de. *Aubrey de Grey at TEDMED 2009*. https://www.youtube.com/watch?v=hgLRhxvRlKg. Accessed 24 Aug. 2025.

Grey, Aubrey D. N. J. de, and Michael Rae. *Ending Aging: The Rejuvenation Breakthroughs That Could Reverse Human Aging in Our Lifetime.* 1st. St. Martin's Press, 2007.

Grist, Hannah, and Ros Jennings. *Carers, Care Homes and the British Media: Time to Care*. Palgrave Macmillan, 2020.

Groen, Rick. "Cloudburst: Two Old Broads Who Can Really Act." *The Globe and Mail*, 8 Mar. 2013, https://www.theglobeandmail.com/arts/film/film-reviews/cloudburst-two-old-broads-who-can-really-act/article9459295/. Accessed 23 Mar. 2025.

Gruen, Sara. *Water for Elephants*. Harper Perennial, 2007.

Gubrium, Jaber F. *Speaking of Life: Horizons of Meaning for Nursing Home Residents*. De Gruyter, 1993.

—. *Living and Dying at Murray Manor*. Expanded pbk. ed. UP of Virginia, 1997.

—. *Analyzing Narrative Reality*. Sage, 2009.

—, and James A. Holstein. "The Nursing Home as a Discursive Anchor for the Ageing Body." *Ageing and Society*, vol. 19, no. 5, 1999, pp. 519–38. journals.cambridge.org/abstract_S0144686X99007448.

Gullette, Margaret Morganroth. *Declining to Decline: Cultural Combat and the Politics of the Midlife*. UP of Virginia, 1997. Age Studies.

—. *Aged by Culture*. U of Chicago P, 2004

—. *Ending Ageism: Or, How Not to Shoot Old People*. Rutgers UP, 2017. Global Perspectives on Aging.

—. *American Eldercide. How It Happened, How To Prevent It.* U of Chicago P, 2024.

Gustavsson, Matilda. "'Nytt rekord för 'Hundraåringen.'" *DN.KULTUR*, 23 July 2014, Online, pp. n.p. https://www.dn.se/kultur-noje/film-tv/nytt-rekord-for-hundraaringen/. Accessed 14 Aug. 2025.

Haber, Carole, and Brian Gratton. *Old Age and the Search for Security: An American Social History*. Indiana UP, 1993.

Harnett, Tove. "Seeking Exemptions from Nursing Home Routines: Residents' Everyday Influence Attempts and Institutional Order." *Journal of Aging Studies*, vol. 24, no. 4, 2010, pp. 292–301. https://doi.org/10.1016/j.jaging.2010.08.001. Accessed 24 Aug. 2025.

Harper, Sarah. "Contesting Later Life." *Contested Countryside Cultures: Otherness, Marginalisation, and Rurality*, edited by Paul J. Cloke and Jo Little, Routledge, 1997, pp. 180–96.

Harris-Kojetin, Lauren, et al. *Long-Term Care Services in the United States: 2013 Overview*. National Center for Health Statistics. National Health Care Statistics Reports 1, https://www.cdc.gov/nchs/data/nsltcp/long_term_care_services_2013.pdf. Accessed 23 Mar. 2025.

Hartswick, Nathan. *The Great Nursing Home Escape: A Comedy in One Act*. Heuer, 2012.

Hartung, Heike. *Narrating Age: Ageing, Gender and Genre in Anglophone Literatures*. Habilitationsschrift, Universität Potsdam, 2013.

—. *Ageing, Gender and Illness in Anglophone Literature: Narrating Age in the Bildungsroman*. Routledge, 2016. Routledge Interdisciplinary Perspectives on Literature.

—, and Roberta Maierhofer. "Introduction." *Hartung and Maierhofer, Narratives*, pp. 5–18.

—, editors. *Narratives of Life: Mediating Age*. Lit, 2009. Aging Studies in Europe 1.

Harwood, Ronald. *Quartet & Equally Divided*. Faber & Faber, 1999.

Hays, Edward. "Turning Old Age's Prison into a Time of Forgiveness and Gratitude." *National Catholic Reporter Online*, 23 Mar. 2025, vol. 2013, pp. n.p. ncronline.org/news/people/turning-old-ages-prison-time-forgiveness-and-gratitude. Accessed 05 Nov. 2025.

Hazan, Haim. *The Limbo People: A Study of the Constitution of the Time Universe Among the Aged*. Routledge, 1980. International Library of Anthropology.

—. *Old Age: Constructions and Deconstructions*. Cambridge UP, 1994.

—. "The Home over the Hill: Towards a Modern Cosmology of Institutionalization." *Journal of Aging Studies*, no. 16, 2002, pp. 323–44.

—. "Beyond Dialogue: Entering the Fourth Space in Old Age." *Valuing Older People: A Humanist Approach to Ageing*, edited by Ricca Edmondson and Hans-Joachim von Kondratowitz, Policy, 2009, pp. 91–104.

Henderson, J. Neil. "The Culture of Care in a Nursing Home: Effects of a Medicalized Model of Long Term Care." *The Culture of Long Term Care: Nursing Home Ethnography*, edited by J. Neil Henderson and Maria D. Vesperi, Bergin & Garvey, 1995, pp. 37–54.

Hepburn, Janet. *Flee, Fly, Flown*. Second Story Press, 2013.

—. *Janet Hepburn Interview Part 2: Flee, Fly, Flown: Youtube Video*. 2013, https://www.youtube.com/watch?v=WhcwHX-NRp4. Accessed 24 Aug. 2025.

Hepworth, Mike. *Stories of Ageing*. Open UP, 2000.

—. "Images of Aging." *Handbook of Communication and Aging Research*, edited by Jon F. Nussbaum and Justine Coupland, Taylor & Francis, 2004, 3–30.

Hess, Linda, and Annika Ullmann. "Queer Theory and Narrating Age Outside the Norm of (Re-)Productive Adulthood." *Lipscomb and Swinnen*, Palgrave, pp. 121–39.

Holstein, Martha, and Thomas R. Cole. "The Evolution of Long-Term Care in America." *The Future of Long-Term Care: Social and Policy Issues*, edited by Robert H. Binstock et al., Johns Hopkins UP, 1996, pp. 19–47.

Hoving, Isabel. "Gardening in the Jungles of Post-Coloniality: Representing Multiculturality and Hybridity." *Bridges Across Chasms: Towards a Transcultural Future in Caribbean Literature*, edited by Bénédicte Ledent, L3- Liège Language and Literature, English Dept., Université de Liège, 2004, pp. 211–19.

—. "Moving the Caribbean Landscape: *Cereus Blooms at Night* as Re-Imagination of the Caribbean Environment." *Caribbean Literature and the Environ-*

ment: Between Nature and Culture, edited by Elizabeth M. DeLoughrey et al., U of Virginia P, 2005, pp. 154–68. New World Studies.

Howells, Coral Ann. *Contemporary Canadian Women's Fiction: Refiguring Identities*. 1st ed. Palgrave Macmillan, 2003.

Huffington Post. "D-Day Veteran Stages Escape from Nursing Home." *Huffington Post Canada*, 16 June 2017, https://www.huffpost.com/archive/ca/entry/d-day-veteran-escapes-nursing-home-to-commemorate-invasions-70t_n_5460358. Accessed 23 Mar. 2025.

Hutcheon, Linda. "'Shape Shifters': Canadian Women Novelists and the Challenge to Tradition." *A Mazing Space: Writing Canadian Women Writing*, edited by Shirley. C. Neuman and Smaro Kamboureli, Longspoon; NeWest, 1986, pp. 219–27.

Ignatieff, Michael. *Scar Tissue*. Penguin, 2006.

Jameson, Fredric. *The Political Unconscious: Narrative as a Socially Symbolic Act*. Cornell UP, 1981.

Jamieson, Anne, et al., editors. *Critical Approaches to Ageing and Later Life*. Open UP, 1997.

Jamieson, Sara. "Mourning in the Burned House: Margaret Atwood and the Modern Elegy." *Canadian Poetry*, no. 48, 2001, pp. 1–23. canadianpoetry.org/volumes/vol48/jamieson.html. Accessed Oct. 31, 2025.

Johnson, Julia, et al. *Residential Care Transformed: Revisiting 'the Last Refuge'*. Palgrave Macmillan, 2012.

Johnson, Todd. *The Sweet By and By*. HarperCollins, 2009.

Jonasson, Jonas. *The Hundred-Year-Old Man Who Climbed Out Of The Window And Disappeared*. Hyperion, 2012.

Jones, Kenneth. "John Mighton's *Half Life*, About Memory, Identity and Love, Gets World Premiere in Toronto Feb. 22." *Playbill*. 2005, playbill.com/article/john-mightons-half-life-about-memory-identity-and-love-gets-world-premiere-in-toronto-feb-22-com-124284. Accessed 23 Mar. 2025.

Kainradl, Anna-Christina, and Ulla Kriebernegg. "'They Say We Messed It up. Killing the Planet with Our Own Greed': Alternswissenschaftliche Überlegungen zu einem Generationengerechten Klimadiskurs in Margaret Atwoods 'Torching the Dusties.'" *Limina*, vol. 3, no. 1, 2020, pp. 166–91. https://doi.org/10.25364/17.3:2020.1.8. Accessed 24 Aug. 2025.

Katz, Michael B. "Poorhouses and the Origins of the Public Old Age Home." *The Milbank Memorial Fund Quarterly. Health and Society*, vol. 62, no. 1, 1984, pp. 110–40.

Katz, Stephen. *Disciplining Old Age: The Formation of Gerontological Knowledge*. UP of Virginia, 1996.

—. *Cultural Aging: Life Course, Lifestyle, and Senior Worlds*. Broadview, 2005.

—. "Hold on! Falling, Embodiment, and the Materiality of Old Age." *Corpus: An Interdisciplinary Reader on Bodies and Knowledge*, edited by Monica J. Casper and Paisley Currah, 1st ed., Palgrave Macmillan, 2011, pp. 187–205.

—, editor. *Ageing in Everyday Life: Materialities and Embodiments*. Policy Press, 2018.

—, and Toni Calasanti. "Critical Perspectives on Successful Aging: Does It 'Appeal More Than It Illuminates'?" *The Gerontologist*, vol. 55, no. 1, 2014, pp. 26–33. Oxford Academic, https://doi.org/10.1093/geront/gnu027. Accessed 24 Aug. 2025.

—, and Kevin McHugh. "Age, Meaning, and Place: Cultural Narratives and Retirement Communities." Cole et al., *Guide*, pp. 271–92.

Kearns, Robin A., and Gavin J. Andrews. "Placing Ageing: Positionings in the Study of Older People." Andrews and Phillips, *Ageing*, pp. 13–23.

Keats, John. "Endymion." *Complete Poems*, edited by Jack Stillinger, 9th ed. Belknap Press of Harvard UP, 2003, 65.

—. "Ode to a Nightingale." *Complete Poems*, edited by Jack Stillinger, 9th ed. Belknap Press of Harvard UP, 2003, pp. 279–82.

Keen, Suzanne. "A Theory of Narrative Empathy." *Narrative*, vol. 14, no. 3, 2006, pp. 207–36.

Klees, Barbara S., et al. *Brief Summaries of Medicare & Medicaid Title XVIII and Title XIX of the Social Security Act*. Department of Health and Human Services, 1 Nov. 2014.. https://www.cms.gov/Research-Statistics-Data-and-Systems/Statistics-Trends-and-Reports/MedicareProgramRatesStats/Downloads/MedicareMedicaidSummaries2014.pdf. Accessed 24 Aug. 2025.

Kontos, Pia. "Resisting Institutionalization: Constructing Old Age and Negotiating Home." *Journal of Aging Studies*, vol. 12, no. 2, 1998, pp. 167–84. https://doi.org/10.1016/S0890-4065(98)90013-5. Accessed 24 Aug. 2025.

—. "Multi-Disciplinary Configurations in Gerontology." Andrews and Phillips, *Ageing*, pp. 24–35.

—. "Rethinking Sociability in Long-Term Care: An Embodied Dimension of Selfhood." *Dementia*, vol. 11, no. 3, 2012, pp. 329–46. https://doi.org/10.1177/1471301211421073. Accessed 24 Aug. 2025.

Krasner, James. "Accumulated Lives: Metaphor, Materiality, and the Homes of the Elderly." *Literature and Medicine*, vol. 24, no. 2, 2005, pp. 209–30. Johns Hopkins UP, https://doi.org/10.1353/lm.2006.0008. Accessed 24 Aug. 2025.

—. *Home Bodies: Tactile Experience in Domestic Space*. Ohio State UP, 2010.

Kriebernegg, Ulla. "Ending Aging in the Shteyngart of Eden: Biogerontological Discourse in a *Super Sad True Love Story*." *Journal of Aging Studies*, vol. 27, no. 1, 2013, pp. 61–70. https://doi.org/10.1016/j.jaging.2012.10.003. Accessed 24 Aug. 2025.

—, and Jason Danely. "Geronticide." "*No Future* Lexicon," edited by Matthew Wolf-Meyer, *Public Books*, 2025, https://www.publicbooks.org/no-future-lexicon-geronticide/. Accessed 22 Aug. 2025.

Kristeva, Julia. *Powers of Horror: An Essay on Abjection*. Columbia UP, 1982.

Kübler-Ross, Elisabeth. *On Death and Dying: What the Dying Have to Teach Doctors, Nurses, Clergy and Their Own Families*. 40th anniversary ed. Routledge, 2009.

Kunow, Rüdiger. "The Coming of Age: The Descriptive Organization of Later Life." *Representation and Decoration in a Postmodern Age*, edited by Alfred Hornung and Rüdiger Kunow, Winter, 2009, pp. 295–309. *American Studies V. 94*.

—. "Chronologically Gifted? 'Old Age' in American Culture." *Amerikastudien / American Studies*, vol. 56, no. 1, 2011, pp. 23–44. https://doi.org/10.2307/23317637. Accessed 24 Aug. 2025.

—. "Aging Between Two Cultures: Migrants and Old Age." *C.IAS Brown Bag Lunch Series*, 7 Nov. 2012, Graz.

Kutzleben, Milena von, et al. "A Conceptual Framework for the Ethical Analysis of Moral Conflicts in Migrant Live-in Care." *Frontiers in Psychiatry*, vol. 15, 2025, api.semanticscholar.org/CorpusID:275454230.

Laderman, David. *Driving Visions: Exploring the Road Movie*. 1st ed. U of Texas P, 2002.

Lalonde, Jeremy. "Narrative Community in Edna Alford's *A Sleep Full of Dreams*." *Studies in Canadian Literature / Études en littérature canadienne*, vol. 29, no. 2, 2004, pp. 84–101. journals.hil.unb.ca/index.php/SCL/article/view/12750/13698. Accessed 31 Aug. 2025.

Lansdale, Joe R. *Bubba Ho-Tep*. 1st trade ed. Night Shade Books, 2003. Kindle.

Larson, Leslie. *Breaking Out of Bedlam: A Novel*. Broadway Paperbacks, 2010.

Laslett, Peter. *A Fresh Map of Life: The Emergence of the Third Age*. First Harvard paperback edition. Harvard UP, 1991.

Laurence, Margaret. *The Stone Angel*. U of Chicago P, 1993 [1964].

Laws, Glenda. "The Land of Old Age: Society's Changing Attitudes Toward Urban Built Environments for Elderly People." *Annals of the Association of Amer-*

ican Geographers, vol. 83, no. 4, 1993, pp. 672–93. https://doi.org/10.1111/j.1467-8306.1993.tb01960.x. Accessed 24 Aug. 2025.

—"Spatiality and Age Relations." Jamieson et al., *Critical*, pp. 90–100.

Lefebvre, Henri. *The Production of Space*. Reprint. Blackwell, 1991.

Leibing, Annette. "Divided Gazes: Alzheimer's Disease, the Person Within, and Death in Life." *Thinking About Dementia: Culture, Loss, and the Anthropology of Senility*, edited by Annette Leibing and Lawrence Cohen, Rutgers UP, 2006, pp. 240–68.

Levine, Carol. *Planning for Long-Term Care for Dummies*. Wiley, 2014.

Life, Patricia. *Long-Term Caring: Canadian Literary Narratives of Personal Agency and Identity in Late Life*. PhD Dissertation, University of Ottawa, 2014, https://ruor.uottawa.ca/items/7c2e9492-d150-4147-ade4-23eab2a9c05d. Accessed 23 Mar. 2025.

Lin, Xiaodong, et al. "Towards Cultural Landscapes of Care." *Health & Place*, vol. 78, 2022, p. 102909. https://doi.org/10.1016/j.healthplace.2022.102909. Accessed 24 Aug. 2025.

Lindquist, Lee A., and Robert M. Golub. "Cruise Ship Care: A Proposed Alternative to Assisted Living Facilities." *Journal of the American Geriatrics Society*, vol. 52, no. 11, 2004, pp. 1951–54. https://doi.org/10.1111/j.1532-5415.2004.52525.x. Accessed 24 Aug. 2025.

Lipscomb, Valerie Barnes, and Aagje Swinnen, editors. *The Palgrave Handbook of Literature and Aging*. Palgrave Macmillan, 2024.

Löschnigg, Maria. *The Contemporary Canadian Short Story in English: Continuity and Change*. Wissenschaftlicher Verlag Trier, 2014. *Cultures in America in Transition* 7.

Luddington, Alice V. "Betty Friedan: Now She's Making Waves in the *Fountain of Age*." *Interviews with Betty Friedan*, edited by Janann Sherman, UP of Mississippi, 2002, pp. 147–52. *Conversations with Public Intellectuals*.

Lustbader, Wendy. *Counting on Kindness: The Dilemmas of Dependency*. Simon & Schuster, 1991.

Maedo, Gregg. *Nursing Home Design – the Biggest Mistakes Made Today: Blog*. 2012, https://www.gmaarch.com/post/nursing-home-design-the-biggest-mistakes-made-today. Accessed 23 Mar. 2025.

Magnin, Joyce. *Blame It on the Mistletoe: A Novel of Bright's Pond*. Abingdon, 2011.

Maierhofer, Roberta. "American Studies Growing Old." *Crossing Borders: Interdisciplinary Intercultural Interactions*, edited by Bernhard Kettemann and Georg Marko, Gunter Narr, 1999, pp. 255–68.

—. "Desperately Seeking the Self: Gender, Age, and Identity in Tillie Olssen's *Tell Me a Riddle* and Michelle Herman's *Missing*." *Educational Gerontology*, vol. 25, no. 2, 1999, pp. 129–41. https://doi.org/10.1080/036012799267918. Accessed 24 Aug. 2025.

—. "Crossing (Age) Lines and Negotiating Difference: Narrative Bonds in American Fiction." *Expanding Circles, Transcending Disciplines, and Multimodal Texts. Reflections on Teaching, Learning and Researching in English and American Studies*, edited by Bernhard Kettemann and Georg Marko, Narr, 2003, pp. 249–61. *AAA – Arbeiten Aus Anglistik Und Amerikanistik* 20.

—. *Salty Old Women: Eine anokritische Untersuchung zu Frauen, Altern und Identität in der amerikanischen Literatur*. Die Blaue Eule, 2003.

Massey, Doreen. *Space, Place and Gender*. Polity, 1994.

May, Vivian M. "Dislocation and Desire in Shani Mootoo's *Cereus Blooms at Night*." *Studies in the Literary Imagination*, vol. 37, no. 2, 2004, pp. 97–122.

—. "Trauma in Paradise: Willful and Strategic Ignorance in *Cereus Blooms at Night*." *Hypatia*, vol. 21, no. 3, 2006, pp. 107–35. https://doi.org/10.1111/j.1527-2001.2006.tb01116.x. Accessed 24 Aug. 2025.

Mayer, Ruth. "'Just Driving': Contemporary Road Novels and the Triviality of the Outlaw Existence." *Space in America: Theory, History, Culture*, edited by Klaus Benesch and Kerstin Schmidt, Rodopi, 2005, pp. 369–84.

McDowell, Linda. *Gender, Identity, and Place: Understanding Feminist Geographies*. U of Minnesota P, 1999.

—, and Joanne P. Sharp, editors. *Space, Gender, Knowledge: Feminist Readings*. Arnold; J. Wiley, 1997.

McHugh, Kevin. "Generational Consciousness and Retirement Communities." *Population, Space and Place*, vol. 13, no. 4, 2007, pp. 293–306. https://doi.org/10.1002/psp.448. Accessed 24 Aug. 2025.

—. "Movement, Memory, Landscape: An Excursion in Non-Representational Thought." *GeoJournal*, vol. 74, no. 3, 2009, pp. 209–18. https://doi.org/10.1007/s10708-008-9222-0. Accessed 24 Aug. 2025.

McKenzie, Ashley, director. *Rhonda's Party*. 2010. Performance by Marguerite McNeil and Karine Vanasse, Ashley McKenzie, 2010, Online.

Mehrotra, Chandra, et al. *Aging and Diversity: An Active Learning Experience*. 2nd ed. Routledge, 2009.

Middleton, Thomas, et al. *The Old Law*. Edited by Catherine M. Shaw. Garland Pub, 1982. *Garland English Texts, no. 4*.

Mighton, John. *Half Life*. Playwrights Canada Press, 2005.

Mitchell, David. *Cloud Atlas*. Sceptre, 2003.

Moggach, Deborah. *These Foolish Things: A Novel*. Chatto & Windus, 2004.

Moore, Jim. *They Should Live so Long*. Authors' Choice, 2001.

Mootoo, Shani. *Cereus Blooms at Night*. Grove, 2009 [1996].

Moss, Hilary, and Desmond O'Neill. "Aesthetic Deprivation in Clinical Settings." *The Lancet*, vol. 383, no. 9922, 2014, pp. 1032–33. https://doi.org/10.1016/S0140-6736(14)60507-9. Accessed 24 Aug. 2025.

Müller, Gabriele. "The Aged Traveler: Cinematic Representations of Post-Retirement Masculinity." Hartung and Maierhofer, *Narratives*, pp. 149–65.

Munro, Alice. "Spelling." *Night Light: Stories of Aging*, edited by Constance Rooke, Oxford UP, 1986, pp. 83–96.

—. "The Bear Came over the Mountain." *Hateship, Friendship, Courtship, Loveship, Marriage: Stories*. McClelland & Stewart, 2001, pp. 275–323.

Murphy, James J., III. *The Nursing Home*. L & J Pub., 2009.

National Post. "Cloudburst, Reviewed: Olympia Dukakis Cusses Her Way to a Lesbian Love Story Crowd-Pleaser." *National Post*, 7 Mar. 2013, https://nationalpost.com/entertainment/movies/cloudburst-reviewed-olympia-dukakis-cusses-her-way-to-a-lesbian-love-story-crowd-pleaser. Accessed 23 Mar. 2025.

New Model Army. "Vagabonds." *Youtube*, https://www.youtube.com/watch?v=yJjjohHBvDg. Accessed 31 Aug. 2025.

Nicol, Marc, and Nick Craven. "My Great Escape, by Bernard the D-Day Rascal: 'I Was Naughty but I Had to Be There'... For the First Time, Britain's Favourite Runaway Tells His Full Amazing Story." *The Daily Mail Online*, 7 June 2014, vol. 2014, Online, https://www.dailymail.co.uk/news/article-2651658/For-time-Britains-favourite-D-Day-runaway-Bernard-Jordan-tells-amazing-story.html. Accessed 23 Mar. 2025.

Nussbaum, Martha C. *Poetic Justice: The Literary Imagination and Public Life*. Beacon Press, 1995. *The Alexander Rosenthal Lectures 1991*.

—. *Cultivating Humanity: A Classical Defense of Reform in Liberal Education*. Harvard UP, 1997.

Older Adults: LGBTQ Films. *Programsforelderly*. https://www.programsforelderly.com/documentaries-gay.php. Accessed 23 Mar. 2025.

Olssen, Mark. *Michel Foucault: Materialism and Education*. Bergin & Garvey, 1999. *Critical Studies in Education and Culture Series*.

O'Neill, Margot. *Mistreated Nursing Home Residents 'Better Off in a Concentration Camp'*. 2013, https://www.abc.net.au/news/2013-07-16/shocking-claims-elderly-being-mistreated-in-nursing-homes/4821492. Accessed 23 Mar. 2025.

Osachoff, Margaret Gail. "Intoxication: Book Review." *Canadian Literature*, no. 95, 1982, pp. 165–68.

Owusu, Prince, et al. "Equity and Diversity in Nursing Home Care: Lessons from Canada and Sweden." Armstrong and Braedley, *Care*, pp. 117–36.

Parks, Jennifer A. *No Place Like Home? Feminist Ethics and Home Health Care*. Indiana UP, 2003.

Peace, Sheila M., et al. *Environment and Identity in Later Life*. Open UP, 2006. *Growing Older*.

—. "Social Interactions in Public Spaces and Places: A Conceptual Overview." *Environmental Gerontology: Making Meaningful Places in Old Age*, edited by Graham D. Rowles and Miriam Bernard, Springer, 2013, pp. 25–49.

Peck, M. Scott. *A Bed by the Window: A Novel of Mystery and Redemption*. Arrow Books, 1994.

Perrakis, Phyllis Sternberg, editor. *Adventures of the Spirit: The Older Woman in the Works of Doris Lessing, Margaret Atwood, and Other Contemporary Women Writers*. Ohio State UP, 2007.

Peterson, Peter G. "Gray Dawn: The Global Aging Crisis." *Foreign Affairs*, January/February, 1999, .

Quarrington, Paul. *King Leary*. Anchor Canada ed. Anchor Canada, 2007 [1987].

Quill and Quire. *Flee, Fly, Flown Reviewed on Quill and Quire*. 2013, https://www.quillandquire.com/review/flee-fly-flown/. Accessed 23 Mar. 2025.

Radley, Gail. *The Golden Days*. Puffin Books, 1992.

Radović, Stanka. *Locating the Destitute: Space and Identity in Caribbean Fiction*. U of Virginia P, 2014.

Ray, Ruth E. *Endnotes: An Intimate Look at the End of Life*. Columbia UP, 2008.

Roberts, Shari. "Western Meets Eastwood: Genre and Gender on the Road." *The Road Movie Book*, edited by Steven Cohan and Ina Rae Hark, Routledge, 1997, pp. 45–69.

Robledo, Luis Miguel Gutiérrez, et al. "The State of Elder Care in Mexico." *Current Translational Geriatrics and Experimental Gerontology Reports*, vol. 1, no. 4, 2012, pp. 183–89. https://doi.org/10.1007/s13670-012-0028-z. Accessed Aug. 31, 2025.

Roca, Paco. *Wrinkles*. Knockabout 2015.

Rooke, Constance. "Old Age in Contemporary Fiction. A New Paradigm of Hope." *Handbook of the Humanities and Aging*, edited by Thomas R. Cole et al., 1st ed., Springer, 1992, pp. 241–57.

Roth, Philip. *Everyman*. 1st Vintage International ed. Vintage International, 2007, c2006.

Rowe, John W., and Robert L. Kahn. *Successful Aging*. Pantheon Books, 1998.

Rowles, Graham D., and Miriam Bernard, editors. *Environmental Gerontology: Making Meaningful Places in Old Age*. Springer, 2013.

—., and Habib Chaudhury. "Between the Shores of Recollection and Imagination: Self, Aging, and Home." Rowles and Chaudhury, *Home*, pp. 3–18.

—, editors. *Home and Identity in Late Life International Perspectives*. Springer, 2005.

Rubinstein, Robert L., and Kate de Medeiros. "Home, Self, and Identity." Rowles and Chaudhury, *Home*, pp. 47–62.

Russo, Mary. *The Female Grotesque: Risk, Excess, and Modernity*. Routledge, 1995.

Rutherford, Jonathan. "The Third Space. Interview with Homi Bhabha." *Identity: Community, Culture, Difference*, edited by Jonathan Rutherford, 1st ed. 1990, repr., Lawrence and Wishart, 1998, pp. 207–21.

Ryvicker, Miriam. "Preservation of Self in the Nursing Home: Contradictory Practices Within Two Models of Care." *Journal of Aging Studies*, vol. 23, no. 1, 2009, pp. 12–23. https://doi.org/10.1016/j.jaging.2007.09.004. Accessed 31 Aug. 2025.

Sandick, Phil. *Amigoland, by Oscar Casares: Book Review*. *Fiction Writers Review*. 2010, fictionwritersreview.com/review/amigoland-by-oscar-casares/. Accessed 23 Mar. 2025.

Sandlin, Tim. *Jimi Hendrix Turns Eighty*. Thorndike Press, 2007. Thorndike Press Large Print Laugh Lines.

Sarton, May. *As We Are Now: A Novel*. 1st ed. Norton, 1973.

Scharff, Virginia. *Taking the Wheel: Women and the Coming of the Motor Age*. 1st pbk. ed. U of New Mexico P, 1992.

Scheidt, Rick J. "The Tip of the Spear." *Gerontologist*, vol. 53, no. 3, 2013, pp. 516–17.

Schotland, Sara. "Forced Execution of the Elderly: Old Law, Dystopia, and the Utilitarian Argument." *Humanities*, vol. 2, no. 2, 2013, pp. 160–75. https://doi.org/10.3390/h2020160. Accessed 31 Aug. 2025.

Scotten, Neil. *Half Life. A Workbook for Teachers and Students Prepared for the Centaur Theatre Company*. 2008.

Seidler, Miriam. *Figurenmodelle des Alters in der deutschsprachigen Gegenwartsliteratur*. Narr, 2010.

Shakespeare, William. *Richard II*. [New Penguin Shakespeare ed.]. Penguin, 2008.

Shapiro, Joseph P. *No Pity: People with Disabilities Forging a New Civil Rights Movement*. 1st ed. Times Books, 1993.

Shield, Renée Rose. *Uneasy Endings: Daily Life in an American Nursing Home*. Cornell UP, 1988. *Cornell Paperbacks*.

Shields, Rob. "Henri Lefebvre." *Key Thinkers on Space and Place*, edited by Phil Hubbard and Rob Kitchin, 2nd ed, Sage, 2011, pp. 279–85. Kindle.

Simonsen, Peter. *Livslange liv: Plejehjemsromaner og pensionsfortællinger fra velfærdsstaten*. University of Southern Denmark Studies in Scandinavian Languages and Literatures, no. 118, Syddansk Universitetsforlag, 2014.

Slettedahl Macpherson, Heidi. *Women's Movement: Escape as Transgression in North American Feminist Fiction*. Rodopi, 2000. *Costerus 128*.

Small, Helen. "Care Noir: Before and After COVID-19." Lipscomb and Swinnen, *Palgrave*, pp. 177–95.

Smith, Ali. "Introduction." *The Hearing Trumpet*. By Leonora Carrington. Penguin, 2003 [1974].

Smith, David Barton. *Long-Term Care in Transition: The Regulation of Nursing Homes*. BeardBooks, 2001.

Snaith, Helen. "Dystopia, Gerontology and the Writing of Margaret Atwood." *Feminist Review*, vol. 116, no. 1, 2017, pp. 118–32. https://doi.org/10.1057/s41305-017-0068-5. Accessed 31 Aug. 2025.

Soja, Edward W. *Thirdspace: Journeys to Los Angeles and Other Real-and-Imagined Places*. Blackwell, 1996.

—. *Postmodern Geographies: The Reassertion of Space in Critical Social Theory*. Verso, 1989.

Sontag, Susan. "The Double Standard of Aging." *Saturday Review*, 1972, September 23, 1972, pp. 29–38. https://www.unz.org/Pub/SaturdayRev-1972sep23-00029?View=PDF. Accessed 23 Mar. 2025.

South London and Maudsley NHS Foundation Trust. *Bethlehem Royal Hospital – Our History*. South London and Maudsley NHS Foundation Trust. 2014, https://www.slam.nhs.uk/about-us/art-and-history/our-history/prior-to-1600. Accessed 05 Nov. 2025.

Soyka, Amelie. *Raum und Geschlecht: Frauen im Road Movie der 90er Jahre*. Peter Lang, 2002.

Span, Paula. "They Still Don't Want to Live with You." *The New York Times*, 20 June 2012, Online, https://newoldage.blogs.nytimes.com/2012/06/20/they-still-dont-want-to-live-with-you/. Accessed 23 Mar. 2025.

Sparks, Nicholas. *The Notebook*: A Novel. Warner Vision, 1998 [1996].

Springer, Marlene. "As We Shall Be: May Sarton and Aging." *Frontiers: A Journal of Women Studies*, vol. 5, no. 3, 1980, pp. 46–49. https://doi.org/10.2307/3346510. Accessed 05 Nov. 2025.

Stafford, Philip B., editor. Gray Areas: Ethnographic Encounters with Nursing Home Culture. 1st ed. School of American Research Press, 2003. School of American Research Advanced Seminar Series.

—. Elderburbia: Aging with a Sense of Place in America. Praeger, 2009.

Stahl, Michael J. "Joint Commission on Accreditation of Healthcare Organizations (JCAHO)." *Encyclopedia of Health Care Management*, edited by Michael J. Stahl, Sage, 2004, p. 315. https://sk.sagepub.com/ency/edvol/healthcare management/chpt/joint-commission-accreditation-healthcare-organiza tions. Accessed 23 Mar. 2025.

Stevens, Al. *Nursing Home Ninjas*. Five Star, 2013.

Stout, Janis P. *The Journey Narrative in American Literature: Patterns and Departures*. Greenwood, 1983.

Stowe, James D., and Teresa M. Cooney. "Examining Rowe and Kahn's Concept of Successful Aging: Importance of Taking a Life Course Perspective." *The Gerontologist*, 2014, https://doi.org/10.1093/geront/gnu055. Accessed 05 Nov. 2025.

Seuss, Dr. *Oh, the Places You'll Go!*. Collins Picture Lions, 2003.

Surrey, Janet L. "The 'Self in Relation': A Theory of Women's Development." *Women's Growth in Connection: Writings from the Stone Center*, edited by Judith V. Jordan, Guilford, 1991, pp. 51–66.

Tem, Melanie. *The Tides*. Leisure Books, 1999. Leisure Horror.

The Eden Alternative. *The Eden Alternative® – Improving the Lives of the Elders*. 2014, http://www.edenalt.org/. Accessed 23 Mar. 2025.

Tisdale, Sallie. *Harvest Moon: Portrait of a Nursing Home*. Holt, 1987.

Tostevin, Lola Lemire. *The Other Sister: A Novel*. Inanna Publications, 2008. Inanna Poetry and Fiction Series.

Tuan, Yi-Fu. "Home." *Patterned Ground: Entanglements of Nature and Culture*, edited by Stephan. Harrison et al., Reaktion Books, 2004, pp. 164–65.

—. *Space and Place: The Perspective of Experience*. 7. print. U of Minnesota P, 2011 (1977).

Twigg, Alan. *Strong Voices: Conversations with Fifty Canadian Authors*. Harbour, 1988.

Twigg, Julia. "Bathing and the Politics of Care." *Social Policy & Administration*, vol. 31, no. 1, 1997, pp. 61–72. https://doi.org/10.1111/1467-9515.00038.

—. "Deconstructing the 'Social Bath': Help with Bathing at Home for Older and Disabled People." *Journal of Social Policy*, vol. 26, no. 2, 1997, pp. 211–32. https://doi.org/10.1017/S0047279497004960. Accessed 31 Aug. 2025.

—. *Bathing-the Body and Community Care*. Routledge, 2000.

—. "The Body, Gender, and Age: Feminist Insights in Social Gerontology." *Journal of Aging Studies*, vol. 18, no. 1, 2004, pp. 59–73. https://doi.org/10.1016/j.jaging.2003.09.001.

—. *The Body in Health and Social Care*. Palgrave Macmillan, 2006.

Uhlenberg, Peter. "Replacing the Nursing Home." *Public Interest*, no. 128, 1997, pp. 73–84.

United States Congress. *Social Security Act: SSAct, Pub.L. 74–271*. 1935, https://www.ssa.gov/history/35act.html. Accessed 31 Aug. 2025.

Urry, John. "Mobility and Proximity." *Sociology*, vol. 36, no. 2, 2002, pp. 255–74. https://doi.org/10.1177/0038038502036002002. Accessed 31 Aug. 2025.

Uteng, Tanu Priya, and Tim Cresswell. "Introduction." *Gendered Mobilities*, edited by Tanu Priya Uteng and Tim Cresswell, Ashgate, 2008, pp. 1–12.

Venema, Kathleen. "Remembering Forgetting: Graphic Lives at the End of the Line." *a/b: Auto/Biography Studies*, vol. 33, no. 3, 2018, pp. 663–86. https://doi.org/10.1080/08989575.2018.1499497. Accessed 31. Aug. 2025.

Vincent, John A. "Ageing Contested: Anti-Ageing Science and the Cultural Construction of Old Age." *Sociology*, vol. 40, no. 4, 2006, pp. 681–98. https://doi.org/10.1177/0038038506065154.

Waltner-Toews, David. "A Sunny Day in Canada." Anthologized in 1979 in *Fiddlehead Greens. One Foot in Heaven*, 1st US edition 2006. Coteau Books, 2005, pp. 239–61.

Warnock, Jeanie E. "'Soul Murder' and Rebirth: Trauma, Narrative, and Imagination in Shani Mootoo's *Cereus Blooms at Night*." Perrakis, *Adventures*, pp. 270–98.

Waxman, Barbara Frey. "From 'Bildungsroman' to 'Reifungsroman': Aging in Doris Lessing's Fiction." *Soundings: An Interdisciplinary Journal*, vol. 68, no. 3, 1985, pp. 318–34.

—. *From the Hearth to the Open Road: A Feminist Study of Aging in Contemporary Literature*. 1. publ. Greenwood, 1990.

—. "Literary Texts and Literary Critics Team Up Against Ageism." Cole et al., *Guide*, pp. 83–104.

Welty, Eudora. "A Visit of Charity." *Literature and Aging: An Anthology*, edited by Martin Kohn et al., Kent State UP, 1992, pp. 331–35. 1.

Wheelwright, Julie. "Exit Lines, by Joan Barfoot: The Rage of the Aged: A Haunting, Disturbing Tale of Growing Old Disgracefully." *The Independent*, 17 Sept. 2008, https://www.independent.co.uk/arts-entertainment/books/reviews/exit-lines-by-joan-barfoot-932884.html. Accessed 23 Feb. 2025.

Whitman, Walt. "Song of the Open Road." *Leaves of Grass*. New American Library, 1980, pp. 123–33. 451-CJ1395.

Wiersma, Elaine C. "'You Can't Turn Back the Clock': Conceptualizing Time After Institutionalization." *Canadian Journal on Aging / La Revue canadienne du vieillissement*, vol. 31, no. 1, 2012, pp. 73–85. https://doi.org/10.1017/S0714980811000572. Accessed 31 Aug. 2025.

—, and Sherry L. Dupuis. "Becoming Institutional Bodies: Socialization into a Long-Term Care Home." *Journal of Aging Studies*, vol. 24, no. 4, 2010, pp. 278–91. https://doi.org/10.1016/j.jaging.2010.08.003. Accessed 31 Aug. 2025.

Wilkening, Hartmut. "Michel Foucaults Panoptismus." *Räume in der Kunst: Künstlerische, kunst- und medienwissenschaftliche Entwürfe*, edited by Sabiene Autsch and Sarah Hornäk, transcript, 2010, pp. 83–96.

—. *Foucault Project in Nursing Home Building*. 24 Jan. 2011, https://www.hartmutwilkening.de/Hartmut_Wilkening/Foucault_project_in_nursing_home_building.html. Accessed 23 Mar. 2025.

—. "Frage ad Foucault / Vrij Geestig." E-mail received by Ulla Kriebernegg, 29 Mar. 2015.

Wilkins Freeman, Mary E. "A Mistaken Charity." *A Humble Romance*. Girlebooks, 2014 (1887), pp. 234–49.

Williams, Leigh Anne. *Atwood's Tales: Margaret Atwood*. 2014, https://www.publishersweekly.com/pw/by-topic/authors/profiles/article/64151-atwood-s-tales-margaret-atwood.html. Accessed 23 Mar. 2025.

Wohlmann, Anita. *Metaphor in Illness Writing: Fight and Battle Reused*. Edinburgh UP, 2022.

Woodward, Kathleen M. "May Sarton and Fictions of Old Age." *Gender and Literary Voice*, edited by Janet M. Todd, Holmes & Meier, 1980, pp. 108–24. *Women & Literature 1*.

—. "Instant Repulsion: Decrepitude, the Mirror Stage, and the Literary Imagination." *Kenyon Review*, vol. 5, no. 4, 1983, pp. 43–66.

—. *Aging and Its Discontents: Freud and Other Fictions*. Indiana UP, 1991.

—. "Performing Age, Performing Gender." *NWSA Journal*, vol. 18, no. 1, 2006, pp. 162–89.

—. "A Public Secret: Assisted Living, Caregivers, Globalization." *International Journal of Ageing and Later Life*, vol. 7, no. 2, 2012, pp. 17–51. https://doi.org/10.3384/ijal.1652-8670.1272a2. Accessed 31 Aug. 2025.

Wyatt-Brown, Anne M. "The Coming of Age of Literary Gerontology." *Journal of Aging Studies*, vol. 4, no. 3, 1990, pp. 299–315. https://doi.org/10.1016/0890-4065(90)90029-8. Accessed 31 Aug. 2025.

—. "Resilience and Creativity in Aging: The Realms of Silver." Cole et al., *Guide*, pp. 55–82.

Yahnke, Robert E. "Representations of Aging in Contemporary Literary Works." *Generations*, vol. 17, no. 2, 1993, pp. 83–86.

Zeilig, Hannah. "The Uses of Literature in the Study of Older People." Jamieson et al., *Critical*, pp. 39–48.

Zieleniec, Andrzej Jan Leon. *Space and Social Theory*. Sage, 2007.

Filmography

24 Stunden. Directed by Harald Friedl, Mischief Films – Verein zur Förderung des Dokumentarfilms KG, 2024, 100 min. Distributed by Polyfilm Betriebs GmbH. Film-Institut – Austrian Film Institute, https://www.filminstitut.at/filme/24-stunden. Accessed 24 Aug. 2025. polyfilm.at+9Österreichisches Filminstitut+9Ös

Almost Home. Directed by Brad Lichtenstein and Lisa Gildehaus, 371 Productions, 2006. DVD. Almost Home, https://www.almosthomedoc.org.

Arrugas [Wrinkles]. Directed by Paco Roca, Perro Verde Films, 2011. DVD.

Away from Her. Directed by Sarah Polley, performance by Gordon Pinsent, et al., 2007, DVD.

Bonnie and Clyde. Directed by Arthur Penn, performances by Warren Beatty and Faye Dunaway, Warner Brothers, 1967.

Cloudburst. Directed by Thom Fitzgerald, performances by Brenda Fricker and Olympia Dukakis, Emotion Pictures / Sidney Kimmel Entertainment, 2011. DVD.

Gen Silent. Directed by Stu Maddux, Mad Stu Productions, 2010. DVD.

Iris. Directed by Richard Eyre, performances by Judi Dench, Kate Winslet, Jim Broadbent, and Hugh Bonneville, Miramax Films and BBC Films, 2001. IMDb, https://www.imdb.com/title/tt0280778/. Accessed 24 Aug. 2025.

It Is Not Over Yet. Directed by Louise Detlefsen, Hansen & Pedersen Film og Fjernsyn, 2021.

Mâine Mă Duc – Tomorrow I Leave. Directed by Maria Lisa Pichler and Lukas Schöffel, Sixpackfilm, 2024.

Memee. Directed by Evelyn Verschoore. Cinnamon Entertainment, 2010, DVD.

Penelope. 371 Productions. 2014, 371productions.com/non-fiction/penelope-the-documentary. Accessed 23 Mar. 2025.

Plan 75. Directed by Chie Hayakawa, performances by Chieko Baisho, Hayato Isomura, and Stefanie Arianne, Happinet Phantom Studios / Urban Factory, 2022.

Quartet. Directed by Dustin Hoffman, performances by Maggie Smith, Tom Courtenay, Billy Connolly, and Pauline Collins, Momentum Pictures, 2012. DVD.

Rhonda's Party. Directed by Ashley McKenzie, performances by Marguerite McNeil and Karine Vanasse, Grassfire Films, 2010.

Robot and Frank. Directed by Jake Schreier, written by Christopher D. Ford, Dog Run Pictures, 2012. DVD.

Room 335. Directed by Andrew Jenks, Hemi Productions and HBO Box Office, 2006. iTunes.

Runaway Train. Directed by Andrei Konchalovsky, performances by Jon Voight, Eric Roberts, and Rebecca De Mornay, Cannon Group, 1986. DVD.

The Best Exotic Marigold Hotel. Directed by John Madden, performances by Judi Dench, Bill Nighy, and Maggie Smith, Fox Searchlight Pictures, 2011.

The First of May. Directed by Paul Sirmons, SHO Entertainment in association with John B. Goodman, 1999. IMDb, https://www.imdb.com/title/tt0132160/. Accessed 24 Aug. 2025.

The Great Escape. Directed by John Sturges, performances by Steve McQueen, James Garner, and Richard Attenborough, Mirisch Company, 1963. DVD.

The Greyed Escape. Directed by Jeremy Dehn, 21 Sept. 2007, https://vimeo.com/77169678. Accessed 23 Mar. 2025.

The Hundred-Year-Old Man Who Climbed Out of the Window and Disappeared. Directed by Felix Herngren, performance by Robert Gustafsson, Lionsgate / Music Box Films, 2013.

The Mayor: Live It Up, at 88. Directed by Jared Scheib, Life Waltz Productions, 2011. DVD.

The Notebook. Directed by Nick Cassavetes, performances by Gena Rowlands and James Garner, New Line Cinema, 2004. IMDb, https://www.imdb.com/title/tt0332280/. Accessed 24 Aug. 2025.

The Savages. Directed by Tamara Jenkins, performances by Laura Linney, Philip Seymour Hoffman, and Philip Bosco, Fox Searchlight Pictures, 2008. DVD.

The Stone Angel. Directed by Kari Skogland, performance by Ellen Burstyn, Buffalo Gal Pictures and Skogland Films, 2007. IMDb, https://www.imdb.com/title/tt0847897/. Accessed 24 Aug. 2025.

Thelma & Louise. Directed by Ridley Scott, performances by Susan Sarandon and Geena Davis, Pathé Entertainment, 1991.

Torching the Dusties. Directed by Marlene Goldman and Philip McKee, performances by Claire Coulter, Eric Peterson, and Aris Tyros, Filmcoop Inc., 2019.

Up. Directed by Pete Docter and Bob Peterson, performance by Ed Asner and Christopher Plummer, Pixar Animation Studios, 2009. DVD.

Index

D